GALEN

GALEN

ON RESPIRATION AND THE ARTERIES

— ◆ —

An edition with English translation
and commentary of *De usu respirationis*,
An in arteriis natura sanguis contineatur,
De usu pulsuum, and
De causis respirationis

DAVID J. FURLEY AND

J. S. WILKIE

PRINCETON UNIVERSITY PRESS
1984

PREFACE

This book originates from translations of Galen's treatises on blood flow and the arteries made for teaching purposes in University College London by J. S. Wilkie. Collaboration with David J. Furley, of the Greek Department of the same college, began in the 1960s, and continued—with many interruptions—after he moved to Princeton University in 1966.

The three longest treatises are all concerned with the linked subjects of blood flow and respiration, and all are concerned with the defense of Galen's theory against the earlier theory of Erasistratus. They clearly belong together. They are important documents in the history of physiology, especially in the development of Harvey's theory of the circulation of the blood. So far as we know, they have not previously been translated as a whole into English or any other modern language; we hope the present book will make a contribution of some use to teaching and research in the history of biology.

The Greek text presented here is newly edited. *De usu respirationis* was last edited, with a new collation of the more important manuscripts, by R. Noll in 1915. We have checked his work, and made some changes in the text, mainly because of our different interpretation of the argument. *An in arteriis* was last edited by F. Albrecht in 1911. We have the advantage over him in having access to an Arabic translation based on an earlier and better Greek text than any of the surviving Greek manuscripts or editions. The changes we have been able to make as a result of this are far-reaching. *De usu pulsuum* has not been edited since the very imperfect edition of Gottlob Kühn (1822). We have collated the surviving Greek manuscripts afresh, without much profit; improvements have again been made possible by the discovery of an Arabic translation, and again the changes we have made are significant.

We have added a newly edited text of the short work transmitted with Galen's other writings under the title *De causis respirationis*, with a translation and commentary.

The style of our translations is deliberately somewhat archaic, on the ground that the treatises will take their place in the history of biology more naturally in that guise than in what is obviously twentieth-century English. It is our hope that clarity is not impaired.

Text, translation, and commentary are a product of two of us working together; the introductory essays are contributed by each of us individually, according to his area of specialization. Most of the work was completed before we had access to the book by C.R.S. Harris, *The Heart and the Vascular System in Ancient Greek Medicine* (Oxford: Clarendon Press, 1973). We have revised some passages and added references after reading this; but since we have entered in more depth into several issues treated summarily in Harris's book, we believe there is still some use in adding our contribution to the history of this subject.

It is a pleasure to acknowledge help from several persons and institutions: to Mr. Vivian Nutting, Mr. George Pope, Professor Heinrich von Staden, and Professor Phillip DeLacy for many extremely useful criticisms and suggestions; to Professor P. M. Daniel and Professor Sir Andrew Huxley for various communications; to Dr. M. C. Lyons and Professor Fadlou Shehadi for help with the Arabic manuscripts; to Mr. David Blank for reading some of the Greek manuscripts; to Mr. George Ryan for checking parts of the penultimate typescript; to Professor Arthur Hanson for help in preparing the indexes; to the director of the American Academy at Rome for providing a place for collaborative work in 1968; and to the National Science Foundation for funds for research and travel.

Marginal notations in the Greek text refer as follows: A = Albrecht; N = Noll; K = Kühn IV, except for *De usu pulsuum*, which refers to Kühn V.

[J. S. Wilkie died in 1982, before seeing the page proofs of this book.]

CONTENTS

INTRODUCTION

I. THEORIES OF RESPIRATION BEFORE GALEN

a. Empedocles, the Sicilian School, and Plato

Most of the work of the early Greek *physiologoi* is lost. It must count, therefore, as a piece of good luck that one early theory of respiration was described in a surviving work of Aristotle, and that his description was supported by a direct quotation of twenty-five consecutive lines of hexameter verse. Empedocles was the author; Aristotle quotes him in his *De respiratione*, Ch. 7, 473 b 9 (fr. 100 of Empedocles, in Diels-Kranz *Fragmente der Vorsokratiker*). The date of Empedocles' work cannot be determined exactly, but 450 B.C. is probably correct within a margin of ten or fifteen years.

> Thus do all things breathe in and out: for all, there are tubes of flesh, left by the blood, *stretched over the outermost part of the body*, and over the mouths of these *the exterior surface of the skin* is pierced through with close-set furrows, in such fashion that blood lies hidden within, but a clear path for air is cut through by these channels. When the delicate blood runs away from these, air seething with fierce flood rushes in; when it flows back, it breathes out in return.

The italicized phrases, translated unambiguously above, are ambiguous in Greek, as will be explained. But one thing is clear and undisputed: in Empedocles' theory, blood and breath move in the same vessels of the body—"tubes of flesh, left by the blood" in the sense that the blood that they contain regularly flows out of them, leaving room for air to enter. They are alternately filled with blood and breath. It is of great importance for the understanding of Greek physiology to observe that from the earliest recorded theory the two systems of blood flow and respiration were linked. If we are to understand the conceptual framework of Greek theory, we must put aside the modern notion that the only link between them is the oxygenation of the blood in the lungs.

But what exactly was the physiology and anatomy of blood and breath as conceived by Empedocles? This is a very difficult question

3

to answer because of the ambiguities referred to above.[1] The chief difficulty is the word "$\dot{\rho}\iota\nu\hat{\omega}\nu$" in the fourth line: it is translated above as "skin," but it may also mean "nostrils," and there is some evidence to show that Aristotle, our sole source for the fragment, understood it in this latter sense.[2] In classical Greek prose, "$\dot{\rho}\iota\nu\hat{\omega}\nu$" would normally be interpreted as "nostrils." It is possible, with ingenuity, to make some sense of the opening lines on the assumption that Empedocles used the word in that sense. The words "$\pi\dot{\nu}\mu\alpha\tau o\nu$ $\kappa\alpha\tau\dot{\alpha}$ $\sigma\hat{\omega}\mu\alpha$," translated above as "over the outermost part of the body," can be read as "deep inside the body,"[3] and "$\dot{\rho}\iota\nu\hat{\omega}\nu$ $\ddot{\epsilon}\sigma\chi\alpha\tau\alpha$ $\tau\dot{\epsilon}\rho\theta\rho\alpha$," translated above as "the exterior surface of the skin," can be read as "the furthest ends of the nostrils."[4] On this interpretation, Empedocles asserts that tubes of flesh lead from deep inside the body to the back of the nostrils, and where these tubes meet the nostrils there are perforations so small that air can pass through but blood cannot.

In my opinion, this view must be rejected. There is no such set of perforations at the back of the nostrils, nor has any supporting evidence of belief in them been found in other Greek writers.[5] The trachea, which is the likeliest candidate for a "tube" leading from deep inside the body to the nostrils, is not normally filled with blood, nor is there any reason why Empedocles should have thought it was. Moreover, this is a forced interpretation of the Greek phrase "$\pi\dot{\nu}\mu\alpha$-$\tau o\nu$ $\kappa\alpha\tau\dot{\alpha}$ $\sigma\hat{\omega}\mu\alpha$," and this way of reading the lines makes poor work of the simile of the clepsydra that follows.[6]

[1]From the twenties of this century to the fifties there was fairly general agreement on the interpretation of this fragment, but since 1957 there has been nothing but controversy. See my "Clepsydra," and Timpanaro Cardini ("Respirazione"), Booth ("Empedocles"), Lloyd (*Polarity*, pp. 328–33), Guthrie (*History* II), Bollack (*Empédocle* III, 470–501), Seeck ("Empedocles"), and O'Brien, ("Simile"). For details see the Bibliography.

[2]This is disputed, however, by Bollack, *Empédocle* III, 481.

[3]So Guthrie, *History* II, 220, following Booth.

[4]So Guthrie again.

[5]Seeck, p. 50 n. 1, quotes Galen *De instrumento odoratus* (K II 867). Galen speaks of "sieve-like bones" that conduct some of the breath from the nostrils to the brain. But there is no evidence that Empedocles knew of the theory of breathing into the brain.

[6]For further discussion of the simile and defense of the "skin-breathing" interpretation, see my article "Clepsydra", reprinted (1975) with a postscript. For criticisms of this view, see Booth "Empedocles," G.E.R. Lloyd (*Polarity*

It is much more probably that we have in this fragment a theory of breathing through pores in the skin. The "tubes of flesh" are simply the blood vessels, some of which are indeed "stretched over the outermost surface of the body," just under the skin. "Over their mouths," according to Empedocles, the skin is pierced with small holes, through which breath but not blood can pass. As blood withdraws from the surface, so breath enters, and as blood returns, breath leaves through the same pores.

It is likely that Empedocles chose the ambiguous word "ῥινῶν" deliberately. If he had wanted a nonambiguous word for "skin," "δέρματος" could have been substituted without any other change in the hexameter. The skin, in his theory, is functioning like the nose, an obvious and undisputed organ of respiration, and he uses a pun to draw attention this claim.[7]

The notion that blood vessels "breathe" through pores in the skin is an integral and quite important part of Galen's theory of blood flow and respiration, as we shall see.[8] By Galen's time it was a theory of some precision: the arteries draw in air through the skin in diastole and expel waste through the skin in systole, and this process is part of the system that maintains moderate heat in the body. It is said that skin-breathing is a characteristic feature of Sicilian medical doctrine,[9] and we shall see in later paragraphs that there is evidence for attributing it to Philistion and Diocles, as well as to Plato, who adopted much from the Sicilians. There are some grounds, however, for thinking that the doctrine spread to other schools, even before the time of Galen. Jaeger attributes it to Aristotle,[10] but I have found no evidence for it, and some evidence against it.[11] Galen finds no inconsistency in attributing to Erasistratus the view that air is emptied out

---

pp. 328ff.), and O'Brien ("Simile"; he has however not understood it). Bollack also defends skin-breathing.

[7]I reached this conclusion when I read Booth's reply to my article. Independently, W. J. Verdenius (see Guthrie, *History* II, 220 n. 3), and J. Bollack (*Empédocle*, III, 481) have come to the same conclusion. Bollack suggests that the pun begins with "στομίοις," the "mouths" of the vessels, in line 3.

[8]Introduction, II. See also Harris, *The Heart*, p. 282.

[9]W. Wellmann, *Sikel.*, p. 71; Jaeger, *Diokles* 214; Harris, *The Heart*, pp. 17–18.

[10]*Diokles*, p. 214.

[11]See below, section d, for Aristotle's theory of the blood vessels.

of the body after passing through the arteries—presumably through pores in the skin, as in his own theory, although he does not say so.[12] Anonymus Londinensis attributes skin-breathing to Hippocrates;[13] so Wellmann's view, based on *De morbo sacro*, that the Coan school denied skin-breathing may need qualification.[14] But we will return to these controversial matters below, in the sections of this Introduction that deal with the various schools.

It must be observed that Empedocles' theory of respiration was not intended as a purely physiological theory, in any sense. Breath was either identical with or closely related to one of the four cosmic elements that formed the basis of his whole world picture. Blood, according to fragment 98, is made of these four elements, and "blood around the heart in men is thought" (fr. 105). There is evidence that the proportions of the mixture were crucial to thinking.[15] So it is a reasonable conjecture that breathing was supposed to serve the purpose of preserving the right balance, in some way, between the elements in the blood. It is possible that the balance was especially a matter of the right heat,[16] but the evidence is not conclusive. In the present context, however, we need go no further into the speculations of Empedocles.

Philistion, mentioned by Galen in *De usu respirationis* 1 (K IV 471), along with Diocles, as maintaining that respiration is for the sake of the preservation of the innate heat, is relatively unknown except for the account of his theories given by the medical papyrus called Anonymus Londinensis.[17] In date he was contemporary with Plato.

In a summary of Philistion's views on the causes of disease, Anonymus Londinensis says he divided the causes into three classes: the elements, through excess of one of their "powers"; the condition of our bodies; and external causes. He explains the second of these: "The condition of our body is a cause of disease in the following way. When, he says, the whole body breathes well and the breath passes through unhindered, health is the result. For breathing (ἀναπνοή)

---

[12] *De usu respirationis* 2 (K IV 482).
[13] vi 14–31: see § c below.
[14] W. Wellmann, *Sikel.*, 71.
[15] Theophrastus, *De sensibus* 10.
[16] See Bollack, *Empedocle* I, 245.
[17] References are given to the edition by my former teacher, W.H.S. Jones.

takes place not only by way of mouth and nostrils, but also over all the body" (xx 42–47, transl. Jones). It has been argued[18] that this is not sufficient evidence to attribute skin-breathing to Philistion, but that seems unnecessarily sceptical; it is only the belief that skin-breathing is an eccentric doctrine that would suggest looking for another interpretation.

At least there can be no doubt that Plato's *Timaeus* includes skin-breathing in its physiological doctrine, and that breathing is closely connected with blood flow as in Empedocles.

In *Timaeus* 79 b1–e9, the explanation of breathing begins from the proposition that there is no void space into which a thing may move. Hence the air expelled by breathing out displaces its neighbor, and that displaces *its* neighbor, until the last in the circular chain replaces the air that was breathed out. That is to say, air enters the chest and lungs *through the skin* to replace the air breathed out through the nose and mouth, and when this air leaves again and moves outward through the body, by a circular thrust it pushes air in through the nose and mouth. Having thus set out the general principle, Plato gives a causal explanation. The natural heat of the body, harbored in the blood and the vessels ($\phi\lambda\acute{\epsilon}\beta\epsilon\varsigma$), has a natural tendency to seek the company of its kin outside the body. There are two directions it can take to the outside, one "by way of the body" ($\kappa\alpha\tau\grave{\alpha}\ \tau\grave{o}\ \sigma\hat{\omega}\mu\alpha$), the other by way of the mouth and nostrils. When it moves toward one of these exits, it pushes air around into the other; that which goes out is cooled, that which enters is warmed, and this change in heat causes a reversal of flow.

The physiology of the *Timaeus* closely connects blood flow, respiration, and nutrition. Food in the stomach is worked on by the heat of the body and thus transformed into blood (80 d), with which the blood vessels are filled. The blood is washed around the body so as to nourish all its parts by the respiratory movement of air in the blood vessels. Respiration is caused mechanically, then, by the movement of "fire" toward its like, and the cooling action brought about by this motion, which puts it into reverse. The reciprocating motion causes air to be first introduced into the vessels of the body and then expelled by the same route; inspiration through the mouth and nos-

[18]By Seeck, "Empedocles," pp. 50–52.

trils takes place at the same time as expiration through the pores of the skin, and vice versa.[19] The reciprocating motion of the air in the vessels moves the blood, and thus nourishes the body.

There are two particularly striking features of this theory, both of which are significant in the history of Greek physiology. First, blood is regarded quite unambiguously as food. This was an *idée fixe* among Greek thinkers, and was probably more than anything else responsible for their failure to understand that the blood circulates through the body and returns to its starting point. The idea survives intact in Galen, who had "his mind firmly rooted in the older notion that blood is a sort of warm nourishing soup in which all the parts are amply bathed."[20] Second, it will be noticed that the heart plays no part in Plato's account of the distribution of blood. It is the movement of the air that moves the blood, not the pumping action of the heart. The heart is indeed mentioned in the *Timaeus* as "the fountain of the blood that courses over all the limbs," and as the "knot of the vessels" (70a–b). This is not, however, in the context of nutrition, but of functions of the three parts of the soul. The heart is the center of the *thymos* or spirited part; when appropriate messages reach the heart from the rational part of the soul, the *thymos* boils, and the emotional message, "felt along the blood," as we might say, is carried to all the limbs. This must imply that the heart is at the focal point of all the vessels, so that it has lines of communication to them all. There seems to be also a suggestion, not fully developed, that the heat of the *thymos* is a cause of the movement of blood outward from the heart. But it would be a mistake to regard Plato as having taken a position in the controversy that developed later among biologists as to whether the heart is the "origin" of the blood vessels. Plato's account of the anatomy of the blood vessels is quite fanciful, and bears little relation to scientific knowledge, ancient or modern.

We have now mentioned three theories of blood flow and respiration, of which the last is reported in more detail than the others. Whether or not they are all the same theory, handed down from Empedocles to Philistion and Plato, is not clear.[21] There is no reason to think that Empedocles held the Platonic theory of the tripartite

[19] It is a curious feature of this theory that it allows no role to the contraction and expansion of the thorax.

[20] Hall, *Studies*, p. 404.

[21] Harris, *The Heart*, p. 119, regards them as essentially the same.

soul, and he could hardly therefore have written in just the same way about the heart as the seat of the *thymos*. Though it has been strongly denied, it is probable that Empedocles' theory of breathing included the notion of reciprocal breathing in and out through the skin and the nose and mouth. There is also nothing inconsistent, in the fragments of Empedocles and Philistion, with the *Timaeus* theory of heat as the cause of the reciprocal motion.

It is interesting that Galen criticizes the "circular thrust" theory of Plato's *Timaeus* at some length in his *De placitis Hippocratis et Platonis* VIII 9 (K V 713–16). Plato attributed everything to pushes instead of to attraction (ὁλκή), and this was a great mistake, in Galen's view. He quotes three examples of attraction to show what he means: a man can suck water up through a tube by sucking the air out of the tube first; babies suck milk from the breast; bellows draw in air when expanded. The thorax, likewise, on expanding, draws in air from outside through the nose and mouth, and the arteries on expanding draw in air from outside through the skin. (Attraction, ὁλκή, is one of Galen's favorite concepts, and we shall say more about it below, in connection with his criticism of Erasistratus.)[22] Galen adds two more criticisms. Plato ignores the element of choice in breathing, which is obvious, since one can hold one's breath at will; and he also ignores the lack of synchronization between respiration and pulse. Galen thus assumes that breathing through the skin is Plato's explanation of the observable pulse in the arteries—a doubtful assumption.

b. Diogenes of Apollonia

Brief mention should be made here of one more of the pre-Socratic philosophers: Diogenes of Apollonia (probably not the Cretan Apollonia but the Milesian colony on the Pontus), who lived some time in the mid-fifth century B.C., perhaps a little later than Empedocles. He is not, indeed, a central or essential figure in the background to the dispute between Erasistratus and Galen which forms the chief subject of this book, because his theories did not have much of a following. But he has two claims to a mention here: he is the author of the earliest surviving Greek anatomy of the blood vessels (if we discount Aristotle's brief mention of the mysterious Syennesis of Cyprus in

[22] Below, pp. 28–30.

Historia animalium III 2, 511 b 24ff.), and he attached truly astonishing properties to the air that he supposed to be distributed by the vessels.

His anatomy of the vessels is recounted in the Aristotelian *Historia animalium* III 2, 511 b 30ff. No distinction is made between arteries and veins: the word used throughout is *phlebes*. There is no mention of the pulse. Nothing is said about the function of the vessels in this passage, and very little about the contents: the description occurs in the context of an account of blood, however, and it appears to be assumed that their business is the distribution of blood. What is striking is that the heart plays no special role. Aristotle includes Diogenes among those who place the origin of the vessels in the head (513 a 11), but the quoted description seems to have them originate vaguely in the middle. The main feature of Diogenes' vascular anatomy is a pair of major vessels, one left and one right, with big or little branches spreading to all parts, and a pair of smaller vessels passing from the head through the neck and going down the arms to the hands alongside the major ones. Although this doubling is not clearly maintained in the rest of the passage, it may suggest that Diogenes "had observed, without knowing it, the double system of veins and arteries" (Harris, *The Heart*, p. 25).

It is not Aristotle but the doxographer Aëtius who shows that the blood vessels in Diogenes' theory, as in Empedocles', contain air as well as blood: "Whenever the blood, being distributed to the whole [body], fills the vessels and forces the air contained in them out into the chest and the belly underneath, sleep occurs and the thorax is warmer. If *all* of the airy matter leaves the vessels, death ensues" (Aëtius V 24, 3; DK 64 A 29). According to Theophrastus (*De sensibus* 39–43), Diogenes held that the senses function by virtue of the entrance of air into the vessels, and that pleasure and pain result from the right and wrong mixture, respectively, of air with blood. Simplicius adds (*Physics* 153.13ff.) that "thinking takes place when the air along with the blood occupies the whole body through the vessels." This sounds like an abbreviated account of a modification of Empedocles' idea that "blood around the heart in men is thought." We have Diogenes' own words, finally, to the effect that the outside air is itself the source of thought and life, not only for men and animals but for the whole cosmos.

The outside air, then, enters the body not only in respiration (*anapneonta* in fr. 4) but also through the sense organs, and it brings with it life, sense perception, pleasure, and thought, which it conveys to the body by its passage, along with the blood, in the vessels. It is not merely the active cause of these things: it actually possesses them itself, in some fashion, and imparts them to the body.

c. Hippocrates and the Hippocratic Corpus

The problem of the relation between the collection of texts handed down from antiquity as the work of Hippocrates and the historical Hippocrates is too well known to need more than a mention here.[23] We will consider three topics, without attempting to put together a consistent historical account: first, the doctrine about breathing attributed to Hippocrates by the writer known as "Anonymus Londinensis"; second, Galen's view of Hippocrates' theory of respiration and blood flow; and third, doctrines on these subjects to be found in extant Hippocratic treatises.

The medical papyrus referred to now as Anonymus Londinensis has a section on the aetiology of diseases according to various authorities. There is reason to think this section goes back to Menon, the pupil of Aristotle who was the author of a medical work (a "collection," $\sigma\upsilon\nu\alpha\gamma\omega\gamma\acute{\eta}$), now lost, but sometimes mentioned by classical authors. According to Galen[24] this was attributed to Aristotle, and Anonymus purports to quote from Aristotle, not Menon.

He says that "Aristotle" attributes to Hippocrates the doctrine that diseases are brought about by "breaths" ($\phi\hat{\upsilon}\sigma\alpha\iota$—winds, gales) which arise from the residues of undigested food.

What moved Hippocrates to adopt these views was the following conviction. Breath (pneuma), he holds, is the most necessary and the supreme component in us, since health is the result of its free, and disease of its impeded passage. We in fact present a likeness to plants. For as they are rooted in the earth, so we too are rooted in the air, *by our nostrils and by our whole body.*[25] At least we are, he says, like those plants which are called "soldiers." For just as they, rooted in the moisture, are carried now to this moisture and now

[23]See Edelstein, "Hippocrates" and "Genuine Works"; Diller, "Stand"; and Harris, *The Heart*, pp. 29–96.
[24]K XV 25.
[25]My italics.

to that, even so we also, being as it were plants, are rooted in the air, and are in motion, changing our position now hither now thither. If this be so, it is clear that breath (pneuma) is the supreme component. (VI 14–31, trans. Jones)

This strange passage gives us some authority for attributing to Hippocrates the view that human beings depend on the surrounding air for life and health in the same sort of way that plants depend on the soil in which they are rooted. The special comparison with the water plant called "soldier" is presumably to meet the objection that human beings do not remain stationary in one place, as most plants do; he finds a plant with movable roots, so to speak. Notice the phrase italicized, which suggests that Hippocrates too held a theory of skin-breathing.[26]

Galen praises Hippocrates for his understanding of breathing.[27] He is fond of quoting from Hippocrates, with approval, an expression found in *Epidemics* VI: "the whole body breathes in and out." In *De usu respirationis*[28] he quotes it in support of his own doctrine that the arteries breathe through the skin, the brain through the nostrils, and the heart through the lungs. So it appears that Galen might have attributed skin-breathing to Hippocrates, even though it is impossible to find any certain confirmation of it in the *Corpus Hippocraticum*. In his *De placitis* II he quotes from Hippocrates the saying: "The source of nourishment of pneuma is the mouth, the nostrils, the wind-pipe, the lung, and the rest of the transpiration (διαπνοή)."[29] The word "transpiration" need not refer to skin-breathing; it may mean only the distribution of pneuma through the body.

There are several features relevant to respiration and blood flow that Galen finds to admire in Hippocrates. In his view, Hippocrates is on the whole sound on the "use" of respiration, believing as Galen does that it is for the replenishment of psychic pneuma and for cooling the innate heat.[30] He is sounder than both Plato and Erasistratus

---

[26]Compare this phrase: "κατά τε τὰς ῥῖνας καὶ κατὰ τὰ ὅλα σώματα" with xx 45: οὐ γὰρ μόνον κατὰ τὸ στόμα καὶ τοὺς μυκτῆρας ἡ ἀναπνοὴ γίνεται, ἀλλὰ καθ' ὅλον τὸ σῶμα (on Philistion).

[27] *De difficultate respirationis* II, K VII 826.

[28]Chapter 5 § 4. below

[29]K V 281; see Hippocrates, *Alim.* xxx (L IX 108).

[30] *De usu respirationis* 1.

on the subject of "attraction" (ὁλκή).[31] He believes, as Galen does, that the source of the veins is the liver, not the heart,[32] and that the pulsating dynamis flows from the heart along the coats of the arteries.[33] He believes, as Galen does, in the direct replenishment of the psychic pneuma by the intake of air into the brain.[34]

It is not possible to extract a consistent physiology from the extant *Corpus Hippocraticum* — indeed, such a thing is not to be expected, in view of the variety of date and purpose among the various treatises. There are, however, a few salient points that may be mentioned here.

The theory that in respiration through the nostrils air goes directly to the brain occurs in *De morbo sacro*, one of the earlier treatises. The writer makes no distinction between veins and arteries, but asserts that pneuma is carried by the vessels (φλέβες) all over the body.[35]

> The brain is the most powerful organ of the human body, for when it is healthy, it is an interpreter to us of the phenomena caused by the air, as it is the air that gives it intelligence. Eyes, ears, tongue, hands, and feet act in accordance with the discernment of the brain; in fact the whole body participates in intelligence in proportion to its participation in air. To consciousness the brain is the messenger. For when a man draws breath into himself, the air first reaches the brain, and so is dispersed through the rest of the body, though it leaves in the brain its quintessence, and all that it has of intelligence and sense. If it reached the body first and the brain afterwards, it would leave discernment in the flesh and the veins, and reach the brain hot, and not pure but mixed with the humor from flesh and blood, so as to have lost its perfect nature. (*Morb. Sacr.* 19, trans. Jones)

It will be seen that the anatomy is primitive and that Galen in fact takes over rather little of the author's peculiar theory.

The treatise *De flatibus*, a rhetorical exercise on the virtues of pneuma, refers to pneuma as nutriment (τροφή),[36] but since it is nutriment for heat in the body, it is not perhaps very remote from

[31] *De placitis* VIII 8 (K V 708).
[32] *De placitis* VI (K V 580).
[33] *De usu pulsuum* 4.
[34] *De usu partium* VIII 6 (K III 649–51).
[35] *Morb. Sacr.* 7.
[36] *Flat.* 3 (L VI 93). See also *Carn.* (L VIII 592).

the theory of Aristotle and Galen that breathing maintains the innate heat at a moderate temperature. However, no clear theory emerges from the text. It appears that blood and pneuma are combined in the vessels (again, there is no distinction between veins and arteries);[37] but the author is not interested in explaining how they got there, in what proportions, how they move, and so on.

The Hippocratic treatise that bears most interestingly on our topic is *De corde*. The author knows of the heart valves, and for this reason is usually dated after Erasistratus. Like Galen, and unlike Erasistratus, he thinks of the valves as only more or less cutting off backward flow: the pulmonary artery takes blood to the lungs for their nourishment, but also brings air in, "but not very much," from the lungs to the right side of the heart.[38] Since this is likely to be a third-century treatise, however, it will be more profitable to turn now to Aristotle and Erasistratus, who play much more significant roles in this history.[39]

d. Aristotle

i. *The Use of Respiration in Aristotle's Theory*

The main importance of Aristotle for this piece of history is his emphasis on the cooling function of respiration, which is also the mainstay of Galen's theory.

Like Galen, he argues against the view that breath is some kind of substance whose consumption is necessary for the vital heat.[40] He uses different arguments from Galen, of course. If this were so, he says, it should be true of all animals, since they all have vital heat; and he claims to have shown earlier, against Democritus and others, that not all animals breathe.[41] Second, we know that it is food that

---

[37] *Flat.* 14 (L VI 111).

[38] *Cord.* 12 For discussion of this treatise, see Hurlbutt, "Peri kardies"; Lonie, "The Heart"; and Harris, *The Heart*, pp. 83–96.

[39] It may be worth mentioning that in the late 1930s excited voices were raised announcing the discovery of a theory of the circulation of the blood in the *Corpus Hippocraticum*. But excitement was premature: the texts will not bear this interpretation. For a critical examination of the relevant texts, see Diller "Blutkreislauf," and Abel "Blutkreislauf".

[40] *PN* 473 a 3–15.

[41] 470 b 28–471 b 29.

generates heat, he says, and third, if breath were a kind of food, we should have an unparalleled case of the input of food and the output of excrement proceeding by the same route.

The natural heat that is a prerequisite for life may be destroyed, Aristotle says, in two ways: by extinction or by exhaustion.[42] All fire, of which the natural heat is one kind, is extinguished by meeting with excessive cold, or by being scattered. It is exhausted, on the other hand, if the heat becomes too great for the supply of fuel. It is to prevent the latter that some cooling device is necessary for life. Just as a charcoal fire without a through draught quickly goes out, even though there is a plentiful supply of fuel,[43] so heat will build up round the heart so much that the fuel cannot maintain it if there is no breathing to cool it down.

The relation between natural heat and ordinary fire in Aristotle's theory requires more careful examination. There is an interesting passage in the *De generatione animalium* II 3 in which he shows that natural heat cannot be simply identified with fire. The principle of life is soul, and since new life is generated from semen, semen must contain whatever substance it is that forms the material basis of soul. This is what we call "the hot" ($\tau\grave{o}$ $\kappa\alpha\lambda o\acute{v}\mu\epsilon\nu o\nu$ $\theta\epsilon\rho\mu\acute{o}\nu$); it is not fire or a "power" like that; it is the pneuma that is contained in the foamy stuff of the semen. The heat of the sun and the heat of animals have generative power, but ordinary fire does not. Hence, "the heat in animals is not fire and does not get its principle ($\dot{\alpha}\rho\chi\acute{\eta}$) from fire."[44]

In *De partibus animalium* II 7 he is after a different distinction. He objects that some thinkers identify soul with fire, whereas it would be better to say that soul "exists in some such body" (such as fire—$\dot{\epsilon}\nu$ $\tauο\iotaο\acute{v}\tau\wp$ $\tau\iota\nu\iota$ $\sigma\acute{\omega}\mu\alpha\tau\iota$ $\sigma\upsilon\nu\epsilon\sigma\tau\acute{\alpha}\nu\alpha\iota$).[45] The reason is that this substance, "the hot," is suitable for assisting the soul's activities, especially providing nourishment (that is, "concocting" food into blood, which is the body's proper nourishment) and causing motion. In this

---

[42] 474 b 13-24.

[43] 470 a 7-12; see also Theophrastus, *De igne* 11.

[44] 736 b 30-737 a 7. It may be observed that the Stoics make the distinction rather differently in their well-known theory of "creative fire" ($\pi\hat{v}\rho$ $\tau\epsilon\chi\nu\iota\kappa\acute{o}\nu$). For translation and commentary on this chapter of Aristotle, see Balme, *De partibus animalium*, pp. 62-65, 158-65.

[45] 652 b 9. The opponent is Democritus; see *De anima* 403 a 4.

passage Aristotle still leaves room for a distinction between natural heat and ordinary fire, by his use of the expression "some such body." Elsewhere he is less careful, and speaks of "the fire inside" or "natural fire."[46]

The juxtaposition of the heat of the sun with animal heat, in *De generatione* II 3, raises some interesting questions.[47] The heat of the sun, in Aristotelian theory, is a perplexing subject. In *De caelo* II 7, where he considers the subject directly, he maintains that the sun, the planets, and the stars are made of their own peculiar element, not of fire as others thought, and their light and heat is due to their friction with the inner sphere of air.[48] "Air" is what he says: but according to the cosmology of the *De caelo* there is not even any contact between air and the heavenly spheres, since they are separated by the sphere of fire. The explanation usually put forward is that the fiery element iself is ignited by friction with the heavenly bodies, and in turn fires the air under it. Whatever the exact explanation may be, the heat of the sun appears to be a kind of heat that does not consume fuel and is creative rather than destructive. Aristotle goes out of his way to refute the popular theory that the sun is fueled by moist exhalations from below,[49] and he does not suggest an alternative fuel. Animal heat is certainly similar in that it is not destructive, and accordingly its relation to its fuel is somewhat different from that of ordinary fire. It does not work exactly as the sun does, because it needs fuel—namely, food. But it does not destroy the fuel, as ordinary fire does; on the contrary, it "concocts" the food taken into the stomach, and turns it into vapor, which then rises to the heart where it is made into blood.[50]

Natural heat is like ordinary fire in that it has waste products. There is some analogy, for instance, between cinders and ash, the waste products of fire, and animal excrement and bile.[51] I have not, however, found any mention in Aristotle of the "smoky wastes" that in Galen's theory are expelled by breathing out. He mentions that

[46] 473 a 4, 474 b 12.

[47] 737 a 1ff.; see Balme's commentary, pp. 163–65.

[48] *De caelo* II 7; see also *Meteor.* I 4, 341 b 12–23.

[49] *Meteor.* II 2, 354 b 33–355 a 32.

[50] 456 a 30ff.; also *PA* II 4, 666 b 24. At 473 a 11–12, Aristotle speaks of food as the fuel for natural heat.

[51] *PA* II 2, 649 a 25.

the expired air is warmer than the inspired air,[52] but that of course is merely because it has been warmed by its contact with the heat of the heart or the blood in the lungs.

The passage in which Aristotle compares the generative power of the sun's heat and animal heat also contains a reference to "the element of the stars." The pneuma in animals, which is what we call "the hot," is said to be analogous to this.[53] This is a tantalizing sentence, which suggests a much larger fabric of doctrine—but there is notoriously little elsewhere in Aristotle to supply it.[54]

It is not easy to make a consistent whole of Aristotle's theory. Just as there is some mystery attending the relation between natural heat and the element of the heavenly bodies, so we are left with an unsolved problem with regard to the function of air in breathing. It is to cool the natural heat of the heart—but in Aristotle's scheme air is a warm element.[55] Perhaps air is cool relatively to fire, but Aristotle never explains this.

ii. *Aristotle's View of the Heart*

So much for biochemistry (if it is permissible to use this term). To turn now to the organs concerned with respiration in Aristotle's theory, we must first observe that the heart is one of them. Whether the reason was the observation of anatomical connections (the pulmonary artery and veins) between the heart and lungs, or the fact that breathing and the beating of the heart change in similar ways, or the intimate connection between breathing and the heartbeat as signs of life, or some combination of all of these, the idea that the heart is an organ of respiration was established early in the history of Greek physiology and was still strongly entrenched in Galen's theory.

At the end of his *De respiratione*, Aristotle summarizes three types of motion of the heart, all of them due in some way to heat: they are palpitation (πήδησις), pulsation (σφυγμός), and breathing (ἀναπνοή). We can postpone the first two for the moment. In its breathing capacity, the heart is like a bronze smith's bellows. Increasing

[52] *PN* 472 b 34.

[53] *GA* II 3.

[54] For discussion and bibliography, see P. Moraux, "Quinta Essentia," especially 1205–07 and 1213–15, and Balme's commentary *ad loc.*

[55] *GC* II 3, 330 b 4.

heat in the heart causes it to expand and rise up, and this causes the surrounding parts to expand as well. As with bellows, the expansion causes air to flow in from outside. This cools the heat, the heart subsides again, and the air, now warmed by its contact with the interior heat, is expelled.[56]

In this description, Aristotle does not say explicitly whether the cooling air is supposed to flow into the heart itself, or only into the lungs that surround the heart. He does say, however, that the simile of the bellows fits both heart and lungs,[57] and he also remarks[58] that the heart has communications ($\sigma\acute{u}\nu\tau\rho\eta\sigma\iota\varsigma$) with the lungs; in contrasting air-cooled with water-cooled creatures he remarks that air gets easily to the source of heat in the heart.[59] This seems to mean that air does enter the heart as well as the lungs. But the respiratory motion is apparently all one; the heart expands, through increasing heat, and thus causes expansion in the lungs, and the air is drawn into the lungs and the heart. This theory is to be distinguished from those that attribute the expansion of the lungs to another cause, and think of the *pulse* as the heart's breathing motion.[60]

Pulsation, Aristotle says,[61] is like boiling, which takes place "when that which is moist is pneumatized by heat; it rises because its volume ($\acute{o}\gamma\kappa o\varsigma$) becomes greater.... In the heart, the swelling, because of the heat, of the moisture which is continually coming in from the food produces pulsation, as it rises against the exterior coat of the heart.... And the blood vessels ($\phi\lambda\acute{e}\beta\epsilon\varsigma$) all pulsate, and all at the same time, because they are all dependent upon ($\mathring{\eta}\rho\tau\mathring{\eta}\sigma\theta\alpha\iota$) the heart. It moves them continually, and therefore they move contin-

---

[56] *PN* 480 a 16–b 12. For a fuller discussion of Aristotle's doctrine, see Harris, *The Heart*, pp. 121–76, especially pp. 160–73.

[57] *PN* 480 a 22.

[58] *PN* 478 a 26.

[59] *PN* 478 a 23.

[60] As Harris remarks (p. 164), this doctrine "would appear on the face of it to establish a one-to-one relation between pulse-rate and the rate of drawn breaths, which it is somewhat difficult to believe that Aristotle could have believed to be the case." Difficult, indeed! Perhaps we are to think of the heartbeat as involving only an incomplete return to unexpanded size, so that there is a gradual expansion of heart and lung through several heartbeats, until the inspired air causes complete contraction again. But I have found no evidence for this idea.

[61] *PN* 479 a 30 ff.

ually, and at the same time as each other, when it moves them." Thus the heating of the blood in the heart produces pneuma, just as the heating of any liquid does; the expansion of volume causes the heart to pulsate, and the heart causes its connected blood vessels to pulsate.

This pneuma is not to be confused with the breath drawn in from outside in the breathing process. It is natural pneuma ($\sigma\upsilon\mu\phi\upsilon\tau\grave{o}\nu$ $\pi\nu\epsilon\hat{\upsilon}\mu\alpha$), which is continually created and renewed inside the body so long as there is heat and life. It is the vehicle of soul, and as such is responsible for reproduction and movement.[62]

It is an extraordinary feature of Aristotle's account of these matters that he does not give any final cause for pulsation. Apparently he has nothing to say about the use of the pulse; it appears to be just a necessary accompaniment of the work of the natural heat in the heart in making blood out of food. In fact, he links it with the first in his list of motions of the heart—palpitation—which he recognizes as pathological. He does not, of course, think of pulsation as pathological, but even so he begins by comparing it with the throbbing of an abscess.[63]

This brings us to the major function of the heart in Aristotle's biological theory. The soul is the organizing principle of all the functions of an animal, and it must have a single central location:

The constitution of an animal must be regarded as resembling that of a well-governed city-state. For when order is once established in a city there is no need of a special ruler with arbitrary powers to be present at every activity, but each individual performs his own task as he is ordered, and one act succeeds another because of custom. And in the animals the same process goes on because of nature, and because each part of them, since they are so constituted, is naturally suited to perform its own function; so that there is no need of soul in each part, but since it is situated in a central origin of authority over the body, the other parts live by their structural attachment to it and perform their own functions in the course of nature. (*De motu animalium* 10, 703 a 29–b 2, trans. Forster)

[62]See Jaeger, "Pneuma"; Peck, ed., *GA*, App B, pp. 576–93; and Balme, *De partibus animalium*, pp. 160–65.
[63] *PN* 479 b 26.

The heart is the center of the natural heat of the body. As such it is the primary cause of nutrition—that is to say, of the process of "concocting" the food into blood, which is the true nutriment of the body. But also, and more importantly, it is the controlling center of all sensation and movement in the body. Aristotle wrote before the discovery of the nerves. He was convinced of the necessity of some central focus for all sensory processes, and found a suitable anatomical pattern in the heart and the vessels that spread all over the body from it.[64]

On the anatomy of the heart itself, Aristotle was primitive and obscure. He asserted that it has three chambers, and he had no knowledge of the valves.[65]

iii. *Aristotle on the Blood Vessels*

Aristotle makes no distinction between veins and arteries, but uses the same word, φλέβες, for both. The word is commonly translated "blood vessels," for obvious reasons, although this translation has the disadvantage of making Aristotle's assertion[66] that the φλέβες are contrived by nature for holding blood into an analytic proposition, which it is not.

Blood is the "final nutriment" of the living body;[67] that is to say, blood is the last stage through which food goes, after being taken into the body by the mouth, before being consumed by the parts of the body. This nutriment, without which continuing life is impossible for those animals that have blood, is distributed all over the body and to all its parts by the vessels.

The "starting point" (ἀρχή) of the vessels is the heart. This point is elaborated in *PA* III 5. The sensory soul in every animal is a unity,

---

[64]Not all of Aristotle's works locate the soul unambiguously in the heart. This is one of the criteria that have been used to arrive at a relative dating of his writings. See especially Nuyens, *Évolution*, and Ross, ed., *PN*, with my review of the latter.

[65]For further discussion of the difficulties in his description, see D'Arcy Thompson's translation of *HA* III 3, and Platt, "Aristotle on the Heart." There is a useful essay on the whole subject of Aristotle's theory of the heart by James Rochester Shaw (1972).

[66]*PA* III 5, 665 b 14.

[67]*PA* II 3, 650 a 34 and elsewhere.

and must be located in a single part, which must also be the source of heat. But this source is the cause of the blood's heat and fluid nature. "So because the ἀρχή of sensation and that of heat are in one single part, the blood originates from a single source too; and because of the unity of the blood, the vessels also originate from a single source."[68]

From the heart, the blood passes through the vessels to provide the material out of which the body is made and maintained.

> The system of blood-vessels in the body may be compared to those of water-courses which are constructed in gardens: they start from one source, or spring, and branch off into numerous channels, and then into still more, and so on progressively, so as to carry a supply to every part of the garden. And again, when a house is being built, supplies of stones are placed all alongside the lines of the foundations. These things are done (a) because water is the material out of which the plants in the garden grow, and (b) because stones are the material out of which the foundations are built. In the same way, Nature has provided for the irrigation of the whole body with blood, because blood is the material out of which it is all made. (*PA* III 5, 668 a 14–22, trans. Peck)

In addition to their primary function as distributors of nutriment, the vessels play other parts in Aristotle's theory, although they are much less explicitly described.

There is one definite statement that the passage of food from the stomach to the heart is by way of the blood vessels. Aristotle refers to a lost work *On Nutrition*, and briefly summarizes its contents in his discussion of *Sleep and Waking*:

> Evidently, the animal must first get nutrition and increase at the time when it gets sensation; and the final nourishment for animals with blood is blood and for bloodless animals the analogous substance; and the place of blood is the blood vessels, whose source is the heart (this is clear from the dissections). So, as the nourishment enters from the outside into the places that are to receive it, exhalation takes place into the blood vessels, and there it changes and is made into blood and moves toward the source [that is, the heart]. (*PN* 456 a 32–b 5)

[68] 667 b 28–31.

21

This account of how the nutriment is transferred from the digestive organs to the heart is not supplanted by any other in Aristotle's work, so far as I have observed; yet it is strictly inconsistent with his often repeated statement that blood originates only in the heart.[69] Among many obscurities in his physiology, this is one of the most striking. Literal consistency may be saved by supposing that the "exhalation" as it passes through the vessels is only potentially blood, and requires the action of the heart to actualize it. But there is nothing to explain how the exhalation moves through the same vessels through which blood moves in the opposite direction, from the heart, nor of how it gets into the heart, which also sends blood out into the vessels.[70]

There is some evidence, very sketchy and inconclusive, that Aristotle thought of the blood vessels as channels conveying messages from the sense organs to the heart and from the heart to the muscles that bring about bodily movement. He said clearly that it is not the blood itself that has the function of sensation,[71] although it is necessary for sensation: bloodless parts are insensitive. But there are hints that it is pneuma that conveys both sensory messages and motor impulses, and that the pneuma may be contained in the blood vessels along with the blood.[72]

e. Praxagoras, Philotimus, Herophilus

Praxagoras of Cos—a fellow countryman of Hippocrates—lived in the second half of the fourth century.[73]

It has become accepted doctrine that Praxagoras was the first to distinguish clearly between arteries and veins. Galen expressly says

[69] *PA* III 4, 666 b 24: "as we have said many times."

[70] Galen faces a similar problem in *De usu partium* IV 19 (K III 336): how does "useful blood" flow back through the same vessels through which anadosis to the liver takes place? His answer is the powerful force of attraction (*holke*). See May, *Usefulness*, p. 242, n. 101.

[71] *PA* III 4, 666 a 17–18.

[72] These hints are developed rather fully by Peck, ed., *GA*, pp. 586–93. For a more cautious account, see F. Solmsen, "Nerves," 169–78.

[73] There is an edition of "fragments" (they are really *testimonia*) of Praxagoras and Philotimus by Fritz Steckerl. The collection is useful, but the interpretation is frequently unconvincing.

that Praxagoras, like Erasistratus, supposed the arteries to carry pneuma, not blood.[74] In a lengthy discussion near the beginning of his *De placitis Hippocratis et Platonis*, Galen describes Praxagoras' strange theory that the smaller arteries turn into *nerves*.[75] He especially attacks this notion because it makes the nervous system originate in the heart: so it is likely that Praxagoras made the arterial system originate there. Praxagoras recognized pulsation, although he did not distinguish it, except quantitatively, from other movements of the arteries.[76] But he differed from Erasistratus and Galen about what made the arteries pulsate. It was not pneuma pumped from the heart that expanded the arteries, as Erasistratus thought, but a special pulsating power in the arteries themselves; this power was not, as Galen held, transmitted from the heart through the coats of the arteries, but was the special property of the arteries.

It seems well enough established, then, that Praxagoras did indeed, unlike Aristotle, distinguish veins from arteries. Whether he was the first to do so is more problematical, since Galen remarks casually that Praxagoras' father Nicarchus had some of the same views in this area.[77] Since fathers have been known to learn from their sons, this is hardly sufficient ground for accusing Aristotle of ignoring the medical knowledge of his time, on the assumption that Nicarchus must have worked out the difference before Aristotle wrote his biological works.[78]

The surviving evidence does not say that Praxagoras made the distinction between arteries and veins on anatomical grounds—that is to say, because of the observation of a difference in the coats of veins and arteries. On the contrary, it suggests, without proof, that the distinction grew from a theoretical demand for different vessels to convey blood and pneuma. Possibly this was due to the increased importance of pneuma in such works as Aristotle's *De motu animalium*, in which it plays a major part in his account of voluntary motion.[79] Pneuma figured largely in Praxagoras' theory: in *De usu respi-*

---

[74]Galen *De plenitudine* 11 (K VII 573) = fr. 85 Steckerl; *De dignoscendis pulsibus* IV 3 (K VIII 950) = fr. 9 Steckerl.

[75] *De placitis Hippocratis et Platonis* I 7 (K V 189–200) = fr. 11 Steckerl.

[76]Galen *De pulsuum differentiis* IV 3 (K VIII 723) fr. 27 Steckerl.

[77]K VII 573; see note 74 above.

[78]So Fredrich, p. 57 ff.

[79]See *De motu animalium* ch. 10, with Essay no. 3 in Martha C. Nussbaum's edition.

rationis 2 Galen mentions that he took breathing to be for the sake of nourishing the psychic pneuma.[80]

Philotimus, one of Praxagoras' pupils, need not delay us: he is mentioned just because he is referred to, twice, in the following treatises of Galen.[81] The first mentions that he joined Praxagoras in the belief that we breathe to restore the psychic pneuma, the second that he agreed with Praxagoras, Herophilus, and others that the arteries are filled not just from the heart but "from everywhere." Most of the testimonia collected by Steckerl concern diet; we hear nothing else of importance for the theory of respiration and blood flow.

Praxagoras' pupil Herophilus of Chalkedon, who worked in Alexandria, as Erasistratus is also usually supposed to have done,[82] and at approximately the same time as Erasistratus, was a figure of great importance in the history of anatomy and medicine.[83] Some of his advances in knowledge came from dissection of the human body, which had not been possible for his predecessors; if the famous report of Celsus is to be believed, he and Erasistratus were permitted to practice vivisection on criminal prisoners.[84] He is generally credited with the discovery of the nervous system, and he recognized its origin as the brain.[85] As we have seen, Praxagoras had begun to speak of the nerves as channels of pneuma attached to the arterial system. Herophilus dissociated them from the arteries, and for the first time clearly distinguished arteries both from nerves and from veins. According to Galen, he declared that arteries have coats six times as thick as veins.[86]

---

[80] See Introduction, II.

[81] *De usu respirationis* 2, near the end, and *An in arteriis* 8. According to the Greek manuscripts I have looked at, his name was Philotimus; and so he appears, for instance, in Kühn's edition of Galen. Steckerl, in his edition of the "fragments," unaccountably fails to discuss his name. Modern editors are confident that his name was Phylotimus; see Kaibel's edition of Athenaeus (Teubner), p. xli. I have decided to adopt the spelling of our Greek manuscripts.

[82] See below, Introduction, I f.

[83] A new edition of the fragments and testimonia is being prepared by Heinrich von Staden. For the time being, see the account of Herophilus in Harris, *The Heart*, pp. 177–95.

[84] Celsus, *De medicina*, prooemium.

[85] See Solmsen, "Nerves," pp. 185–88.

[86] *De usu partium* VI 10 (K III 445).

Not all was clear, however. Praxagoras appears to have regarded all the vessels originating from the left side of the heart as arteries: they were all part of the system that distributed pneuma to the body. All the vessels attached to the right side were veins, and distributed blood. (In this he was followed by Erasistratus, but not, it appears, by Herophilus). This distinction did not produce the same result as the distinction by thickness of the coats: the pulmonary artery (to use its modern name) has the coats of an artery but belongs to the right side of the heart, and the pulmonary vein has the coats of a vein but belongs to the left side of the heart. The Praxagorean/Erasistratean distinction was allowed to prevail: the standard procedure, used also by Galen, was to call the pulmonary artery "the arterial vein" and the pulmonary vein "the veinlike artery."

There is an explicit statement, however, that Herophilus did not follow Praxagoras' lead: "Herophilus calls the thickest and greatest vein that goes from the heart to the lung [that is, the pulmonary artery] an artery. For the state of affairs at the lung is opposite to the rest: the veins here are strong and closest in nature to arteries, while the arteries are weak and closest in nature to veins." (Rufus of Ephesus, *De nominibus partium* 162).[87]

It seems that Herophilus differed from Praxagoras also on the contents of the arteries: not pneuma only, but blood as well. There is an explicit statement of Herophilus' view, and a criticism of it, in the papyrus known as Anonymus Londinensis (XXVIII 46–XXIX 34). Herophilus held that nutriment (τροφή) is contained both in the veins and in the arteries—and in fact more of it is contained in the arteries, because the pulse causes them to absorb more. He is then criticized for not realizing that the hollow of the veins is actually larger than that of the arteries, and that the pulse will cause the arteries to contain less than the veins, because more is squeezed out by the contraction of the arteries. This report uses the word "nutriment" (τροφή), not "blood." But although Herophilus regarded air drawn in by breathing as the nutriment of the psychic pneuma, it can hardly be this theory that is referred to by Anonymus Londinensis.

[87] Quoted by Harris, *The Heart*, p. 179—but he takes it as evidence that Herophilus adopted the Praxagorean/Erasistraten practice, instead of the opposite. So do Sieveking, "Herophilus," col. 1106, and May, *Usefulness*, p. 26. But Rufus quite plainly says he called the big vein ἀρτηρίαν, and not ἀρτηριώδη.

The "nutriment" carried by the veins is certainly blood, and the dispute concerns the quantity of nutriment in veins and arteries, not its substance.

Galen reports that Herophilus, among others, claimed that the arteries draw in "from everywhere," and not just from the heart, as Erasistratus supposed.[88] That means, presumably, that the expansion of the artery in pulsation causes an intake of matter—both blood and pneuma—through both ends of the artery and through "pores" in the coats. It is a proposition that cannot be consistent with the Erasistratean theory that pulsation is caused by the pumping of pneuma from the heart; so we may take it that Herophilus shared Praxagoras' view of the nature of pulsation—namely, that it is a property of the arteries themselves.

Herophilus wrote much about the pulse, and studied its variations most carefully; Galen refers to him more often in this connection than in any other. But the details of his theories need not concern us here.

Some mention should be made of his theory of breathing, which included a peculiar four-stroke account of the action of the lungs.[89] The first diastole of the lungs draws in air from outside, the first systole thrusts the air into the thorax (not into the heart); the second diastole draws the used air from the body, the second systole expels it to the outside. Like the Otto cycle in an internal combustion engine, this model appears to necessitate valves of some kind. Galen reports that Herophilus wrote about the valves of the heart, although he was not, says Galen, as clear on the subject as Erasistratus was.[90] But no such details are reported about the respiration processes.

f. Erasistratus

In the works that follow in this volume, Galen regards Erasistratus as his chief opponent. To understand his position fully, it would be necessary to know in detail the reasoning with which Erasistratus defended his theory of the function of respiration and the arteries. Unfortunately, none of the works of Erasistratus survives. There is some significant information in the book of Anonymus Londinensis,

[88] *An in arteriis* 8 (K IV 732).
[89] Aëtius *Placita* IV 22, 3 = Ps.-Galen *Historia philosophiae* K XIX 318.
[90] *De placitis Hippocratis et Platonis* I 10 (K V 206).

but by far the biggest source of knowledge of his theories is Galen himself.[91] Followers of Erasistratus were active in Galen's own time, and he attacks them in his writings as his own personal opponents. We do not find dispassionate historical acounts of Erasistratus' views; on the contrary, although Galen shows a high regard for his abilities as compared with others, he habitually writes contentiously and even sarcastically about him. Consequently our knowledge of Erasistratus' system is full of gaps and uncertainties.

The Erasistrateans claimed that their master associated with the philosophers of the Peripatos,[92] and especially with Theophrastus.[93] His theories are commonly thought to borrow from those of Strato of Lampsacus, Theophrastus' successor as head of Aristotle's school from about 287 to 269 B.C. We shall look into these relationships later.[94] Erasistratus worked in Alexandria;[95] his dates cannot be determined more accurately than the first half of the third century.

Around the time of Erasistratus there was an important advance in knowledge of the anatomy of the heart: the discovery of the valves and their functions. Galen observes that Erasistratus wrote accurately about the valves, whereas his contemporary Herophilus wrote carelessly.[96] Perhaps it was Erasistratus who discovered the valves and their functions.[97] At all events, with this discovery the Aristotelian theory of a single direction of flow through all the vessels away from the heart became impossible to hold. It was clear that blood flowed into the right side of the heart from the vena cava, and out of the heart toward the lung through what was called the "arterial vein" (that is, the pulmonary artery), and that whatever it was that filled

---

[91] Galen was probably in possession of some of Erasistratus' books. Kühn's index (XX, 228) says that none of his books survived to Galen's time, but this seems to be a wrong inference from a counterfactual at *De venae sectione* 5 (K II 71). See Harris, *The Heart*, p. 195.

[92] Galen, *De nat. fac.* II 4 (K II 88).

[93] Galen, *An in arteriis* 7 (K IV 729).

[94] Below, pp. 34–35.

[95] P. M. Fraser argues that the evidence placing Erasistratus and his school in Alexandria is weak, and that he probably worked in Antioch; see his "Career of Erasistratus,", pp. 518–37. But this is rejected by Harris, *The Heart*, pp. 177–78.

[96] *De placitis Hippocratis et Platonis* I 10 (K V 206). See also *De usu pulsuum* 5 (K V 166).

[97] See Abel, "Blutkreislauf" p. 133, Wilson, "Erasistratus," etc.

the left side of the heart came from the lung through the "veinlike artery" (that is, the pulmonary vein) and went from the heart out into the body through the aorta and the whole arterial system.

Erasistratus placed the blood-making faculty in the liver, not the heart.[98] From the liver it flowed over the whole of the body through the venous system to provide nourishment for all the parts of the body, including the heart. From the right side of the heart it flowed to the lungs, to provide nourishment for them.

The theory held that air is drawn into the lungs in breathing, and most of it is expelled by the same route. The air is drawn in by the expansion of the thorax, which would otherwise create a vacuum: this is an important theoretical point, to which we shall return. While the air is in the lungs, it can be drawn into the heart in *its* movement of expansion, the diastole, through the veinlike artery. When the heart contracts, the air is prevented from returning to the lungs by the valve, and instead it is forced out by the heart through the arteries to the rest of the body. As it is forced out by the heart, it causes an expansion of the arteries. Thus the pulsation of the heart is the active cause of the movement of pneuma, but the pulsation of the arteries is caused by the movement of pneuma, and the systole of the heart is simultaneous with the diastole of the arteries.

When Galen asks "What is the use of breathing?" and classifies answers according to whether they name the substance or a quality of the breath, Erasistratus naturally belongs to those who name the substance.[99] For healthy life, the arteries must be filled with pneuma, and they are kept full by the respiratory work of the lungs and heart. Anonymus Londinensis attributes to Erasistratus the thesis that both blood and nutriment are "material" ($\H{\upsilon}\lambda\eta$), which is required to replace that which is expended.[100] Galen says he made blood, nutriment and breath "a factor in producing natural activities."[101] There is no inconsistency between these two accounts: both blood and breath are materials necessary for life and both must be present in the body, but only blood makes the actual fabric of the body.

It is pneuma that works the muscles in Erasistratus' theory, including those that work unconsciously, like the muscles of the stomach in

[98]Erasistratus' views about blood are also discussed in Introduction, II.
[99] *De usu respirationis* 1 (K IV 473).
[100]xxii 49.
[101]K XIV 697: συνεργὸν εἰς τὰς φυσικὰς ἐνεργείας.

digestion. Erasistratus distinguishes between vital pneuma and psychic pneuma, and locates the center of the former in the left side of the heart, and the latter in the head. Both, apparently, were replenished from the heart by respiration.

Although Galen does not mention it in his discussion of Erasistratus, Anonymus Londinensis explains that Erasistratus' theory also allotted a cooling function to breathing: "The breath, cold to begin with, is exhaled warm, inasmuch as it is borne through warm bodies. Of course the inhaling takes place, he says, with a view to reducing the excessive heat about the heart, and to prevent its becoming solid and burning up our bodies" (xxiii 36–42, trans. Jones).

Warm air is exhaled from the lungs via the mouth and nostrils, together with moisture.[102] Some of the inhaled air, however, passes into the heart and from the heart into the arteries. Once it has entered the arteries it cannot return through the heart, because of the valves. It is not consumed by the body like food or fuel, but has to circulate through it and eventually, it appears, pass out again through the skin. Anonymus Londinensis is again the authority: "Now from these places [the reference is not quite clear] it is borne into the individual arteries, and it is also borne into the cavities [κοιλώματα], and similarly into the pores [? ἀραιώματα] all over the body, then it passes through the natural pores in the flesh to the outside" (xxiii 18–23, trans. Jones). It would appear from this that skin-breathing is a feature of Erasistratus' theory, too.

However, there is some doubt about the theory here. In his polemic against Erasistratus, Galen raises the objection that all the essential pneuma may theoretically escape from the system whenever the skin is punctured, since the skin itself contains as one of its elements very small branches of the arterial system.[103] From this it seems that the arterial system as a whole is like the inner tube of a tire, which must be unpunctured if it is to function. How can this be the case, if pneuma is all the time escaping from the arteries by way of the natural pores in the skin?

The answer is probably that Galen is being tendentious. Erasistratus certainly believed that pneuma escaped from the arteries, unnaturally and pathologically, in the case of wounds. It is perfectly possible

---

[102] Anonymus Londinensis xxiv 13.
[103] *An in arteriis* 4 (K IV 712).

to combine this proposition with the assumption of a natural flow of pneuma through the arteries and out of the whole system at its natural vents. All that is required is some concept of a measured flow. Galen's notion of a kind of balloon that collapses at a pinprick is a polemical exaggeration—although not a totally unjustified one, as we shall see.[104]

There was much controversy in antiquity about what is the *arche* of the veins and arteries. The concept of *arche* is an ambiguous one, and it is impossible to translate the word into English with the same kind of ambiguity. "Origin" is perhaps the nearest, since it preserves at least the ambiguity between a temporal and a spatial meaning. One of the possible interpretations of the statement that the origin (*arche*) of the veins is the heart is that the veins grow from the heart in embryonic development; another is that they are channels for a flow that begins from the heart, related to it as a river is to its source. But the Greek *arche* has another element in it—the notion of control or direction; the verb *archein* means both "to begin" and "to rule." In this sense, to say that the heart is the *arche* of the veins is to say that the veins are subordinate to the heart, that their function is in some way directed or controlled by the heart.

Galen discusses the question of the *arche* of the various "powers" that control animal life in the sixth book of his *De placitis Hippocratis et Platonis*. Aristotle and Theophrastus, he says, believed that they all come from the heart, whereas Hippocrates and Plato thought there were three separate *archai*—brain, heart, and liver. Galen's own view is closest to the latter: the brain is the *arche* of the nervous system, the heart of the arteries, the liver of the veins. The heart is not the source of the arterial system in the sense in which a river has a source, because the flow is through the heart, from the "veinlike artery" (the pulmonary vein) and into the aorta. A better model than a river is the seed of a tree, which puts out both roots and a trunk: the veinlike artery is like the roots, the aorta is like the trunk.[105] The model of a seed might suggest that it is the temporal sense of *arche* that is dominant here, but Galen makes it clear that this is not the only or the primary sense. "Just as plants draw in all their food through the roots, so the heart draws in air from the lung through

---

[104] Below, p. 37.
[105] K V 525.

the arteries already mentioned" (that is, the veinlike arteries; note that it is air that the heart draws in, even in Galen's theory; more on this below). The heart is the *arche* of the powers that regulate the whole arterial system.[106]

With this established, Galen discusses the *arche* of the veins, and it is in this connection that he writes about the theory of Erasistratus. Erasistratus held that the heart is the *arche* both of the arteries and the veins. Galen's chief objection is based on the anatomy of the valves, which, he emphasizes, Erasistratus himself understood and explained.[107] The valves ensure that there is only one exit from the heart in the venous system, and that is the arterial vein, which leads only to the lungs.[108] If the heart were the *arche* it ought to be responsible for distributing the blood over the whole body, not just to the lungs. Moreover, it was not open to Erasistratus, Galen says, to escape by saying that the heart is the *arche* of the power that controls the veins. He could not say this, because he had denied it of the arteries; Galen's own view is that the heart transmits a power through the coats of the arteries, but Erasistratus said that pulsation was merely the effect of pneuma being forced through them by the heart. Galen goes on to consider and reject another possible interpretation of Erasistratus, that the heart is the origin of the veins in the embryo; but we need not pursue the argument.[109]

What did Erasistratus mean when he said that the heart was the *arche* of the veins as well as of the arteries? Galen's criticism that the valves make nonsense of this thesis appears at first sight to be a good one, because the distribution of blood to the whole body, which is the function of the veins, has not been shown to be due to the heart. Modern writers on Erasistratus have usually not faced this question,[110] and it is a difficult one. It seems probable that the answer lies in

[106] K V 525: ἀρχὴ τῶν διοικουσῶν αὐτὰς δυνάμεων.

[107] K V 548ff.

[108] K V 551.

[109] K V 555ff.

[110] An exception is I. M. Lonie ("Erasistratus"). But I disagree with his conclusions. He thinks, rightly, that Galen found Erasistratus obscure on this question, but adds, wrongly, that there was a sect of Erasistrateans who held that blood is distributed to the whole body via the vena cava from the heart, in spite of the valves. The crucial sentence (522.10–12 Mueller; K V 533–34) is not a statement of the theory, but one of Galen's alternative interpretations of it.

Erasistratus' mechanical system. Galen himself gives a clear pointer, although he does not follow it up: "Matter, he [Erasistratus] says, does not flow into it [the heart] of its own accord (αὐτομάτως), as into some lifeless receptacle, but the heart itself, when it expands, draws it in like a bronze smith's bellows and fills up the expansion."[111] This principle is applied to *anadosis*, that is, the distribution of nutriment, again in Erasistratus' theory, in *De nat. fac.* II 1. The heart is thus the cause of motion of the blood in the veins that lead to itself: perhaps Erasistratus thought this was sufficient to explain the motion of blood in *all* the veins, and therefore of the nutrition of the whole body, but this can only be conjectured.[112] The heart draws matter into itself, in Erasistratus' theory, through the principle of filling a vacuum. this is a keystone in the structure of his physiology, and one that excites Galen's scorn. The whole concept must be examined closely.

IN MANY areas of his physiology, Erasistratus used the concept of "following into what is emptied" (πρὸς τὸ κενούμενον ἀκολουθία). This is a clumsy translation, but it is as well to stay with it at least initially, because the principle needs to be carefully distinguished from others.[113]

The principle itself is perfectly simple, and familiar under the Latin name *horror vacui*. In nontechnical terms, it asserts that if a substance is removed from a container with rigid walls, then another substance must enter to take its place.

There had been many years of speculation on this subject when Erasistratus wrote. We have mentioned[114] Plato's theory of circular

---

[111] K V 549.

[112] *De nat. fac.* II 1 = K II 76 makes it clear that the contraction of the veins played some part in Erasistratus' theory. Perhaps this assisted the pumping action of the heart in some way.

[113] It is not clear whether τὸ κενούμενον is the substance emptied out (as in *An in arteriis*, often) or the place that is being emptied (as in *An in arteriis* 5.12 and 7.5; K IV 710 and 713). If it were the substance, one would expect the dative to be used rather than πρός with an accusative. On the other hand, if it were the place, why not εἰς, rather than πρός? In either case, note the *present* participle: nothing is emptied, ever, but is only in the process of being emptied.

[114] Introduction I a. According to Aristotle, *De respiratione* 471 a 1, the principle was already used by Anaxagoras and Diogenes of Apollonia in explaining how fish breathe.

thrust (περίωσις), used in his explanation of the processes of breathing. After developing that explanation, he remarks that the same theory explains other phenomena: "There are, moreover, the flowing of any stream of water, the falling of thunderbolts, and the attraction (ὁλκή) of amber and of the lodestone at which men wonder. There is no real attraction in any of these cases, but proper investigation will make it plain that there is no void, and that the things in question thrust themselves around, one upon another" (Plato, *Timaeus* 80 b–c, trans. Cornford, slightly adapted).

In this passage, Plato is plainly taking sides in a controversy. We have evidence in surviving texts for the later stages of this dispute. Galen and other medical writers used the concept of *attraction* (ὁλκή) to refer to the power of certain organs, tissues, and so on to draw toward themselves certain specific substances: for example, the power of the kidneys to attract urine. The suction exerted by "what is emptied" is quite different from this. "What is emptied," whether it is a place, bounded by the inner surface of the container, or the substance that is being removed, is qualitatively neutral and attracts whatever is contiguous. Galen criticizes Erasistratus sharply on his use of this principle to explain the secretion of urine in *De nat. fac.*, and makes it quite clear that it is totally different from his "attraction."

The principle of *horror vacui* (let us now call it that) may thus take two forms: it may either stop with the notion of suction, or it may go on to reduce the apparent suction to pushes, by the theory of circular thrust. It is not entirely clear which version Erasistratus adopted, but I have not observed any positive evidence of the circular thrust theory. In both its forms the principle is different from attraction (ὁλκή) as used by Galen.

In ancient explanations of the principle of *horror vacui* it is usually stated that there cannot be in nature a massed empty place (κενὸς ἀθρόος τόπος): for example, in *An in arteriis* 3. This qualification was necessary because of another theory, widely held in antiquity, that void spaces occur in nature dispersed throughout matter in the form of invisibly small "bubbles." This is called "dispersed void" (κενὸν διεσπαρμένον or παρεσπαρμένον), as opposed to massed void. Dispersed void was introduced into the theory of matter as an explanation of compression, the model being a sponge. It also played a part, obviously enough, in explaining the penetration of apparently solid matter by heat or sound.

This theory has nothing to do with the principle of *horror vacui*, although it is not inconsistent with it. One who certainly used both was Hero of Alexandria, in his *Pneumatics*: the Introduction to this work sets out both ideas very clearly. It is usually said that both come to Hero from Aristotle's successor Strato of Lampsacus; and it is also said that Erasistratus took over both ideas from the same source. But these attributions ought not to be accepted uncritically; the evidence is complex and even contradictory.

A doctrine of dispersed void could be a hindrance to the use Erasistratus wants to make of *horror vacui*. If dispersed void can explain compression, it can also explain expansion; so in Erasistratus' theory, when pneuma leaks out of a wounded artery, it might be that the dispersed void grows larger, and then the entrance of blood into the arterial system could not be explained by *horror vacui*.[115] In *De usu respirationis* 2, Galen quotes the theory of dispersed void as an objection to Erasistratus' explanation of why one suffocates when breathing is stopped even if the lungs are full of air. If Erasistratus had held this theory of matter, and Galen had known that he did, why did he not raise his favorite cry of "inconsistency"?

Galen mentions that Erasistratus himself drew a distinction between massed void and dispersed void. This is in *De nat. fac.* II 6 (K II 99), where Galen is criticizing an Erasistratean theory of the composition of nerves. Perceptible nerves, the theory said, are composed of three kinds of tissue—vein, artery, and nerve—each imperceptibly small. In that case, Galen objects, the principle of *horror vacui* cannot be available for explaining what happens to these elements:

> For it has power only in the case of perceptibles, not in the case of theoretical entities, as Erasistratus explicitly concedes—saying that he is not putting forward a theory about the kind of void that is dispersed in small portions in bodies, but about that which is clear, perceptible, massed, large, evident, or whatever else you want to call it. Erasistratus himself says that there cannot be a "massed perceptible" void; the other names I have added, from my abundant store of words meaning the same thing, at least on the present topic. (*De nat. fac.* II 6; K II 99)

[115]See below, *An in arteriis* 4.

It seems clear, then, that Erasistratus knew of the theory of inter-spersed void, and apparently reserved his position on it. So far as I can see, he made no use of it himself.

Questions concerning the void were discussed in the Peripatetic school at the time Erasistratus lived. Strato of Lampsacus, third in line as head of the school, wrote a book *On the void* (apparently still available in the sixth century A.D. to Simplicius), and it is likely that Erasistratus learned from this source. But one ought not to accept without reserve the version of these events that has been rather widely accepted in recent years, that the pneumatic theory described in the introduction to Hero's *Pneumatics* is precisely that which was worked out by Strato, and that this is also the theory of Erasistratus.[116] Hero's pneumatic theory contains three elements that may well not have come from Strato's physics: a corpuscular theory of matter, the idea of the "right tension" ($\epsilon \dot{v} \tau o \nu \acute{\iota} a$) of a body which accounts for its elasticity, and the thesis that a massed void, although it does not exist naturally, can be brought about by force.[117] It should be added that Erasistratus' theory of the void has nothing at all to do with the Atomism of Democritus and Epicurus, as has sometimes been claimed.

Whatever may be the true history of the concept of *horror vacui* before Erasistratus, his own use of it is well documented and suffi-ciently clear. He used it in his explanations of appetite,[118] of diges-tion,[119] the secretion of bile[120] and urine.[121] He used it particularly in the theories of blood flow and respiration attacked by Galen in our treatises. It explains how the lungs draw in air from outside through the nose and mouth, and the left side of the heart draws in air from the lungs, and how the right side of the heart draws in blood from

[116]For this account of the history, see H. Diels ("Straton") and Gottschalk (*Strato*). Doubts about Diels' article were expressed by A. Schmekel, and have been given more body in the recent work by M. Gatzemeier. I hope to write more on this elsewhere.

[117]The relevant text of Hero can be found conveniently in Gottschalk's *Strato*: these three elements are at 115.23, 109.4, and 116.5.

[118]K II 104–105.

[119]K II 63.

[120]K II 63.

[121]K II 77.

the veins. If the argument given above is correct, it explains how blood is distributed over the whole body.

All these are natural functions of the body. We also hear much from Galen about *horror vacui* in one pathological situation. Erasistratus had to explain how it is, if the arteries normally contain pneuma, that they appear to contain blood whenever they are pierced or inspected by dissection. His answer is that the act of puncturing an artery for inspection of its contents, or on any occasion, allows the pneuma to escape. The potential vacuum left by the pneuma must then be refilled, and the only available source from which it can be refilled is the supply of blood in the veins. The arteries are connected to the veins at the extremities of both by invisibly small channels called *anastomoses*. This theory anticipates the discovery of the capillaries, but in antiquity it was simply a postulate: it was a necessary postulate not only for Erasistratus and others who believed that the arteries contain only pneuma in their natural state, but also for Galen, because of the well-known obvservation that *all* the blood in an animal can be lost through a wound in just one vessel, whether an artery or a vein.

Galen criticizes Erasistratus' explanation of how blood gets into the arteries in *An in arteriis*, and there is no need to repeat the details here. It is worth noting, however, that there may have been qualifications in Erasistratus' theory that were ignored by Galen. For example, one of Galen's criticisms is that the immediate presence of blood as soon as an artery is punctured must mean that the whole of the pneuma in the arterial system is emptied out before the blood appears. This is an objection that could be met by supposing that some blood is drawn in from nearby anastomoses before all the pneuma is emptied out. Galen asserts in chapter 5 that although some Erasistrateans did suppose this, Erasistratus himself insisted that blood enters first into that part of the arterial system most remote from the wound. It seems possible to doubt Galen's extreme interpretation of this. Of course, since blood is supposed to enter through the anastomoses, which are at the ends of the arteries furthest from the heart, in a sense blood enters at the point furthest from the wound. But this is no reason why blood should not appear at the wound before all the pneuma is emptied from the aorta, the heart, and the rest of the arterial system.

One of Galen's criticisms, in chapter 1, is that the Erasistratean theory does not explain why the pneuma leaves the body when an artery is punctured, and in fact two versions of the theory are available—one that the pneuma has its own source of motion, and the other that it is under pressure from the heart. Erasistratus certainly thought pneuma difficult to contain: that is why the arteries have thick coats. Perhaps he felt no need to explain why pneuma would escape through a leak. It was notoriously the most volatile of all substances in Greek physical theory, and this quality helps to account for its role in Aristotle's physiology, Epicurus' psychology, and Stoic cosmology. Galen is probably on the right track when he suggests that it may move because it is like "aether": we should not think of the highly specialized sense given to this word in Aristotelian cosmology, where it was used by commentators to refer to the element of the heavens, endowed with natural circular motion, but rather of the Stoic use of it, to refer to pure fire, the fourth element, lighter and finer than the other three. Pneuma in the Stoic theory is a mixture of this pure fire and air. There is no reason to think Erasistratus was so precise; but he would probably think of pneuma as something so light and fine that it would naturally escape upward unless contained in some vessel. If so, we are lacking an explanation of the difference between a pathological leak of pneuma from a punctured artery, and the normal escape of pneuma through the pores of the skin, reported by Anonymus Londinensis.[122]

Galen is much closer to being right than Erasistratus about the contents of the arteries, and on the whole he makes a good case. The crucial point in this case, however, is not the experiment of ligaturing an artery in two places and cutting it between the ligatures, showing that portion to contain blood. This was supposed to be the crucial point by William Harvey[123] and many after him, but they were wrong. Erasistratus' theory was not touched by this experiment, since the act of baring the artery in order to ligature it would in his view be enough to cause the presence of blood in any part of the arterial system. This wrong idea was brought about by a mistake in the text, which we have now corrected.[124] Galen's best argument is probably the simplest one: that no one has observed pneuma escaping from a wounded artery.

[122]xxiii 18–23, quoted above, p. 29.
[123]See Introduction, II.
[124]See *An in arteriis* n. 36.

g. The Atomists and Asclepiades

There is very little to be said on this subject.

First, we must repeat that the theory of Erasistratus owes nothing to the atomic physics of Democritus and Epicurus. Diels[125] and Wellmann[126] were wrong about that. The theory of disseminate void, even if Erasistratus held it (which is doubtful, as we have seen), has nothing to do with the Atomists' void. The principle of *horror vacui* used the concept of void to explain motion in a totally different way from the teachings of the Atomists. Finally, Erasistratus' theory of the invisibly small elements that compose the tissues of the body, the *triplokia* of artery, vein, and nerve, is not an atomistic theory.

The only atomistic theory of which Galen takes note in our treatises is that of Asclepiades, of Prusa in Bythinia, who practiced medicine in Rome in the first half of the first century B.C. His writings are all lost. We hear from Galen[127] that he believed the use of breathing to be the restoration of the psyche, which continually changes its substance in a constant flow.[128] This is reasonably consistent with the doctrine of the Epicureans, who believed that the soul contains a "pneumatic" ingredient, and that all physical compounds, which include souls, interchange atoms with their environment in a continual flow.[129] Asclepiades is linked with Epicurus by Galen.[130] However, other features of Asclepiades' theory appear to owe more to Heraclides of Pontus, the pupil of Plato's Academy and of Aristotle, than to Epicurus. He adopted from Heraclides the theory of "jointless masses" ($\check{\alpha}\nu\alpha\rho\mu o\iota$ $\check{o}\gamma\kappa o\iota$)—a theory that remains mysterious because of the unsatisfactory nature of the surviving evidence.[131] These "masses" differ from Epicurean atoms, apparently, in being breakable and in having some sensible qualities.

Asclepiades subscribed to the Atomists' theory of changes: like them, he denied qualitative change and explained it away as addition, subtraction, or rearrangement of particles. He also followed the

[125] "Straton," p. 106.

[126] "Erasistratos," col. 334.

[127] *De usu respirationis* 1-2. See Wellmann's article "Asclepiades."

[128] Sextus *Math.* viii 7 confirms that Asclepiades held some doctrine of the flow of matter.

[129] Epicurus, *Ep.* 1, 46.

[130] For example, *De usu partium*, K I 415, II 135.

[131] See Lonie, *Heraclides.*

Atomists in abandoning teleological explanations in favor of mechanistic ones. Galen attacks both of these features powerfully.[132] However, he regards Asclepiades' theory of the use of respiration as beneath contempt, and we hear nothing of his theory of the arteries in our treatises.

[132] For example, *De usu partium* VI (K I 344ff.), and frequently in *De nat. fac.* I.

II. GALEN AND THE
LATER HISTORY OF THEORIES
OF THE HEART, LUNGS,
AND VESSELS

The three longer tracts here presented deal with problems in the physiology of the lungs and vascular system. At least since the time of Aristotle it had become clear that the lungs and heart are in some way intimately associated; and some special association between the activities of the lungs and those of the arteries was almost certainly accepted by Praxagoras, and was made by Erasistratus a fundamental postulate of his system of physiology.

Our three tracts, therefore, would be seen to belong together, even had Galen not been at pains to connect them by explicit cross-references.

Galen was obliged to be either a follower or a critic of Erasistratus, for in the intervening centuries no physiologist of comparable stature had arisen. It is clear, however, that although Galen set himself to produce a new system of physiology to supersede that of Erasistratus, he was unable to achieve anything better than a reform of the Erasistratean system by a conflation with elements derived from the Aristotelian and Hippocratic writings.

Three elements borrowed from these earlier sources are of central importance in the tracts considered here: first, a firm belief in the reality and great significance of the innate heat, with its need for moderation by the cooling action of air drawn into the body; second, a belief in brain-breathing, that is, the drawing of air directly into the cavities of the brain through the nostrils and the cribriform plates of the skull; third, a belief in the passage of air through fine pores in the skin into the terminal twigs of the arteries.

The first of these elements Galen derives principally from Aristotle himself, though he rejects Aristotle's notion that the brain is a cooling device. What he takes from Aristotle, consequently, is the idea that the lungs exist to cool the heart. Since Aristotle said that the air passes from the lungs into the heart to cool it, Galen is able to conflate Aristotle's theory of cooling with Erasistratus' theory of pneuma supplied from the air: a theory which itself owes something to Aristotle, and perhaps something also to Hippocratic writings.[1] The second element, brain-breathing, seems to be borrowed from *The Sacred Disease*, and reinforced by actual observations of rhythmic movements of the membranes around the brain. This element was not well assimilated in Galen's theoretical system, as will be understood from a consideration of some of his experiments.[2]

The third element, arterial breathing, seems to me to be borrowed from Empedocles, as reported by Aristotle.[3] It is possible that Galen misunderstood this passage, but I cannot myself see any reason to suppose that Empedocles is talking about the lungs, and there seem several reasons to suppose that he is speaking of the arteries. If Empedocles is concerned to explain the action of the lungs, the liquid in the clepsydra has no analogue; and, what is worse, Empedocles' reference to blood in vessels is incomprehensible.

Galen says that Erasistratus did his best anatomical work in his old age.[4] If this is true, it might account for the most striking characteristic of his theory of the vascular system and lungs: the theory is brilliant in conception, and contains a large measure of physiological truth, but it is unsatisfactory when considered anatomically.

Erasistratus considers that there are in effect two vascular systems: the veins, which carry the products of digestion from the alimentary tract to the whole body; and the arteries, which carry to the whole body pneuma, derived from the air in the lungs. Since the pulmonary veins belong to the pneumatic system, they are considered to be arteries;[5] and since the pulmonary artery is supposed to exist to carry nour-

---

[1] *Alim.*, xxix (L IX 98): "The lungs draw a nourishment which is the opposite of that of the body . . . "; xxxi (L 110), "Roots of veins, liver; roots of arteries, heart. Out of these travel to all parts blood and breath . . . "; xlviii (L 116), " . . . For breath too is nourishment."

[2] This will be explained below (Introduction, III a), together with the nature of the movements of the membranes.

[3] *De respiratione* 473 b 9–474 a 6.

[4] ἀκριβεστέρας ἐποιεῖτο τὰς ἀνατομάς. K V 602. ὅτι πρεσβύτης ὢν ἤδη καθ᾽ ὃν χρόνον αὐτοί φασι τὰ τῶν διαιρέσεων αὐτῷ γεγράφθαι βιβλία. K XVIII, 1 86.

[5] *De usu partium* VI, xii (K III 465, 466). See also Daremberg's note, *Oeuvres de Galien*, I, 422, 423. *Anat. Proc.* VII, iv; (K II 597). This is also discussed above, Introduction, I f.

ishment (blood formed from digested food) to the lungs,[6] it is assigned to the venous system. From this classification of the pulmonary vessels arises the awkward terminology *arteria venosa* and *vena arteriosa*, "the artery that resembles a vein" and "the vein that resembles an artery." That it seems natural to give these terms in Latin arises from the circumstance that they persisted not only up to the time of Harvey but even within his own writings (e.g. *De motu cordis* vi).

The cardinal defect of Erasistratus' system is that since the arteries and veins are considered to belong to two quite distinct systems, the structure of the heart is inadequately explained. Only the left side is accounted for in a satisfactory manner, as a pump drawing pneuma from the lungs[7] and driving it into the arteries of the rest of the body, thus causing both the pulse and, by inflation, the shortening of the muscles.[8] What Erasistratus supposed to occur in the right side of the heart, which for him meant exclusively the right ventricle, is an excruciating problem.

When Harvey came to review the whole question of the action of the heart, he noted that his opinion on the causation of the pulse agreed with that of Erasistratus (allowing, of course, for the fact that the fluid pumped by the left ventricle was not the same, being pneuma for Erasistratus, but blood for Harvey): "the erection of the heart ... is the proper movement of the heart as opposed to its relaxation.... At the moment of erection the blood spurts out and the pulse occurs, a fact which is in favour of the contention of Erasistratus and against that of Galen."[9] Erasistratus, however, no less than Galen, was unable to satisfy Harvey's demand for a theory that would take full account of the anatomical symmetry of the two sides of the heart. "Why, I ask, when we see that the structure of both ventricles is almost identical, there being the same apparatus of fibers and braces, and valves, and vessels, and auricles, and in both the same infarction of blood, in the subjects of our dissections, of the like black color, and coagulation—why I ask, should their uses be imagined to be different, when the action, motion, and pulse of both are the same?"[10] In *An in arteriis*, Galen gives his reasons for reject-

---

[6] *Nat. Fac.* II i (K II 77).
[7] *Anat. Proc.* VII iv (K II 597).
[8] Harris, *The Heart*, p. 232.
[9] Whitteridge, *Lectures*, p. 267.
[10] *De motu cordis*, Prooemium.

ing Erasistratus' postulate that the arteries normally contain only pneuma.

Galen is, of course, in the right, and his tract represents a turning point of importance in the history of physiology; but Galen failed to reject the theory of Erasistratus *in toto*; and, instead of a radically new theory, offered a compromise formation in which the original theory is partly rejected and partly emended, and is awkwardly conflated with notions derived from earlier authors.

In the process, most of what is valuable in Erasistratus' theory is lost: the correct interpretation of the valves of the left side of the heart, the clear notion of some simple and direct derivative of the air being carried in large quantities from the lungs to every part of the body, and the seductive hypothesis of the cause of muscular contraction, which explains the air-hunger that follows intense muscular activity. On the other hand, Galen failed to correct the cardinal defect of the whole Erasistratean complex: the mistaken and ineffectual account of the right side of the heart. Galen's theory, in this respect, no doubt effects a simplification; but it is still unable to explain the essential similarity in form of the two sides. The final theory presented by Galen (if it can be dignified with the name of a theory) is thus a jumble of older and newer elements arranged with varying success to form a pattern that is still to some extent, if not largely, Erasistratean.

What Harvey was, by the circumstances of the case, called upon to do was to break up the awkward compromise and to replace it by a unitary theory that would account for the known facts of anatomy, particularly the anatomy of the heart, and would at the same time give a plausible explanation of the presence of blood in the arteries. Harvey found the problem substantially in the state in which Galen had left it.[11] But two important elements had been added in the late sixteenth century to the body of knowledge and belief about the vascular system: good reasons had been adduced for supposing that the blood passes from the right side of the heart to the left through the lungs—not, as Galen had believed, in a thin and sluggish stream, but rapidly and copiously;[12] and the valves in the veins had been

[11] Nearly the whole of Harvey's Prooemium to the *De motu cordis* is a discussion of Galen's own ideas. For an account of the period between Galen and Harvey, see Pagel, *Harvey*.

[12] The work of Realdus Columbus (1516?–1559) is discussed by Harvey in *De motu cordis* vii.

observed and had been well described by Harvey's teacher, Fabricius ab Aquapendente.[13] Both these new elements were, as he fully acknowledged, of great service to Harvey in the elaboration of his theory; but it must never be forgotten that, though they provided valuable hints toward the completion of Harvey's theory, this theory, as a whole, was principally a reinterpretation of facts known to Galen, and is a striking example of a theory produced by reorganization, by *Umgestaltung*.

What we have in the *De motu cordis et sanguinis in animalibus*, first published in 1628, is not the explanation of a theory that had but just arisen in the mind of its author, but the fruit of about nine years of elucidative and confirmatory research after the theory as such had been excogitated.[14] Among the works of Galen referred to implicitly

[13] Hieronymus Fabricius ab Aquapendente (1537–1619). See *De motu cordis* xiii.

[14] If we suppose that Harvey's dedicatory epistle to Dr. Argent was, as is probable, written just before the *De motu cordis* went to the press in 1628, then the statement with which this epistle begins would mean that he had been teaching his "new view of the motion and use of the heart, and of the circulation of the blood" since about 1619. This agrees well with Dr. Gweneth Whitteridge's supposition (*Lectures*, p. xxviii) that the first set of Harvey's Lumleian Lectures was completed in 1619. Dr. Whitteridge states that, when Harvey began to give these lectures in 1616, he had not yet reached the conclusion that the blood circulates (p. xxix); and there is conclusive evidence in the lecture notes themselves that their general text was completed before he had come to this conclusion. He added to his notes, in detail, up to at least 1626; but did not correct those passages in which the Galenic doctrine of blood being supplied to the parts of the body by the veins is accepted. Anyone who has used a set of notes for some years will appreciate that Harvey's failure to correct certain passages does not prove that he accepted in the later years everything that he wrote in the earlier; so there is no inconsistency in believing that his theory was completed late in 1619.

A study of the basic text of Harvey's notes for his Lumleian Lectures seems to put beyond question that he first elucidated the movements of the heart and its functioning, and only later perceived the implications (respecting the circular motion of the blood) of this new understanding of the heart. He told Robert Boyle that the first hint of the true direction of motion of the blood in the veins was given to him by a consideration of the structure of their valves, as described by Fabricius (Robert Boyle, *A Disquisition about the Final Causes of Natural Things*, Section IV, Proposition ii. See, for example, *Works*, London, 1772, vol. 5, p. 427). This illumination was probably received by Harvey late in 1619. The theory, then, insofar as it related to the

44

or explicitly by Harvey in the *De motu cordis*, the three tracts here presented are of the greatest importance. This is already clear from the Prooemium to the *De motu cordis*, which begins:

> As we are about to discuss the motion, action, and use of the heart and arteries, it is imperative on us first to state what has been thought of these things by others in their writings, and what has been held by the vulgar and by tradition, in order that what is true may be confirmed, and what is false set right by dissection, multiplied experience, and accurate observation.
>
> Almost all anatomists, physicians, and philosophers, up to the present time, have supposed, with Galen, that the object of the pulse was the same as that of respiration, and only differed in one particular, this being conceived to depend on the animal, *that*[15] on the vital faculty; the two, in all other respects, whether with reference to purpose or to motion, comporting themselves alike.

The reference here to the content of our tracts would be obvious, even without further consideration; but, in fact, careful search dis-

---

activities of the heart, was certainly present to his mind by 1619; and the completed theory, including that part of it which concerned the movements of the blood, could hardly have been formed much later than that year; for once he had rejected Galen's theory of the heart, and replaced it by his own, the necessary corollary of the circular motion of the blood must soon have forced itself upon his mind, even without the consideration of the valves of the veins.

The whole argumentation of the Lumleian Lectures gives the impression of a man working toward a new theory. The lectures might almost have been written by a Greek anatomist; and it is particularly striking that Harvey is assisted toward a new view of the heart by his knowledge that Aristotle had given the heart, and not the liver, as the *principle* ($\dot{\alpha}\rho\chi\dot{\eta}$) of the veins, as well as of the arteries. The *De motu cordis*, on the other hand, with its innumerable critical observations and experiments, carries the mark of a work carried out over some years, to confirm a theory already formed; and this is exactly how Harvey himself described his book in his dedicatory epistle to Dr. Argent.

[15] I have given the translation of Willis in the Sydenham Society's publication of 1847, except that he has in this place "the respiration," which is a gloss of his own, and certainly a mistake. Franklin (*De motu cordis*, Oxford, 1957) has also bungled the translation in this place; for he has "and differ only in that the former derives from the psychic faculty, the latter from the vital one"; the Latin, as he himself gives it, being "et una re tantum differre, quod haec ab animali, ille a vitali facultate manet."

covers that the passage which has given such trouble to the translators (see note 15) is a direct quotation from the final summary of the *De usu pulsuum*: "breathing and the pulse differ in only one way, in that the one is moved by the psychic power and the other by the vital power." There is, of course, no problem as to the meaning of "the one" and "the other"; for the psychic (or animal) power certainly emanates from the brain, and the vital from the heart.

In the same Prooemium, which is of no great length, the tract *An in arteriis* is referred to explicitly in two places;[16] and there are probably some implicit references, but these are difficult to establish because Galen is apt to say virtually the same thing in two or three different works. However, at least one citation, of which Harvey does not give the precise source, can be referred with confidence to this tract (*An in arteriis* vi; K IV 724); and in this place Harvey gives an interpretation of Galen's procedure which is of some interest: "That it is blood and blood only which is contained in the arteries is made manifest by the experiment of Galen.... The experiment of Galen alluded to is this: 'If you include a portion of an artery between two ligatures, and slit it open lengthwise, you will find nothing but blood'; and thus he proves that the arteries contain blood only." This passage illustrates the confusion caused by the disturbance of sequence of Galen's argument, produced by the inversion of a page of the codex from which the Western manuscripts were copied (see *An in arteriis* 6). Galen's operation which, taken out of its context, can hardly be called "an experiment," was not intended to show "that the arteries contain blood only"; a proposition which, in any case, it would be difficult to reconcile with many of Galen's statements as to what is contained in the arteries.

The operation, as placed in the Western manuscripts, is almost impossible to interpret, and Harvey has made the best of a bad job.

[16]quid itaque respondeant Galeno, qui librum scripsit, natura sanguinem contineri in arteriis, et nihil praeter sanguinem.... Attamen, libro *Quod sanguis continetur in arteriis*, Galeni experimentum in contrarium sic se habet.

III. GALEN'S EXPERIMENTS AND THE ORIGIN OF THE EXPERIMENTAL METHOD

The tracts offered in text and translation should be of great interest to all historians of science, because they contain very clear evidence that the design and the logic of experiments, in the strictest sense of the word, were both well understood in antiquity.

In this place I propose to discuss the experiments reported by Galen in these tracts, and then to point out that he was undoubtedly in possession of the logic necessary for a full understanding of the nature of arguments based upon experiment. Galen was unquestionably a superb anatomist, but from our discussion of some of his experiments it may well be concluded that he was not a great experimentalist; and it appears extremely improbable that he was the first person to conduct well-conceived experiments. We should inquire, therefore, at what time Greek thinkers became aware of the precise formal structure of experiments, and I shall suggest that the experimental method, in the strictest sense, was developed in the third century B.C.[1]

Even if my conclusion be accepted, however, too much importance must not be attached to it. Some of the criticisms we feel inclined to make of Galen as an experimenter would, in all probability, occur to our minds with equal force could we read the treatises of other Greek physiologists. In the tract *An in arteriis natura sanguis contineatur*, we find a failure to understand the hazards of experimentation; a failure, that is, to check with sufficient care the results of experiments, and a failure to understand how meager are the conclusions that can be based upon even the best-conducted experiment if taken in isolation. It is probable that these defects were not peculiar to Galen; and, if

[1] What I have suggested, on rather sketchy evidence, in this essay has now been fully argued and documented by H. von Staden, "Experiment and Experience." That it is still necessary to emphasize the wealth of experimentation in antiquity, however, is shown by a statement in J. G. Landels' excellent book *Engineering in the Ancient World*, p. 193: "There are very few examples of experimental method in Greek science, but it is not true to say that there are none at all."

the Greeks were clearly in possession of that tool called "experimentation," it seems they did not fully appreciate how it should be employed.

a. The Experiments Reported by Galen
in the Three Tracts

It is not unreasonable to ask whether Galen actually performed the experiments he describes, but the evidence seems strongly to favor the assumption that he did. He certainly vivisected animals.[2] His experiments on the nervous system, in particular, carry total conviction as accounts of what he had himself actually done and seen.[3]

The experiment on the dog, reported in the *De usu pulsuum* ii (K V 154) seems entirely convincing. Its result does not seem to be so neatly appropriate to Galen's theories as to suggest a mere *Gedankenexperiment*: indeed, there is every appearance that Galen found the initial result somewhat puzzling. This experiment is of particular interest on account of its two stages, each of which involves the answer to a precise question: first, whether the connection between the heart and the brain is required constantly throughout the life of the animal; second, whether, if the answer to the first question is negative, there is evidence that some substance is supplied by the heart to the brain and stored there so as to be available for activity even when the continuity of the supply is interrupted.

A puzzle arising from Galen's account is why he did not consider the possibility of the brain receiving blood and pneuma from the heart through the vertebral arteries. This question was raised, perhaps for the first time, by Vesalius.[4] That Galen knew of the existence of the vertebral arteries is certain;[5] but he also knew that the

---

[2] If we deny this we have to assume a degree of duplicity on the part of Galen that seems totally incredible. For example, he frequently says that the student must practice on the cadaver before proceeding to vivisection: *Anat. Proc.* VIII, iv and viii; XIV, vii. Particularly striking is his remark, that, in demonstrating to students or to the public, he used pigs "because there is no advantage in having an ape in such experiments and the spectacle is hideous," *Anat. Proc.* VIII, viii (K II 690).

[3] *Anat. Proc.* VIII, i–x (K II 651–706); IX, x–xiv.

[4] *De corporis humani fabrica* VII, xix.

[5] *De usu part.* XIII, ix (K IV 116); *Anat. Proc.* XIII, ix.

terminations of their principal trunks lie in the region of the hind-brain.[6] It is possible, therefore, that he thought these arteries could be disregarded as not supplying anything to the forebrain; for it is at least extremely probable that he believed the forebrain alone to be the material substratum of consciousness.[7] There can be no doubt at all that the operation described by Galen can be performed, and no reasonable doubt that it would have the results described by him. In 1836 Sir Astley Cooper performed the much more radical operation of ligaturing both common carotids and both vertebral arteries in a dog.[8] After the operation, the animal appeared "insensible, or as if intoxicated.... It ran against the leg of the table, or any other body,

[6] *De usu part.* XVI xix (K IV 331).

[7] I do not seriously doubt that this was his opinion; but it is difficult to prove, by brief citations, that it was; since he uses the word ἐγκέφαλον for the whole brain, and κατ' ἐξοχήν (as he says himself in *De usu part.* VIII, xi; K III 666) for the forebrain. He says that the rational soul has its seat in the ἐγκέφαλον, and that it is by means of this organ that we reason (*De usu part.* IX, iv; K III 700); moreover, the cerebellum is much harder than the ἐγκέφαλον (*De usu part.* VIII, xii; K III 671), and the soft is more appropriate to feeling, the hard to action (*De usu part.* VIII v; K III 634). It would seem reasonable to infer that the highest mental processes would require the soft-est organ, and hence would be carried on in the ἐγκέφαλον of *De usu part.* VIII, xii; that is, in the forebrain; and that in the dog consciousness would depend upon this part.

In another passage (*De usu part.* VIII, iv; K III 625ff.) Galen discusses at some length the word ἐγκέφαλον, but there is nothing in this discussion of interest for our present purpose. We note with some interest, however, that Galen recommends the use of the Latin name (τὸ κερέβρον ... τοῦτο γὰρ αὐτὸ ὀνομάζουσι, K III 629) in preference to the Greek; because, he says, not all animals have their brains in their heads. Of considerable historical importance is the fact that Galen rejects (K III 626) Aristotle's invaluable term ἀνάλογον, a term only fully reinstated in the mid-nineteenth century, when the terms "homologue" and "analogue" were introduced to designate, respectively, an organ similar in form or origin to some other organ, but not necessarily having the same function (such as the human hand and the bat's wing); and an organ having the same function, but not the same form or origin as some other organ. I believe this distinction was clear to Aristotle, but it could hardly be explicitly formulated on a basis of adequate compara-tive studies until after the work of the idealist anatomists of the late eigh-teenth and early nineteenth centuries.

[8] *Guy's Hospital Reports*, 1836, 1, 457–60. My attention was drawn to this paper by Professor P. M. Daniel of the Department of Neuropathology of the Bethlem Royal Hospital and the Maudsley Hospital.

without seeing or regarding it." The operation was performed on the 28th of January, and on the 1st of February the animal "was much better: it ate and drank; and from that time gradually recovered. It afterwards became a good house-dog." Sir Astley Cooper kept it for nine months, after which he killed it in order to inject its arteries. The circulation of the brain was found to have been restored by the enlargement of numerous anastomoses. For example, "the left carotid was obliterated from near its origin, but filled with injection above the obliterated part, by the inferior thyroideal artery communicating with the superior, and by the ascending cervical artery from the subclavian, by numerous and large anastomoses, and by an oesophageal artery from one of the intercostals communicating with the superior thyroid artery." These anastomoses would not, of course, be formed *de novo*, but only enlarged in the course of time. Thus in Galen's dog the circulation of the brain could well have been maintained by such anastomoses, together with the vertebral arteries. The tying of the arteries would have diminished the circulation and this diminution could well have been exposed by forcing the animal to exert itself, exactly in accordance with Galen's description.

The experiment with the bladder placed over the boy's head (*De usu resp.* 5), though well conceived, clearly cannot have been correctly conducted. Professor Daniel writes, "I suppose the bladder ... was very stiff and allowed air to seep in round the neck, but it seems most unlikely that the poor child suffered no inconvenience."[9] It may be that the boy was able to breathe in this way for some time, and that Galen then gave up observing and entrusted the further supervision of the experiment to a slave, who allowed the boy to remove the bladder during the greater part of the day.

In the seventeenth century trials were made by members of the Royal Society to discover "how long the same air would serve for respiration without the supply of fresh air." These trials were suggested by Hooke, who made the first of them himself.[10] "He made a trial with a bladder ... and he found, that it served for five inspirations, though with difficulty. He was ordered to try it again, but with a glass." At the next meeting, "Mr. Hooke was ordered ... to pro-

[9] In a letter very kindly sent to me on January 25, 1968.
[10] Birch, *Royal Society*, I, 179.

cure a glass to be made, that might serve instead of a bladder, to make the experiment of respiration."[11]

At the two following meetings a bag was used, and a glass immersed first in cold, then in warm water. From the results we can infer that Hooke's tolerance was rather small, the greatest number of times he was able to respire being twenty-five; whereas Merret respired thirty-six times in the cooled glass and seventy-six times in the bag.[12]

From the use of a bladder for the first trials, and from the experimenters' cooling and warming the glass, it seems clear that Hooke, in thinking of these experiments, was inspired directly or indirectly by Galen.

The experiment of inserting a reed, or bronze tube, into an artery is described at least twice by Galen; once in the *An in arteriis* viii (K IV 733) and once in the *De anatomicis administrationibus* VII, xvi (K II 646ff). These two accounts differ significantly: in that given in the *An in arteriis* it is claimed that the pulse below (that is, distal to) the inserted tube is seen to continue until the ligature is applied, which presses the coat of the artery against the tube; the other account is less clear, but there is certainly no mention of the pulse being observable below the tube at any time. The experiment as described in the *An in arteriis* is much the better of the two, as a demonstration of Galen's contention that the pulse is carried in the coats of the arteries; but it is not easy to see how he could have got the result he claims to have observed. If he used a soft reed, he could have compressed the reed so as to slow down the bloodflow, and this could have the effect of rendering an already diminished pulse invisibly small or absent; but with a bronze tube this could hardly be expected to occur. The other account of the experiment is entirely credible, supposing the tube (or the quill, for he here also speaks of a quill) to have been of very narrow bore; for this could render the pulse imperceptible below the site of the operation; but if the pulse was at no time present below the tube, how can Galen assert that it was the ligature around the tube, and not the tube itself, that stopped the pulse? This experiment is of the greatest historical importance. The account given by Galen in the *De anatomicis administrationibus* implies

[11]Birch, I, 182.
[12]Birch, I, 192, 194.

that the experiment was performed by Erasistratus, who asserted "that the part below the quill is seen moving."[13] Since there is no reason to doubt Galen's testimony, this shows that well-conceived experiments were already being performed by the middle of the third century B.C.

In his introduction to the *De motu cordis*, Harvey discusses this experiment, saying that he has not tried it, but doubts whether it could be performed. In a later work he writes:[14]

This experiment is spoken of by Vesalius, the celebrated anatomist; but neither Vesalius nor Galen says that he tried the experiment, which, however, I did.[15] Vesalius only prescribes and Galen advises it ... not thinking of the difficulties that attend its performance, nor of its futility when done; for indeed ... it supplies nothing in support of the opinion which maintains that the coats of the vessels are the cause of the pulse; it much rather proclaims that this is owing to the impulse of the blood. For the moment you have thrown your ligature around the artery upon the reed or tube, immediately, by the force of the blood thrown in from above, it is dilated beyond the circle of the tube, by which the flow is impeded, and the shock is broken; so that the artery which is tied only pulsates obscurely, being now cut off from the full force of the blood that flows through it, the shock being reverberated, as it were, from that part of the vessel which is above the ligature; but if the artery below the ligature be now divided, the contrary of what has been maintained will appear, from the spurting of the blood impelled through the tube.

---

[13]K II 646–649. Even if we had no direct evidence of the fact, we should have to infer that the hypothesis that the pulse is carried in the walls of the arteries as a result of the transmission of a faculty from the heart must have existed at the time of Erasistratus, for the experiment can refute this hypothesis, but could not directly confirm that of Erasistratus. However, Galen actually tells us that the hypothesis that the pulse is due to a faculty transmitted in the walls was held to be true by both Hippocrates and Herophilus (*De usu pulsuum* iv; K V 164).

[14] *De circulatione sanguis, exercitatio altera ad J. Riolan.* English of R. Willis, *Harvey*, pp. 110–11.

[15]Harvey is mistaken in saying that Galen does not claim to have performed the experiment, for in the *De anatomicis admin.* VII, xvi (K II 645) he referred to "those who had observed my experiment."

This experiment has been performed recently by Professor M. P. Amacher of Los Angeles, whose account of the result agrees closely with Harvey's.[16]

Galen does not set out formally the logic of these three experiments, but that he could have done so had he wished cannot be doubted. Our three tracts give abundant evidence of his awareness of logical forms; and, particularly, the *An in arteriis* is so heavily charged with formalized arguments that in reading it the word "scholastic" inevitably comes to mind. Of great historical interest is the type of logic employed: it is entirely Stoic. It will be remembered that the set of *undemonstrated arguments* most generally approved by the Stoic writers consisted of five forms or schemata:[17]

1. From a conditional and its antecedent infers the consequent as a conclusion.
2. From a conditional and the contradictory of its consequent infers the contradictory of the antecedent as a conclusion.
3. For its first premise has the denial of a conjunction; for its second premise, one of the conjuncts; for its conclusion, the contradictory of the other conjunct.
4. Employing a disjunction (exclusive) as one premise and one of the disjuncts as the other, infers the contradictory of the remaining disjunct as its conclusion.
5. Having an exclusive disjunction and the contradictory of one of the disjuncts as premises, infers the other disjunct as its conclusion.

The second type (*modus tollendo tollens*) may be considered as the most classical form of argument in experimentation; since it is in this form that we present the negation of an hypothesis. Of this form there are several examples in our tracts, and Galen says that even the man in the street knows that "from the conditional and the contradictory of the consequent, the contradictory of the antecedent follows."[18]

Within two chapters (vi and vii) of the *An in arteriis* we find examples of the first, second, and fifth of the Stoic *undemonstrated arguments*.

[16] Amacher, "Galen's Experiment."
[17] Mates, *Stoic Logic*, pp. 67ff.
[18] *An in arteriis* vi.

First form: If the arteries contain blood, then they are not filled with pneuma from the heart.

But they do contain blood.

Therefore they are not filled with pneuma from the heart.

Second form: If the arteries contain blood, and they are expanded through being filled from the heart, then the order of their movements will be destroyed.

But it is not destroyed.

Hence not both: they contain blood, and they are expanded through being filled from the heart.

Fifth form: Either the arteries are expanded through being filled with pneuma from the heart, or they are filled because they are expanded.

But not the first, therefore the second.

Not only does Galen employ the Stoic schemata, but, as we see in the last example, he also uses the Stoic variables. It will be remembered that Aristotle used as variables the letters of the alphabet, whereas the Stoics used ordinal numbers.[19] Moreover, the technical terms used by Galen in discussing his formal arguments are mainly Stoic. Thus in his discussion of the second of the three arguments just quoted (form 2 combined with form 3), he uses συνημμένον (conditional); ἡγούμενον (antecedent); λῆγον (consequent) and συμπέρασμα (conclusion). In the *De usu respirationis* 4 (K IV 494) we find again the word συνημμένον and in that place it appears in conjunction with the word πρόσληψις, the Stoic term for the second premise of argument forms having a conditional for the first premise. All these terms are listed by Benson Mates in his glossary. The only one that is Peripatetic rather than Stoic is συμπέρασμα, for which the preferred Stoic term would be ἐπιφορά.

If we accept the evidence of Galen himself that Erasistratus performed well-designed experiments,[20] the most sensible suggestion as

[19] Almost without exception the variables used by Aristotle stood for classes, whereas the Stoic variables stood for propositions. Bochenski has pointed out that Aristotle sometimes, though rarely, used propositional variables; but the symbols used for these were still letters. See I. M. Bochenski, *A History of Formal Logic* (Indiana: University of Notre Dame Press, 1961), p. 77.

[20] See also the experiment on the weight of a bird before and after feeding, etc., attributed to Erasistratus in Anonymus Londinensis (ed. Jones, p. 127). This, however, is of a different logical form from those referred to above.

to the time at which the experimental method was first clearly, though doubtless not fully, understood would seem to be that it was understood as a result of the combined efforts of philosophers and physiologists during the third century B.C. A necessary condition for clear understanding is that an adequate logic had been, or was being, developed; and this enables us to assert with confidence that understanding of the experimental method would have been impossible before Stoic logic had received at least a preliminary formulation.[21] We may say with some confidence that the development of Stoic logic cannot have begun before about 300 B.C., and that it had reached a high degree of elaboration well before the end of the third century. Some of the *undemonstrated arguments* had probably been recognized by logicians during the lifetime of Erasistratus; but whether his understanding of the refutation of an hypothesis was formal and analytic or only intuitive, is, of course, impossible to decide.

That the early Stoics were interested in physiology cannot well be doubted; but how much their logic owed to the experiments of physiologists, and how much the experiments owed to their logic it is idle to seek to determine. It does, however, seem clear that by 200 B.C. the elements required for the formal understanding of experiments (the logic and the actual performance of well-designed experiments) were present in the Greek world, and that these elements were so combined as to justify a claim that "the experimental method" was explicitly elaborated by that date.

I have said above that I do not wish to claim for any Greek philosopher or physiologist a full understanding of the limitations of the experimental method; an understanding, that is, of the many practical hazards that beset the conduct of a single experiment, and of the multiplicity of considerations that must enter into the evaluation of the result of even the best-conducted experiment. We have seen that Galen was not happy in the conduct of his experiments, and we have also to note that he was either ignorant or clumsy when called upon to evaluate an experiment in its appropriate context. Thus, in discussing the experiment of ligaturing the carotids he should have said

[21] "Aristotle has no word for a conditional statement. He does not use the word ὑποθετικός or make a contrast between hypothetical and categorical statements or syllogisms. The theory of those arguments whose validity depends on the meaning of conditional or other complex sentences was in antiquity the work of the Stoics." (Kneale, *Development*, p. 99.)

explicitly that this experiment can properly be viewed as complete in itself; for it does, at first sight, appear that some premise or premises referring to brain-breathing should have been included in the argument;[22] since the same end-product (psychic pneuma) can be arrived at either by the elaboration of something drawn from the blood or by the elaboration of something derived directly from the air taken in by the brain from the nasal cavities. Further consideration, indeed, does show that the experiment requires no such premises in its argument, because the question to be settled is, "is anything required to be derived from the heart for the brain," and not, "is the production of psychic pneuma entirely dependent upon some pabulum drawn from the blood?" It is difficult, however, to see how Galen can be excused for having omitted all considerations of this kind.

With the experiment of putting a bladder over a boy's head, Galen should have seen that, had the result of the experiment really been as he supposed, it must have followed both that "the substance of the air" is not required in lung-breathing and that it is not required in brain-breathing. Or, if he supposed that the brain could store enough

---

[22]Galen's strange notion that the brain has a respiratory motion of expansion and contraction of its own, independent of the lungs is probably derived from three sources: 1. The statement in Hippocrates *De morbo sacro* X that "when a man takes in breath by the mouth or nostrils, it first goes to the brain." 2. The anatomy of the olfactory organs of the sheep, pig, and so on. For Galen clearly believed that the nasal cavity communicates, through the perforations of the cribriform plate, with the obvious cavity of the olfactory stalk of these animals (a cavity he mistakenly believed to be present also in the human brain), which cavity in turn is in communication with the lateral ventricle. 3. Actually observed movements of the exposed brain. Besides the movements occasioned by the pulse of the arteries in the membranes (often, I think, believed by later anatomists to be the movements referred to by Galen), there may be movements of the same rhythm, though not of the same phase, as those of the lungs. These movements were explained by Haller in the eighteenth century: the brain, he says, swells during each expiration. The positive pressure within the thorax is transmitted along the veins and occasions a swelling of the membranes, so that the brain appears to be breathing within its membranes. It seems to expand as the lung contracts, and to contract as the lung expands (Albrecht von Haller, *The First Lines of Physiology*, Edinburgh, 1779, p. 320).

Galen briefly refers to brain-breathing in *De causis respirationis* (K IV 466), and discusses it at some length in *De usu partium* VIII, vi, vii, x; IX, xvi (K III 650ff., 747ff.).

psychic pneuma to be able to dispense for a whole day with both forms of breathing, he should have said so.

From everything that we know of Galen, however, it would seem that this blindness to the wider context and implications of a particular experiment was his personal failing, and that we need not attribute it to all Greek physiologists indiscriminately. Erasistratus would seem to have been much more aware of the need to preserve a consistent theory, or higher-level hypothesis.

IV. "USE" AND "ACTIVITY"

In the last book of his *De usu partium* Galen gives the following brief characterization of the two notions signified by χρεία and ἐνέργεια: "Thus the activity (ἐνέργεια) of a part differs from its use (χρεία), as I have said,[1] in that the activity is an active motion (κίνησις δραστι- κή), whereas the use is the same as what is commonly called "util- ity" (εὐχρηστία)" (XVII 1; K IV 346). (English translation is difficult here: we have regularly used the word "use" to translate χρεία in this book, and it is impossible to think of a more popular or common word to translate εὐχρηστία.)

The notion of "active change" (κίνησις δραστική) is explained in the *De naturalibus facultatibus* I 2 (K II 7). Galen first divides motion into the two Aristotelian subclasses of qualitative change and local motion. Then he continues:

> We shall devote the whole of the following discussion to asking ... how many and what are the faculties (δυνάμεις) of nature, and what is the effect (ἔργον) that each naturally produces. By effect I mean, of course, that which has already come into exis- tence and has been completed by the activity (ἐνέργεια) of these faculties—for example, blood, flesh, or nerve; and *activity* is the name I give to the active motion (δραστικὴ κίνησις), *faculty* the name I give to the cause of this.
>
> Thus, when food turns into blood, the motion of the food is passive, and that of the vein, active. Similarly, when the limbs change position, the muscle is the mover, and the bones are moved. I call the motion of the vein and the muscle an activity, and that of the food and the bones a symptom and an affection, since the former is altered and the latter are moved.[2]
>
> The activity might be called an effect of nature—for example, digestion, transmission of food, blood production. But the effect is not always an activity; for example, flesh is an effect of nature,

---

[1] See *Methodus medendi* I 6 and II 3 (K X 45–46, 87).

[2] In *De placitis Hippocratis et Platonis* VI 1 (K V 507), Galen makes the distinction simply by saying that the active motion is self-produced, whereas the passive is produced by something else.

but not an activity. Clearly the former term is used in two senses, the latter not.

The concept of "use" he hardly bothers to define, beyond saying that it is equivalent to "utility," as we have seen. "Χρεία means for him," Dr. May writes, "[not function but] rather the suitability or fitness of a part for performing its action, the special characteristics of its structure that enable it to function as it does."[3] Galen observes, at the beginning of his *Use of the Parts*, that use is related to soul:

> For the body is the instrument of the soul, and consequently animals differ greatly in respect of their parts because their souls also differ. For some animals are brave and others timid; some are wild and others tame; and some are, so to speak, members of a state and work together for it, whereas others are, as it were, unsocial. In every case, the body is adapted to the character and faculties of the soul. (*De usu partium* I 2; K III 2)

The notion is plainly related closely to what Aristotle wrote in the *De partibus animalium*, and especially with book IV, chapters 8–11, which Galen himself quotes in this context (I 3; K III 5). In these chapters Aristotle introduces a concept of use that is hardly found elsewhere in his writings, and since he varies the abstract noun χρεία with other cognate words, we can see something of the origin of the idea.

> Being upright by nature, Man has no use for forelegs, and in place of them nature has given him arms and hands. Now Anaxagoras says it is because he has hands that Man is the cleverest of the animals; but reason demands that he get hands because he is cleverest. Hands are a tool, and nature, like a clever man, always allocates a thing to whatever can use it. (*PA* IV 9, 687 a 6)

> [Fish lack tongues.] The reason is that they have little use for a tongue, since they are not able to chew or taste. (*PA* IV 11, 690 b 26)

In these two examples χρεία comes close to meaning "need": the use of a part is just what the animal would feel the need of, if it lacked the part.

---

[3]May, *Usefulness*, I, 9.

[Men and viviparous quadrupeds move their jaw up, down, and sideways; fish, birds and oviparous quadrupeds, up and down only.] The reason is that the latter motion is useful (χρήσιμος) for biting and cutting up, whereas the sideways motion is useful for grinding. So to those that have molars the sideways motion is useful, but to those that do not, it is not useful at all, and hence it is withdrawn from all the latter; for nature does nothing superfluous.

Now all the other creatures move the lower jaw; the river crocodile alone moves the upper. The reason for this is that it has feet that are useless (ἀχρήστους) for seizing and holding, since they are extremely small. So for these uses (χρείας) nature has made their mouth useful (χρήσιμον), instead of their feet. (*PA* IV 11, 691 a 27)

Although Aristotle seldom uses the word χρεία in this way, the idea is, of course, one that is familiar from the whole range of his works on the natural world. As a rule, instead of saying that something has such and such a use, he says it is "for the sake of such and such" (ἕνεκα τοῦ —).

That the terms δύναμις and ἐνέργεια are technical terms of Aristotle's philosophy is too well known to need more than a mention here. Δύναμις in Aristotelian contexts is usually translated as "potentiality" or "potency." The translation "faculty," in Galen, marks his more limited application of the term. Whereas Aristotle employed it to refer to any capacity that exists in a thing for changing into something else, or developing in any way, Galen normally reserves it for the capacities of the natural tissues and organs for doing their regular work. Both Aristotle and Galen make ἐνέργεια a correlative of δύναμις, although in the case of Aristotle, at least, it would be better to put it the other way round, since he is emphatic that the ἐνέργεια has priority, except in the unimportant sense of temporal priority. The working of a δύναμις is its ἐνέργεια. Galen adds that what is produced by the working of the faculty is called its ἔργον ("effect")—but that makes him a little uneasy because it is a rather unnatural limitation on the normal meaning of ἔργον. So he adds (in *De usu partium* XVII 1) that sometimes we also call an ἐνέργεια an ἔργον.

Before proceeding to consideration of the need for two terms, it will be as well to say a few words about their translation. Daremberg

objects to the translation of χρεία by the word *usage*, and argues that
the correct rendering is *utilité*, with this point we need not further
concern ourselves, since it seems to refer only to the niceties of the
French language. His use of *fonction* for ἐνέργεια, however, raises
the question whether we should employ the word "function" to
translate this Greek word into English. Although Liddell and Scott
give "function" for ἐνέργεια in a Galenic and physiological context, it
seems better to avoid this rendering, since it is notorious that modern physiologists employ "function" where earlier authors would
have used "purpose" or "use."

We find that Harvey wrote *usus et actio*, and that these words are
translated by "use and action" by Willis. Conversely, where we read
"function" in Willis, we find that Harvey has in one place *munia* and
in another *officium*, both of which words seem rather to signify purpose or use than activity.[4] Clearly, these few remarks on the usage of
the word "function" would not justify our avoiding the word if we
had no suitable alternative; but the word "activity" seems in every
way appropriate, and does not have the disadvantages of "function."

It may, however, be asked whether there is really any need for the
two terms "use" and "activity." For it seems that modern physiology
has no satisfactory equivalents for them.[5] There is no absolute necessity to employ two words, but it is not difficult to show that it is
convenient to do so and that Galen's use of χρεία and ἐνέργεια is
not a defect in his exposition. We may know a good deal about some
part, process, or product of the body from the one point of view, and
little or nothing from the other. Thus, the fact that saliva digests
starch was known long before any account could be given of the
process by which this digestion is accomplished; in this case, then,
the use was known before the activity could be described. The uses
of the great sense organs are well known, and could be examined in
great detail without any knowledge of their activities; the powers of
discrimination of the eye and ear, for example, can be studied inten-

[4]Harvey, *Works* (trans. Willis), pp. 91, 98, 99. Harvey actually uses the
more recondite word *munia*, rather than *munus*.

[5]Professor Sir Andrew Huxley, F.R.S., informs me that he employs the
terms "function" and "action" in making the distinction made by Galen; but
the distinction is seldom clearly drawn by other biological writers, and when
made presents, I believe, no agreement in usage, as far as the second of the
two notions is concerned.

sively without our being obliged to have recourse to any knowledge of the activities of these organs.

Conversely, we may know a good deal about the activity, without knowing the use. Harvey's study of the circulation of the blood was both novel and entirely satisfactory, as far as it went; but it was limited to the exposition of an activity, of which the corresponding use entirely escaped him; for he was only able to attribute to the circulation a use (the distribution of heat from the heart) that was neither novel nor, as we now see it, acceptable.[6]

A particularly striking instance of a considerable knowledge of the activity preceding by many years any acceptable explanation of the use is furnished by the more recondite sense organs of insects. Consider, for example, the halteres of flies. These organs, which resemble minute drumsticks, are placed just behind the wings; and, in the cranefly they are so obvious that they cannot escape the notice of the most casual observer. Moreover, the apparatus needed to record their vibrations, and to study their muscles and to some extent their nerves, has been available for at least a hundred years; yet an acceptable account of their use was not given till 1948, in a paper by Pringle.[7] It had, indeed, been suggested somewhat earlier that they were "stimulation organs"; but this class of organs, whose concept was based on a self-discrediting theory, has proved to be a mere bag into which was thrown any organ, in appearance sensory, to which no precise sensory function could at the time be assigned.[8]

That Pringle's analysis of the function of the halteres does in fact concern their use can be seen from a brief citation.

A hypothesis to explain the function of the halteres may now be stated:

1. The halteres of Diptera are organs of special sense giving an indication to the fly of rotations in the yawing plane.[9]

[6]This explanation of the use of the circulation was still given by Harvey in 1649, in his *Epistle to John Riolan*.

[7]Pringle, "Gyroscopic Mechanism."

[8]The theory here referred to is that of J. von Uexküll, in his "Studien über Tonus I." His "tonus" is a fluid that is neither physical nor nonphysical; and his "hydrodynamic" model for the nervous system does not, on his own admission, obey the known laws of hydrodynamics.

[9]Pringle, "Gyroscopic Mechanism," p. 377.

Explanations of use and explanations of activity will refer to quite different sets of facts; and this is as true today as it was for Galen.

In the case of the explanations of breathing, the set of facts underlying the explanation of the activity itself divides into two subsets: the passage of something from the outer air into the organism through the lungs;[10] and the movements of bones and muscles by which the lungs are filled and emptied. We may note, in passing, that although Galen could not be expected to deal to our satisfaction with the passage of oxygen into the capillaries of the lungs, his analysis of the activities of the bones and muscles is nothing less than brilliant.

The use of the lungs is explained by specifying the benefit received from their activity by other parts of the body. For Galen the lungs exist for the sake of the heart and, to a lesser extent, of the nervous system; modern physiology sees them as necessary for every part of the body; but both in Greek and in modern physiology the enquiry as to the part played by the lungs in the general economy of the body (their use) is entirely proper, and differs entirely from the enquiry as to their activity or *Wirkungsweise*.

I have said that Galen could not be expected to give an explanation of that part of the activity of the lungs which consists of the passage of gases through membranes. He did see clearly the need for an explanation of this part of the activity; for though he thought that the principal use of the lungs was to cool the heart and their activity corresponding to this use probably did not require the passage of air into the veins of the lungs (to employ the modern anatomical term),[11] yet the secondary use of the lungs was for him one that did depend upon the entry of air into the system, and this activity he explains as a form of digestion (πέψις) or elaboration: the lung digests or elaborates air as the liver elaborates food.[12] In *De naturalibus facultatibus* (I, ii) Galen sets out the general principles of the analysis or explanation of activities. He tells us that an activity is a change (κίνησις) and a change is either a change of quality or of

[10]Something is, of course, passed out also, as Galen very properly believed.

[11]In the classical theory of the lungs, air passes from them into the heart (Aristotle, *HA*, 496 a 30–35), but it is not very clear whether this is necessary for the cooling action of the lung upon the heart. See *De usu partium* VIII, iii (K III 621).

[12]*De usu partium* VII, viii (K III 539, 540).

place (ἀλλοίωσις or φορά). He says that the cause of the change or activity is to be called a faculty (δύναμις); and "so long as we are ignorant of the true essence of the cause which is operating, we call it a faculty."[13] It seems that, at least in the case of the homoeomerous parts of the body, to know "the true essence of the cause" would be to know the exact proportions of the warm, the cold, the moist, and the dry that naturally characterize the part concerned:

> bodies act upon and are acted upon by each other in virtue of the warm, cold, moist, and dry. And if one is speaking of an activity, whether it be exercised by vein, liver, arteries, heart, alimentary canal, or any other part, one will be inevitably compelled to acknowledge that this activity depends upon the way in which the four qualities are blended. (*Nat. Fac.* II, ix; K II 126)

Therefore, if you wish to know which alternative faculties are primary[14] and elementary, they are moisture, dryness, coldness, and warmth, and if you wish to know which ones arise from the combination of these, they will be found to be in each animal of a number corresponding to its *sensible elements*. The name *sensible element* is given to all the homogeneous [homoeomerous] parts of the body, and these are to be detected not by any system, but by personal observation of dissections.... Now the peculiar flesh (ἡ ἰδία σάρξ) of the liver is of this kind as well, also that of the spleen, that of the kidneys, that of the lungs, and that of the heart; so also the proper substance of the brain, stomach, gullet, intestines, and uterus is a *sensible element* of similar parts all through, simple, and uncompounded. That is to say, if you remove from each of the organs mentioned its arteries, veins, and nerves, the substance remaining in each organ is, from the point of view of the senses, simple and elementary. As regards those organs consisting of two dissimilar coats, of which each is simple, of these organs the coats are the elements—for example, the coats of the stomach, esophagus, intestines, and arteries. (*De nat. fac.* I vi; K II 12–13)

[13] *Nat. Fac.* I, iv (K II 9).

[14] This is an awkwardness. Galen has said that we say the cause of an activity is a faculty as long as we are ignorant of "the true essence of the cause"; but there is no reason to suppose that any further and unknown cause is supposed by him to underly the four qualities, so they should not be called faculties.

We are left in no doubt, therefore, as to how the activities of the homoeomerous parts are to be explained or analyzed; but the analysis of their activities is very different from that of the activity of the hand, which is explained by a prolonged exposition of the uses of the parts of the hand: that is, of the hand and forearm, which together form a unit of activity. This appears at first sight confusing, and when Galen says, both with reference to the hand and with reference to the arteries, that it is difficult to discover the uses of the parts without first having understood their activities, we are at first in doubt as to what exactly he can mean.[15] It is quite clear that the two questions, "What is the part for?" and "How does the part work?" are distinct, and that the mode of operation ($\dot{\epsilon}\nu\dot{\epsilon}\rho\gamma\epsilon\iota\alpha$) may be related to the use as final cause, on the one hand, and, on the other, to the elements and faculties as productive causes. This fact suggests a linear scheme of explanation. In the case of such an organ as the eye, we can state first its use, then explain its activity, showing how this activity is related to its use, and can finally show how the matter of which it is composed is related to its activity.[16]

But it would be a mistake to believe that Galen supposed that all analyses of organs or operations should follow this scheme, or even that the scheme itself is complete. Galen was too good a naturalist to believe that no further question could be asked about, for example, vision or hearing; for we could certainly ask what part is played in the life of a particular animal by those modes of vision and of hearing of which it happens to be possessed. "In all animals," he tells us, "Nature has formed the various parts of their bodies in relation to their habits and abilities."[17] Moreover, "use is of three kinds: it is related either to life itself, or to convenience of living, or to the preservation of both."[18] A linear scheme of explanations is thus

---

[15] "First I will remind you that, as has been shown above, we cannot fully ($\kappa\alpha\lambda\hat{\omega}s$) discover the use of a part without first having specified its activity. The activity of the hands is prehension; as is clear, universally recognized and in need of no proof. But there is no general agreement upon the activities of arteries and nerves, muscles and tendons; these activities are not obvious, and so these parts call for longer treatment." (*De usu partium* I, xvi; K III 45–45).

[16] *De usu partium* X, iii and vi (K III 769, 785).

[17] *De usu partium* III, xvi (K III 264).

[18] *De usu partium* VI, vii (K III 435).

possible, its two last terms being, respectively, the activity of the four qualities and the preservation of life (or of "the convenience of living").

Such a linear scheme appears appropriate when we are dealing with parts such as the eye and ear, or the hands and feet, by which the organism as a whole is enabled to survive in a changing environment; but for parts such as the lung or the arteries the linear scheme turns out to be inadequate. In such cases we are concerned with parts whose use relates more immediately to the preservation of particular activities of the body, and we discover that here the explanatory sequence tends to circularity: in the sense that activity is for use, but use may be for some further activity, which again has its use. Thus the activity of the lungs is analyzed partly in terms of the uses of the muscles, bones, and nerves that are responsible for the movements of respiration;[19] and it is the activity of these parts (muscles, etc.) that is explained in terms of the primary qualities; and the use of the lungs is related to the maintenance of activities elsewhere in the body.

Insofar as the activity to which the lungs are of service is, for Galen, the regulation of the innate heat, it might be thought that the chain of explanations must terminate at this point, because the innate heat, as heat, is a primary quality, and, as innate, is very near to being life itself.[20] Yet it is clear that Galen is prepared to assign particular uses to the innate heat, for he tells us "that alteration is effected mainly by the warm principle, and that therefore digestion, nutrition, and the generation of the various humors, as well as the qualities of the surplus substances, result from innate heat; all these and many other points ... were correctly stated first by Hippocrates ... and were in the second place correctly expounded by Aristotle" (*De nat. fac.* II, iv; K II 89–90, trans. Brock). The analysis of the activity of the arteries is less elaborate than that of the lungs, for it is carried out in terms of the primary qualities, which endow the coats

---

[19]Similarly, the activity of the hand was analyzed in terms of the uses of the bones and muscles.

[20]Cf. Harvey: "And this indeed is the principal use and end of the circulation (*praecipuus usus quidam et finis est*) ... to wit, that all parts dependent on the primary innate heat may be retained alive." ("An Anatomical Disquisition on the Circulation of the Blood, to John Riolan." Harvey, *Opera* I, 100; *Works*, p. 98).

of the arteries with the power of contraction, which is evoked by the pulsatile faculty derived from the heart. This faculty is itself a direct consequence of the composition of the peculiar flesh of the heart. The use of the pulse (the pulse is the activity of the arteries) is elucidated like that of respiration, not as being directly concerned with the preservation of life but as serving to maintain the same activities as are maintained by the lungs—the same activities, though not in the same parts of the body.

In spite, however, of the complications of these analytical or ex-planatory schemata, we can always distinguish the causal analysis of the activity of a part from its finalistic explanation. In the case of the lungs the causal analysis is in two stages, of which the first is from one point of view finalistic; in the case of the pulse the analysis is more simple and direct.

It may be helpful to give here Galen's summary of his completed causal analysis of the activity of the pulse, for comparison and con-trast with his finalistic explanation, given in *De usu pulsuum*.

It has been shown in other treatises[21] that all the arteries possess a power [faculty] which derives from the heart, and by virtue of which they dilate and contract.

Put together, therefore, the two facts—that the arteries have this motion, and that everything, when it dilates, draws neigh-boring matter into itself—and you will find nothing strange in the fact that those arteries which reach the skin draw in the outer air when they dilate, while those which anastomose at any point with the veins attract the thinnest and most vaporous part of the blood which these contain, and as for those arteries which are near the heart, it is on the heart itself that they exert their traction. For, by virtue of the tendency by which a vacuum becomes refilled, the lightest and thinnest part obeys the ten-dency before that which is heavier and thicker. Now the lightest and thinnest of anything in the body is firstly pneuma, secondly vapor, and in the third place that part of the blood which has been accurately elaborated and refined. (*De nat. fac.* III, xiv; K II 204, trans. Brock)

[21] *De placitis Hippocratis et Platonis* VI, vii (K V 562); *An in arteriis* 8 (K IV 733–34).

It is abundantly clear that this account of the causes of the pulsation of the arteries, and of the immediate consequences of their expansion, is an explanation of one aspect of the set of events "the pulsations of the arteries"; whereas the conclusion of the treatise *De usu pulsuum*, namely, that its use is the preservation of heat and the restoration of psychic pneuma, constitutes an explanation of another aspect. That the arteries in expanding draw in air and the lightest and thinnest part of the blood is an immediate consequence of pulsation; the preservation of heat and the restoration of psychic pneuma are more remote consequences. Thus it is possible, if one wishes, to consider both explanations as parts of a unitary causal analysis of different aspects or phases of a complex process. In this way one could avoid the scandal so frequently occasioned by finalistic or teleological explanations. But this, I think, would be to gloss over a helpful and quite harmless distinction.

The drawing in of fluids is a necessary consequence of the expansion of the tubes, and one which occurs, for example, when a syringe is filled. This filling of the arteries is, indeed, useful to the animal, but its analysis ends in itself and does not lead us to any further consideration of the working of the machine as a whole; and this is just what is done by relating the expansion of the arteries to the fundamentally important process of respiration.

In his treatise *De usu respirationis*, devoted to respiration and to the part played by this process in the life of the animal as a whole, Galen has much to say that is of value, and which represents an advance, if only a tentative advance, in the development of the science of physiology. Although he could not bring himself to abandon the concept of innate heat, he was working toward the notion of respiration (the word is not here an anachronism) as a form of combustion. His failure to develop the idea in a more satisfactory manner was not due to his teleology, but to the circumstance that the Greeks had never pushed their chemistry beyond a system based on the four elements. The word on which our "chemistry" is based appears, so Partington tells us,[22] for the first time in an edict of Diocletian given in A.D. 296; and the first author who can plausibly be called a chemist was Zosimos of Panopolis, whose *floruit* is given as A.D. 300.

---

[22]Partington, *Chemistry*, p. 20. Liddell and Scott accept Zosimos' etymology, or at least give no other. Partington is here better informed.

The explicit reference to use is inescapable when we consider the organism as a whole, as a system adapted to life in a particular environment and capable of destruction by adverse influences. Darwin, who had no illusions about the infallible and beneficent wisdom of Nature, and who was at pains to point out the imperfections in some of the organs of existing animals, would never have allowed that there is anything objectionable in the notion of utility as such: "natural selection will never produce in a being any structure more injurious than beneficial to that being, for natural selection acts solely by and for the good of each. . . . If a fair balance be struck between the good and evil caused by each part, each will be found on the whole advantageous."[23] The first impression we receive from Galen's "teleology" is, it must be admitted, grotesque; but, when he is not playing the poet or the theologian, he is, as we have seen in this chapter, capable of employing the notion of χρεία with freedom and subtlety, and to very good effect. That his excessive appeal to this principle is sometimes a hindrance to his physiological analysis cannot be denied; but it is often of assistance, and frequently it is merely indifferent to his scientific purpose, neither helping nor hindering it. A full discussion of this subject, with examples, would naturally require a whole book devoted exclusively to it.

[23]Darwin, *Origin of Species*, pp. 162, 163. The discussion of imperfections in parts of animals occurs on pp. 163, 164.

DE USU RESPIRATIONIS

INTRODUCTION

Title

Galen often refers to this treatise under the title "Περὶ χρείας ἀνα-πνοῆς" (e.g. *De placitis Hippocratis et Platonis* II 4; K V 240; *De usu partium* VI 3; K III 441 and XVI 12; K IV 337).[1] It is translated into Latin *De usu respirationis* in the version followed by Kühn, and *De utilitate respirationis* in some others (these are not two different works, as might be suggested by their listing in Durling, "Census").

For the meaning of "χρεία," see Introduction, Section IV, above.

The Text

This work is preserved in three extant Greek manuscripts: Laurentius plut. 74,5 (fourteenth century) f. 94ᵛ–103ᵛ, designated F; Marcianus 281 (fifteenth century) f. 77ᵛ–81ᵛ, designated M; and Parisinus Suppl. Graec. 35 (fifteenth century) f. 132ᵛ–144ʳ, designated P. Rudolf Noll, in preparing his excellent edition of 1915, used photocopies of F and M. (A check on his work, using new photocopies, has led us to make some minor changes in the *apparatus criticus*, on the following lines in Noll's numeration: 2.19; 4.14–15; 5.10; 6.17; 10.5; 13.5; 23.3; 24.4; 24.19; 25.4; 25.12; 27.4; 29.1; 29.20; 30.1; 33.9.) Noll's conclusion was that these two manuscripts are not themselves related as archetype to copy, but are copied from a common archetype. The revisions I have made in Noll's readings are not sufficient to upset this conclusion, which is based also on collations of eight other works of Galen that the two manuscripts have in common.

The readings of P were not included in Noll's *apparatus criticus*, on the ground that it is a copy of F. Noll relied on an unpublished collation of the first two chapters made by J. Mewaldt in 1910, and notes on the rest supplied by P. Boudreaux. I have examined P, and collated about a quarter of *De usu respirationis*. Noll claims (p. x) that where F and M differ, P always goes with F. This is overstated: P agrees with M, against F, at 4.15, 13.5, and 14.10. These readings are all wrong, however, and may be explained as simple copying errors;

---

[1] For a general account of Galen's self-references, see Bardong, *Beiträge*.

so there is no reason to dissent from Noll's conclusion, which is again based on collations of other works contained by these manuscripts, besides *De usu respirationis*. Where F is corrected, P follows its uncorrected readings.

A Latin translation is preserved in many manuscripts and early printed editions. Noll concludes that it is by Niccolò da Reggio, who mentioned that he had translated this work in the preface to his version of Galen's *De flebotomia*. The second Venetian printed edition, of 1502, attributes this translation to Peter of Abano, but Noll thinks the style is clearly that of Niccolò. There are some differences in the text of the various manuscripts and editions; the text designated N in the *apparatus* is the consensus of these texts as determined by Noll (I have not thought it worthwhile to check Noll's reading of the Latin manuscripts). There is reason to think that Niccolò had a better text of the original Greek than is preserved in the surviving Greek manuscripts. Noll argues (p. xxii) that Niccolò's Greek text was in the same tradition as F and M, on the ground that Niccolò has many of the same mistakes that they have. But the argument is unsound: he quotes eight instances, of which six are not mistakes at all.

No Arabic translation has been found yet. According to M. Ullmann, *Die Medizin im Islam*, p. 41, it is mentioned by Ḥunain Mǎ turgǐma nr. 39, and there is a reference to it in Rāzī, *Al-Hāwī*. J.S.W. has found a reference in the Latin translation of *Al-Hāwī* in the British Museum (*Liber dictus Elhavi*, Brescia, 1486), vol. I, lib. VII, p. 29, col. 2. The passage in question is clearly ch. 4.2 (21.1-5 Noll), but it is not a verbatim citation and does not offer evidence about the virtues of the Arabic translation.

We have made a few changes in Noll's text, not because of new evidence but because of a different reading of Galen's argument. Many of these changes are restorations of the manuscript reading, or different suggestions for obviously corrupt passages. The changes in question are at 3.11-12; 6.11; 9.19; 10.4-6; 12.6-7; 12.13; 20.2-3; 21.18; 22.7; 22.12; 23.16-17; 25.3-4; 25.18; 28.3; 28.6-7; 30.17; 31.6-8.

Pages and lines are numbered according to Noll's edition (N). The pages of Kühn's edition are also noted (K).

Summary

Chapter 1

The following views are recorded about the use of breathing:
1. It is the source of the soul (Asclepiades).
2. It nourishes the soul (Praxagoras).
3. It cools the innate heat (Philistion and Diocles).
4. It both nourishes and cools (Hippocrates).
.5. It replenishes the arteries with pneuma (Erasistratus).

These can be grouped under two heads:
A. The use of breathing lies in the substance of air breathed in.
B. It lies in the quality of air.

Which is right?

Chapter 2. Criticism of A

Having breathed in and held the breath, one suffocates.

Erasistratus replies: this is because the heart cannot then draw pneuma from the lungs, since that would create a void.

Opponents reply:

(a) disseminate void is not ruled out;

(b) air may expand;

(c) the heart is still observed to expand when the breath is held.

The Erasistrateans reply to (c): either

(d) the heart draws from the great artery in these conditions; or

(e) it does not expand but oscillates.

Reply to this: (d) ignores the valves; (e) is contrary to observation; both (d) and (e) fail to explain the continuation of the pulse in the arteries.

Further defence of (d): the valves may not prevent the heart from drawing from the artery in unnatural conditions.

Conclusive arguments again the Erasistrateans:

(f) they cannot explain why one cannot relieve suffocation during suspension of breathing by contracting the thorax;

(g) one suffocates more, the more deeply one has breathed in before holding the breath;

(h) the remedy for this suffocation is to breathe *out*.

75

Further discussion of the continuation of the pulse in the arteries during suspension of breathing: If the heart is both forcing pneuma into the arteries and drawing it from them, why is the pulse not doubled in this condition? Do the arteries then draw air in from outside through pores in the skin? If so, what is the use of the thorax and lung?

These arguments refute all who hold proposition A, including Asclepiades, Praxagoras, and Philotimus, as well as Erasistratus.

Chapter 3. Discussion of B

What quality is required from the inspired air? Is it to cool the natural heat? There is evidence for and against this. Is it to fan the innate heat? Or more generally to preserve it?

Analogy of flames: flames require a double motion, towards the fuel and away from it, in balance. Excessive heat increases the outward motion, excessive cold the inward. Blood is the fuel of the innate heat, and breathing, by fanning and cooling, keeps the two motions in balance. Moreover, breathing out discharges smoke.

So we can accept the view that breathing is to preserve the innate heat.

The analogy is persuasive, though not scientific. It explains the rapidity of death from suffocation.

Chapter 4. Further Testing of Thesis That we Breathe to Preserve the Innate Heat

Variations in breathing in various conditions: at the baths, while breathing various vapors, after exercise, in fevers, in childhood and old age, etc.

All these turn out to be consistent with the thesis.

Chapter 5. Nourishment of psychic pneuma

This may be either 1. from air drawn in in breathing (a) via the heart and arteries (so Erasistratus), or (b) directly into the brain from the nostrils (so Hippocrates); or 2. from vapors arising from the blood.

1(a). Erasistratus has been refuted in *De causis pulsuum* [or *De usu pulsuum*?]. The related thesis that the psychic pneuma is nourished by the pneuma contained with the blood in the arteries is refuted by the experiment of ligaturing the carotid arteries.

2 is also made less likely by this experiment.

1(b) must be the major source of nourishment.

1(a) is also refuted by the experiment of fixing a bladder over the mouth and nostrils.

Psychic pneuma is also served by the role of breathing as moderator of the innate heat, both directly via the nostrils, and via the heart, to keep moderate heat in the blood, if the vapors of the blood also nourish the psychic pneuma. The maintenance of moderate heat in the two organs, heart and brain, is vital. The soul is in the brain, either as natural heat, or as pneuma, or as the form of the brain, or as some connected power. Excess of heat, which is prevented by breathing, would be rapidly fatal whichever of these alternatives is the case.

Appendix: Why is it that the quantity breathed out is the same as that breathed in, if the heart takes some of the air breathed in? Generally, vapors are added to the air breathed out; see *De difficultate respirationis*.

Sigla

F = Laurent. gr. 74,5; s. XIV. f. 94^v–103^v
M = Marcian. gr. 281; s. XV f 77^v–81^v
N = versionis Latinae codicum consensus
  p = Parisin. lat. 6865; s. XIV. f. 67^b–70^b
  e = Amplonian. lat. f. 77a; s. XIV. f. 108^a–110^d
  d = Dresdens. lat. Db. 92; s. XV. f. 20^d–24^b

Raro citatur

P = Parisin. suppl. grec. 35; s. XV–XVI. f. 132^v–144

Editiones Graecae

Aldina, Venetiis 1525 vol. III f. 85–88
Basileensis, apud Cratandrum 1538 vol. III p. 159–65
Charteriana, Parisiis 1679 vol. V p. 413–26
Kühniana, Lipsiae 1821–33 vol. IV (1822) p. 470–511
Noll, Marburgensis, 1915

Citantur etiam Cornarii emendationes, quae apud editionis
Aldinae exemplar Jenense inveniri possunt.

ΓΑΛΗΝΟΥ ΠΕΡΙ ΧΡΕΙΑΣ
ΑΝΑΠΝΟΗΣ

1. Τίς ἡ τῆς ἀναπνοῆς χρεία; ὅτι γὰρ οὐχ ἡ τυχοῦσα, φανερὸν ἐκ τοῦ μηδὲ βραχύτατον ἡμᾶς χρόνον δύνασθαι διαρκεῖν ἀπολομένης αὐτῆς. ᾧ καὶ δῆλον ὅτι πρὸς οὐδεμίαν τῶν κατὰ μέρος ἐνεργειῶν, ἀλλ' εἰς αὐτὴν τὴν ζωὴν διαφέρει. ὥσπερ γὰρ,
5 ὅσα γέγονε πρὸς τὸ βαδίζειν, τούτων στερηθέντες εἰς τὸ βαδίζειν βλαπτόμεθα, καὶ ὅσα πρὸς τὸ βλέπειν χρήσιμα, τούτων στερηθέντες οὐ βλέπομεν, οὕτως ὅσα πρὸς τὸ ζῆν ἀναγκαῖα, τούτων /
στερηθέντες ἀποθνήσκομεν.

2. τί ποτ' οὖν τηλικοῦτόν ἐστι τὸ παρὰ τῆς ἀναπνοῆς ἡμῖν
10 χρηστόν; ἆρά γε τῆς ψυχῆς αὐτῆς γένεσις, ὡς Ἀσκληπιάδης φησίν; ἢ γένεσις μὲν οὐχί, θρέψις δέ τις, ὡς ὁ τοῦ Νικάρχου Πραξαγόρας; ἢ τῆς ἐμφύτου θερμότητος ἀνάψυξίς τις, ὡς Φιλιστίων τε καὶ Διοκλῆς ἔλεγον; ἢ καὶ θρέψις καὶ ἔμψυξις, ὡς Ἱπποκράτης; ἢ τούτων μὲν οὐδέν, ἐπιπληρώσεως δ' ἕνεκεν
15 ἀρτηριῶν ἀναπνέομεν, ὡς Ἐρασίστρατος οἴεται; σχεδὸν γὰρ τοσαῦται γεγόνασιν αἱρέσεις περὶ χρείας ἀναπνοῆς, εἰ καί τινες /
τῶν εἰρημένων δοκοῖεν μὴ διαφέρειν, ὥσπερ ἥ τε τῶν λεγόντων ῥώννυσθαι τὴν ἔμφυτον θερμασίαν ὑπὸ τῆς ἀναπνοῆς καὶ ἡ τῶν ῥιπίζεσθαι· διαφέρουσι γὰρ οὐδὲν αὗται τῆς λεγούσης ἐμψύχεσθαι·
5 πλὴν οὐ τὴν λέξιν χρή, ἀλλὰ τὴν διάνοιαν σκοπεῖν, ἥτις ἐν ἁπάσαις ἐστὶ μία· τὴν γὰρ ψύξιν οὐκ αὐτὴν δήπου δι' αὐτήν, ὥσπερ οὐδὲ τὴν ῥίπισιν ἢ τὴν ῥῶσιν, ἀλλ' ὅτι φυλάττουσι τὴν ἔμφυτον θερμότητα, διὰ τοῦτο εἶναί φασι χρησίμους. καὶ εἰ
τοῦτό ἐστι / τὸ κοινὸν ταῖς τρισὶ δόξαις, ἡ φυλακὴ τῆς ἐμφύτου

N1

2 in tit. post ἀναπνοῆς add. βιβλίον Chartier Kühn
3 ὅτι Aldus: ἐστι FM
4 δύνασθαι διαρκεῖν F: om. M: ἀρκεῖν δύνασθαι edd.
5 ἀπολομένης Noll coll. Περὶ χρείας μορίων vol. I p. 56,13. 19 He.: ἀπολλομένης FM Aldus: ἀπολλυμένης Basil. edd.: pereunte N: fort. ἐπεχομένης, cf. p. 3,3 sqq. ὅτι om. M
8 στερηθέντης FM edd.: ablatis N
12 post αὐτῆς hab. ἐστι M edd.: om. FN

ON THE USE OF BREATHING

Chapter 1

What is the use of breathing? That it is not a trifling use is K470 / N1 clear from our inability to survive for even the shortest time after it has stopped. Hence also it is obvious that its importance is not for any particular and partial activity, but for life itself. For just as our walking is impaired in so far as we are deprived of the means of walking, and our seeing, if we lose the where-withal for seeing, so, if what is necessary for life is cut off, / we K471 die.

2. Whatever is the result of breathing that is of such great use to us? Is it the source of the soul itself, as Asclepiades says?[1] Or not its source, but a kind of nourishment for it, as Praxagoras the son of Nicharchus asserts? Or a cooling of the inborn heat, as both Philistion and Diocles affirmed? Or both nourishing and cooling, as Hippocrates has it? Or none of these things: is it rather that we breathe to replenish the arteries, as Erasistratus believes? There have been about so many doctrines of the use of respiration; though, indeed, some / of those we N2 have mentioned do not really appear to differ from one another: for example, the view of those saying that the innate heat is strengthened by breathing, and that of those saying that it is fanned. For these views do not differ from that which says it is cooled, and what matters is not the way of saying something, but what is signified, and this is the same in all.[2] For they do not mean cooling just for its own sake, or fanning or strength-ening; they mean that these processes are useful because they maintain the innate heat. And if this is / what the three doc- K472

---

13 θρέψις *corr.* P; *cf. p. 2,19–25. 10,11–17:* χρῆσις FM: *sed nutritio aut confor-tatio quaedam* N: ῥῶσις *cod. coll. p. 2,2 et 6* ὡς ὁ τοῦ F: ὁ *om.* M *edd.*
14 θερμότητος F: *om.* M: θερμασίας *edd.* ἀνάψυξις] ῥίπισις καὶ ἀνάψυξις Cornarius *coll. p. 2,3 et 6*
N2
7 διὰ τοῦτο] διὰ τοῦτον *Aldus* φασι *Kühn:* φησὶ FM *edd.*

θερμασίας, χαλεπὸς ὁ περὶ πασῶν αὐτῶν γίνεται λόγος καὶ δυσ-
10 διαίρετος, ὅτι ψυχῆς οὐσίαν οὐκ ἴσμεν. εἴπερ οὖν ἐνέργεια μὲν
ψυχῆς ἡ ζωή, μεγάλα δ' αὕτη φαίνεται πρὸς τῆς ἀναπνοῆς
ὠφελεῖσθαι, μέχρι πόσου τὸν τρόπον τῆς ὠφελείας ἀγνοεῖν εἰκός
ἐστιν ἡμᾶς; μέχρις ἄν, οἶμαι, τὴν οὐσίαν τῆς ψυχῆς ἀγνοῶμεν.
ἀλλ' ὅμως τολμητέον τε καὶ ζητητέον τὸ ἀληθές· ἢν γὰρ καὶ μὴ
15 τύχωμεν αὐτοῦ, πάντως δήπου πλησιέστερον ἢ νῦν ἐσμὲν ἀφιξόμεθα.

3. καὶ πρῶτόν γε δύο κεφάλαια πασῶν τῶν εἰρημένων αἱρέσεων ποιησάμενοι πότερον αὐτῶν ἀληθέστερόν ἐστιν εὑρεῖν πει-
ραθῶμεν. ἐοίκασι γὰρ αἱ μὲν εἰς τὴν οὐσίαν ἀποβλέπειν τοῦ
εἰσπνεομένου ἀέρος, αἱ δὲ εἰς τὴν ποιότητα. τὸ μὲν οὖν γεννᾶ-
20 σθαι λέγειν τὴν ψυχὴν καὶ τὸ τρέφεσθαι καὶ τὸ τὰς ἀρτηρίας
ἐπιπληροῦσθαι τὴν οὐσίαν ἐστὶ μόνον αἰτιωμένων, τὸ δὲ ῥιπίζεσθαι καὶ ῥώννυσθαι καὶ ψύχεσθαι, τὴν ποιότητα. καθ' ὃν,
K473   οἶμαι, λόγον καὶ σιτίον ὁ μὲν ὡς / γλυκὺ προσφερόμενος ἢ αὐστηρὸν
ἢ θερμὸν ἢ ψυχρὸν <εἰς> τὴν ποιότητα μόνον, ὁ δ' ὡς τρέφον,
25 εἰς τὴν οὐσίαν ἀποβλέπων αἰτιᾶται. τοῦτ' οὖν πρῶτον διορισώ- /
N3   μεθα, πότερον αὐτῆς τῆς οὐσίας χρῇζομεν τοῦ κατὰ τὴν εἰσπνοὴν
ἑλκομένου ἀέρος ἢ τῆς ποιότητος ἢ ἀμφοτέρων.

2. Ἐπεὶ τοίνυν εἰσπνεύσαντες [μὲν] τῆς μὲν οὐσίας εὐπο-
ροῦμεν, πνιγόμεθα δὲ οὐδὲν ἧττον ἢ εἰ μηδ' ὅλως εἰσεπνεύσαμεν,
5 ἐμφαίνεσθαι δοκεῖ τὸ μὴ δεῖσθαι τῆς οὐσίας. ἀλλὰ πρὸς τοῦθ'
ὁ Ἐρασίστρατός φησιν, ὅτι μηδ' ἕλκειν δύναται τὸν ἐκ τοῦ
πνεύμονος ἀέρα κατὰ τὴν τῆς ἀναπνοῆς ἐπίσχεσιν ἡ καρδία·
φυλάττεσθαι γὰρ τῶν ἀναπνευστικῶν ὀργάνων τὸν ἴσον ὄγκον

---

9 δυσδιαίρετος FM edd.: om. N: δυσδιαίτητος sugg. Noll, cf. p. 12.13 et K. II
881 (οὐδὲ γὰρ οὐδὲ τοῦτο εὐδιαίτητον): sed IV 400 K. legitur χαλεπὴ καὶ
δυσδιαίρετος ἡ μάχη
10 οὐσίαν] οὐσίας M
11 αὕτη Noll: αὐτὴ FM edd.: hec N
14 ἢν Noll: εἰ FM edd,
19 μὲν οὖν] γ' οὖν F
23 ὁ μὲν Aldus: ὃ μὲν FM: qui quidem N   προσφερόμενος ἢ Aldus: προσφερό-
μενον· μὴ FM: qui ... affert vel N
24 εἰς add. Noll: ad pd: om. e et cdd. lat.· ὁ δ' Aldus: ὃ δ' FM: qui vero N
25 ἀποβλέπων Aldus: ἀποβλέπον FM   αἰτιᾶται Noll coll. v. 21: αἴρεται FM
edd.: eligit N (i.e. αἱρεῖται)   τοῦτ' οὖν edd.: τούτου FM: hoc igitur N   διο-
ρισόμεθα FM edd.: determinemus N

trines have in common, namely, maintaining the innate heat, discussion about all the theories becomes troublesome and hard to decide,[3] because we do not know the substance of the soul. If life is the activity of the soul, and life seems to be greatly served by breathing, how long shall we be likely to remain ignorant of the manner of this service? As long, I suppose, as we remain ignorant of the substance of the soul. All the same, we must make so bold as to seek out the truth; even if we do not reach it, we shall certainly come a good deal nearer to it than we are now.

3. Now first, making our own grouping of the schools of thought just mentioned under two heads, let us try to discover which is the more true. Some appear more concerned with the substance of the inspired air, and others with its quality.[4] To speak of the genesis of the soul, or of nourishing, or of filling the arteries, is appropriate only to those who consider the substance as cause; while, on the other hand, to speak of fanning, or strengthening, or cooling, considers the quality; just as he who prefers food as being / sweet or bitter, or hot or cold, K473 considers only the quality as cause, whereas he who takes it as nourishing considers the substance. First, then, let us decide / this: whether we need the substance itself of the inspired air, or N3 the quality, or both?

Chapter 2

Now, having breathed in [and held the breath], we have a plentiful supply of the substance, but we are stifled no less than if we had not breathed in at all; hence, it seems to be apparent that it is not the substance that we need. But to this Erasistratus says that the heart cannot even draw the air out of the lung during the stoppage of breathing, because in these conditions the same volume of expansion is maintained by the organs of

---

N3

2 ἑλκομένου Noll: ἐρχομένου FM edd.: eius qui ... attrahitur N

3 μὲν del. Noll: om. N

8 τὸν ἴσον ὄγκον Aldus: τῶν εἰς ὄγκων, postea in τὸν ὄγκον corr. F: τῶν εἰς ὄγκον M

τῆς διαστάσεως ἐν ταῖς τοιαύταις καταστάσεσιν. εἴπερ οὖν εἵλ-
10 κυσέ τι μέρος ἀέρος ἡ καρδία, κενὸς ἂν ὁ τοῦ μεταληφθέντος
ἐγένετο τόπος· τοῦτο δὲ γένεσθαι ἀδύνατον. ἵν' οὖν μὴ γένηται
<τι> ἀδύνατον, οὐδὲ μεταλήψεσθαί φησι τὴν ἀρχήν. δεῖ γάρ, ἵνα τι

K474 μεταληφθῇ, μὴ μόνον εἶναι τὸ ἕλξον, ἀλλὰ καὶ τὸ με/ταδῶσον·
οὐ μεταδίδωσι δ' ὁ θώραξ, τὸν ἴσον ὄγκον <φυλάττων> τῆς δια-
15 στάσεως· οὐδ' οὖν οὐδ' ἡ καρδία δύναται μεταλαμβάνειν, ἀλλ'
ἐπιχειρεῖ μὲν ὡς ἔμπροσθεν, ἀνύει δ' οὐδέν· κἀντεῦθεν τὸ πνίγεσθαι. ἐπεὶ τοίνυν, ἵν' ἑλκύσῃ τι τοῦ ἀέρος ἡ καρδία, συγχωρεῖν
χρὴ τὸν θώρακα, συγχωρεῖ δ', ἡνίκ' ἂν μεταβάλλῃ τὴν διάστασιν,
μεταβάλλει δ' εἰσπνεόντων ἢ ἐκπνεόντων, τηνικαῦτα ἡ καρδία
20 μεταλήψεται.

2. ταυτὶ μὲν ὁ Ἐρασίστρατος. οἱ δ' ἀντιλέγοντες αὐτῷ
πρῶτον μέν, <ὅτι> οὐδ' ἀπέδειξέ που μηδ' ὅλως παρεσπάρθαι τοῖς
σώμασί που κενόν, ἀλλ' ὅτι μὴ ἀθρόον, ὑπομιμνήσκουσιν, ἔπειτα δ',
εἰ καὶ τοῦτο συγχωρηθείη, τὸ μηδ' ὅλως ἐν τῷ κόσμῳ μηδαμοῦ /
N4 παραπεπλέχθαι κενόν, ἀλλ' οὔ τι γοῦν ἀδύνατον εἶναί φασι τὴν
αὐτὴν οὐσίαν χεομένην τε καὶ πάντη τεινομένην μείζονα τὸν
πρόσθεν τόπον ἐπιλαμβάνειν, καὶ τρίτον, ὅτι τοῖς ἐναργέσιν ὁ
λόγος αὐτοῦ μάχεται· λέγει μὲν γάρ, ὡς οὐχ ἕλκει κατὰ τὰς
5 ἐπισχέσεις τῆς ἀναπνοῆς ἡ καρδία τὸν ἐκ τοῦ πνεύμονος ἀέρα·
K475 τούτῳ δ' ἕπεται τὸ μὴ δια/στέλλεσθαι τὴν καρδίαν (οὐδὲ γὰρ
ἐνδέχεται κατ' αὐτὸν διαστέλλεσθαι μέν, μηδὲν δ' ἕλκειν· κενὸς
γὰρ ἂν οὕτω γένοιτο τόπος)· εἰ δ' οὐ διαστέλλεται, δῆλον ὡς
οὐδὲ κινεῖται· ἀλλὰ μὴν φαίνεται κινουμένη· τὸ ἐναντίον ἄρα
10 τοῦ πρώτου περαίνεται, τὸ τὴν καρδίαν ἕλκειν ἐν ταῖς ἐπισχέσεσι
τῆς ἀναπνοῆς τὸν ἀέρα.

3. πρὸς δὲ ταῦθ' οἱ Ἐρασιστράτειοι πάλιν ἀμφισβητοῦσι

10 μεταληφθέντος FM: καταληφθέντος edd.
11 δὲ γενέσθαι Furley: δὲ (εἰ postea add.) ἐγένετο F: δὲ εἰ ἐγένετο M
12 <τι> Furley
13 μεταδῶσον F: μεταδοῦν M edd.: μεταδιδοῦν Kühn
14 οὐ corr. P et Aldus: ὁ FM: καὶ P   μεταδίδωσι δ' Noll: μεταδίδωσιν FM:
μεταδίδωσιν δὲ edd.   τὸν ἴσον ὄγκον Aldus: τὸν εἰς ὄγκων F: τῶν εἰς ὄγκον
M: cf. v. 8   φυλάττων] om. FM: add. corr. P: post διαστάσεως add. Aldus:
equalem molem servans dimensionis N
18 ἡνίκα FM edd.: ἡνικ' ἂν Mewaldt
22 πρῶτα FM edd.: corr. Noll   ὅτι add. Cornarius: quoniam N   ἀπέδειξέ postea
in -ξέν mut. F: ἀπέδειξάν M Aldus: ἀπεδεῖξαι (sic) Basil.: ἀποδεῖξαι Chartier
Kühn: ἐπέδειξέν Cornarius: demonstravit N

breathing. Hence, if the heart had taken some part of the air, the place of the air that was taken would have become empty; and that is impossible.[5] So that, therefore, the impossible may not happen, he says that it [the heart] will not even take any of it in the first place. For that something may be taken, it is not enough that there should be something that will attract, but there must also be / something that will give; and the thorax K474 does not give, retaining as it does the same volume of expansion; neither, therefore can the heart take; but it tries, as it did before, and gets nothing, and hence the suffocation. Since, then, in order that the heart may take some of the air, the thorax must cooperate, and when it changes its expansion it does cooperate, and it changes by breathing in or breathing out, it is then that the heart will take up air.

2. So far Erasistratus. But his opponents recall that, in the first place, he has nowhere proved that void is not at all interspersed anywhere in solid bodies, but only that it is not present *en masse*;[6] and second, that even if this be conceded, namely, that void is nowhere at all / interwoven in the universe, even N4 so, they say, it is not impossible for the same substance, relaxing and stretching in all directions, to take up a greater space than formerly; and third, that his opinion is in conflict with what is evident to the senses. For he says that the heart does not draw air from the lungs when the breath is held; and it follows from this that the heart is not / expanded (for it is not K475 possible according to him that it should expand, yet draw in nothing; for an empty space would thus arise); and if it does not expand, clearly it does not move. But it evidently does move; so the conclusion is the contradictory of the original thesis, namely, that the heart does draw in air when the breath is held.

3. But again the Erasistrateans[7] argue against this view, at-

---

N4

1 ἀλλ᾽ εἴτι γ᾽ οὖν ἀδύνατ᾽ ἄν *postea in* ἀλλά τοι γ᾽ οὖν ἀδύνατον *mut.* F: ἀλλά τοι γοῦν ἀδύνατον M *Aldus:* ἀλλά τοι γ᾽ οὐκ ἀδύνατον *a Basil. edd.:* ἀλλ᾽ οὔ τι γοῦν ἀδύνατον *Noll:* non tamen impossibile N

4 λέγει μὲν γὰρ ὡς οὐχ FM: βλέπομεν γὰρ ὡς *edd.:* videmus enim quoniam (*om.* non) N

6 τούτῳ *et* τό μή FM: τοῦτο *et* τῷ (*om.* μή) *edd.* hoc autem sequitur (*om.* non) N γὰρ *del.* F: *hab.* M *edd.*

περί τε χύσεως καὶ συστολῆς τὰ ἐναντία κατασκευάζειν πειρώμενοι καὶ περὶ τῆς τοῦ κενοῦ παραπλοκῆς, καὶ ὡς ἡ μὲν καρδία
15 παρὰ μὲν τοῦ πνεύμονος οὐδὲν ἕλκει τηνικαῦτα, παρὰ δὲ τῆς μεγάλης ἀρτηρίας, ᾗ πρόσθεν ἐχορήγει. τινὲς δὲ οὐδὲ διαστέλλεσθαι καὶ συστέλλεσθαι λέγουσιν αὐτήν, ἀλλ᾽ οἷον κραδαίνεσθαι. τὰ μὲν γὰρ ὑπὸ τῶν περὶ τὸν Ἀσκληπιάδην εἰρημένα κάλλιον εἶναί μοι δοκεῖ παραλιπεῖν, ἄτοπά τε φανερῶς ὄντα καὶ
20 τῶν προσηκόντων ἐλέγχων ὑπ᾽ Ἀθηναίου τετυχηκότα.

4. διττὴν οὖν ἀνάγκη πρὸς αὐτοὺς γενέσθαι τὴν ἀντιλογίαν, πρὸς μὲν τοὺς παρὰ τῆς ἀρτηρίας <ἕλκεσθαι τὸν ἀέρα λέγοντας> /
N5 ἀντιλέγοντας τὴν [διὰ] τῶν ὑμένων ἐπίφυσιν [ἦν] κωλύουσαν, ὡς
K476 αὐτὸς ὁ Ἐρασί/στρατος εἴρηκε, πρὸς δὲ τοὺς κραδαίνεσθαι μόνον, ὅτι παρὰ τὸ φαινόμενον λέγουσι (φαίνεται γὰρ ἐν μέρει διαστελλομένη τε καὶ συστελλομένη), κοινὴν δ᾽ αὖ πρὸς ἀμφοτέ-
5 ρους, τὴν πασῶν τῶν ἀρτηριῶν κίνησιν ὁμοίως γινομένην κατά τε τὴν ἀναπνοὴν καὶ τὴν ἐπίσχεσιν.

5. ἡ μὲν οὖν περὶ χύσεως οὐσίας ζήτησις εἰς ἀπέραντον μῆκος λόγων ἑκατέροις ἐκπίπτει. πρὸς δὲ τὸ μὴ δύνασθαι παρὰ τῆς μεγάλης ἀρτηρίας ἑλκύσαι τι τὴν καρδίαν διὰ τὴν τῶν ὑμένων
10 ἐπίφυσιν ἀπολογούμενοί φασι περὶ τῆς κατὰ φύσιν οἰκονομίας ταῦτ᾽ εἰρηκέναι τὸν Ἐρασίστρατον, οὐ περὶ τῆς βιαίου καὶ παρὰ φύσιν· ἐπειδὴ γὰρ ἀναγκαῖόν ἐστι διαστελλομένην ἑλκύσαι τὴν καρδίαν, ὅταν μὲν ἐκ τοῦ πνεύμονος ἕλκειν ἔχῃ, παρὰ τῆς μεγάλης ἀρτηρίας μὴ λαμβάνεσθαι κωλυόντων τῶν ὑμένων·
15 ὅταν δ᾽ ἀπορῇ τῆς ἐκ τοῦ πνεύμονος χορηγίας, τηνικαῦτα ἐκ

---

13 κατασκευάζειν F: σκευάζειν M *edd.*
14 τοῦ *om.* FM
15 prius παρὰ] περὶ *sed corr.* F   παρὰ δὲ] παρὰ δέ τοι F: παρὰ μέντοι M
16 ᾗ] ἡ *in* ἡ *mut.* F: ᾗ M *Aldus Basil.: corr. Cornarius Chartier*
18 περὶ τὸν Ἀσκληπιάδη *edd.* (-δην *Kühn*): ἐν τῷ μιλτιάδη FM: qui circa Asclepiadem N
20 ὑπ᾽ Ἀθηναίου *Noll (coll. Gal. VII 165. 615 sq. K. De elem. sec. Hippocr. p. 35,20 He.):* ὑπὸ Ἀσκληπιάδους F: ὑπὸ Ἀσκληπιάδου M *edd.:* ab Asclepiade N: ὑπὸ Μηνοδότου *H. Schöne (ap. Diechgräber, Die gr. Empirikerschule, p. 213)*
21 αὐτοὺς *Noll:* γε τοὺς F: γε τούς M *Aldus Basil.:* γε τούτους *Chartier Kühn:* hos N
22 ἕλκεσθαι τὸν ἀέρα λέγοντας *om.* FM: *add. Aldus:* qui ... trahi aerem dicunt N

tempting to establish the contrary of these opinions about expansion and contraction and an interwoven void; they say that at the time in question the heart indeed draws nothing from the lungs, but it does draw from the great artery, to which previously it gave supplies. But some say that the heart does not actually expand or contract, but only oscillates, as it were. As for the things said by the school of Asclepiades, I think them better passed over in silence, being clearly foolish, and having received the appropriate refutation from (?) Athenaeus.[8]

4. So the reply to these views must be twofold: first, against those who say that the air is drawn from the artery, / in contra- N5 diction of the fact that the membranous outgrowths [the valves] prevent this, as / Erasistratus himself said;[9] and second against K476 those who say there is only an oscillation, that they speak against the observable facts; for it can be perceived to expand and contract by turns; moreover there is an objection common to both groups, namely, the movement of all the arteries occurring similarly during both inspiration and holding breath.[10]

5. The inquiry concerning the stretching of the substance degenerates into an endlessly inconclusive disquisition on both sides. However, against the impossibility of the heart's drawing anything from the great artery, on account of the membranous outgrowths, they say in defense that Erasistratus only meant it to be understood as impossible in the natural course of things, not that it was impossible that it should happen by violence and against nature; for since it is inevitable that the heart on expanding should draw in something, whenever it is able to draw from the lungs, it receives nothing from the great artery, because the valves prevent it; but whenever it is without the supply from the lung, then it draws back something from the

---

1 διὰ del. Cornarius: om. N   ἦν FM: del: Aldus   ὡσαύτως FM: corr. Aldus

4 κοινὴ FM edd.: corr. Kühn

7 ἡ μὲν οὖν περὶ Aldus: εἰ μὲν οὖν ἡ FM   χύσεως FM: χήσεως Aldus: σχή-σεως Basil.: recte iam Cornarius Chartier   εἰς ἀπέραντον Noll: εἶτα τὸ πέραν τό FM: εἰς τὸ ἀπέραντον edd.

8 λόγων Noll: λό . . et λόγ . compendiose FM: λόγου edd.: sermonum N

10 ἐπίφυσιν] ἔκφυσιν F

13 ὅταν Aldus: ὁποία FM   ἔχῃ] ἔχει FM edd.: corr. Kühn

τῆς μεγάλης ἀρτηρίας ἀντισπᾶν βιαζομένην τοὺς ὑμένας. περὶ
δὲ τῆς τῶν ἀρτηριῶν κινήσεως ὁμοίως ἔν τε ταῖς ἀναπνοαῖς καὶ
K477   ταῖς ἐπισχέσεσι γιγνομένης οὔ φασι χρῆναι / θαυμάζειν οἱ Ἐρα-
σιστράτειοι· τοσοῦτον γὰρ μόνον παραλλάττειν αὐτὴν τῆς ἐν
20   τῷ κατὰ φύσιν διοικήσεως, ὅτι μὴ παρὰ τοῦ πνεύμονος, ἀλλὰ
παρὰ τῆς μεγάλης ἀρτηρίας ἡ καρδία τὴν ὁλκὴν τοῦ πνεύματος ποιησαμένη πάλιν εἰς ἐκείνην ἐπιπέμπει· καὶ διὰ τοῦτό
φασι πνίγεσθαι τὸ ζῷον, ὅτι τῆς παρὰ τοῦ πνεύμονος ἐστέρηται
χορηγίας.

25   6. τὰ μὲν δὴ πρὸς ἑκατέρων ἀντιλεγόμενα τοιαῦτα τετύ-
χηκεν ὄντα, καὶ πρὸς τούτοις ἔτι τὸ μήπω μὲν εἰρημένον, <εἰρη- /
N6   σόμενον> δὲ νῦν ἰδίᾳ καὶ χωρὶς τῶν ἄλλων, ὅτι μοι δοκεῖ περαίνειν ἐναργέστατα <τὸ προκεί>μενον. ἐν μὲν γὰρ δὴ ταῖς ἐπισχέσεσι τῆς ἀναπνοῆς τί τὸ κωλῦόν ἐστιν ἕλκειν μὲν τὴν καρδίαν ἐκ τοῦ πνεύμονος ἀέρα, συστέλλεσθαι δὲ τὸν θώρακα
5   πεφυκότα γε δὴ τοῦτο πάσχειν; εἰ μὲν γὰρ μήτε διαστῆναι
μήτε συνιζῆσαι δυνάμενον ὄργανον ἦν, ἴσως ἄν τινα νοῦν εἶχε
τὸ πρὸς Ἐρασιστράτου λεγόμενον. ἐπειδὴ δὲ κατ' αὐτὸν
ἐκεῖνον συστέλλεσθαι δύναται, τί κωλύει καὶ νῦν εἰς τοσοῦτον
συνιζάνειν [καὶ νῦν] αὐτόν, εἰς ὅσον ὑπὸ τῆς καρδίας ἐκκενοῦται;
K478 / 10   τά τε γὰρ ἄλλα καὶ διὰ μυῶν ὑπὸ τῆς τοῦ ζῴου / προαιρέσεως
κινεῖσθαί φησιν ὁ Ἐρασίστρατος τὸν θώρακα· καὶ τί νῦν
χαλεπὸν θλῖψαι πανταχόθεν αὐτὸν τοῖς μυσὶ μετὰ τοῦ κωλῦσαι
τὴν ἄνω[θεν] κένωσιν, ὅπερ ἐν ταῖς καλουμέναις τοῦ πνεύματος
καταλήψεσιν κἂν ταῖς ἀποπατήσεσιν γίγνεται; πανταχόθεν γὰρ ἐν
15   ταῖς τοιαύταις ἐνεργείαις θλίβομέν τε τὸν θώρακα καὶ συστέλ-
λομεν βιαίως κλείσαντες τὸν ἄνω πόρον τῆς τραχείας ἀρτηρίας,
<ὡς> μηδὲν δι' αὐτῆς κενοῦσθαι. ὡς εἴγε μὴ μόνον θλίψαιμεν,

---

22 τε πέμπει FM: τε del. Aldus: ἐπιπέμπει Noll coll. p. 33,6   διὰ τοῦτό Noll: δι'
αὐτό τε FM: δι' αὐτό γέ edd.: propter hoc N
23 τῆς om. F
26 εἰρησόμενον om. FM: add. inter ἄλλων et ὅτι ab Aldo edd.: ibidem hab.
dicendum N
N6
1 δὲ νῦν FM: νῦν δὲ edd.: nunc autem N
2 ἐναργέστατα τὸ προκείμενον Noll (coll. De elementis sec. Hipp. p. 5,26 sq. He.
De sententiis Hipp. et Plat. p. 328,6 Mü.): ἐναργέστατε μένον FM: ἐναργέστατον μόνον edd.: ἐναργέστατον μὲν ὄν Noll, Berl. phil. Woch. 33 (1913) col.
1247: evidentissimum existens N

great artery, forcing the valves. And that the motion of the arteries is the same when breathing as when holding the breath, the disciples of Erasistratus say, is in no way / surprising: for K477 the motion differs from what happens in the natural ordering of things only in that the heart does not draw from the lung, but having made a draught of pneuma from the great artery sends it back again into it; and they say that the animal suffocates precisely because it has been deprived of the supply from the lung.

6. These then are the things said by the two opponents; and in addition, there is one thing not previously stated but now / to be stated by itself apart from the rest, because by itself it N6 seems to me to prove the proposition quite conclusively. In the stoppage of breathing, what is it that prevents the heart from drawing air from the lungs, and the thorax from contracting, made as it is by nature to do just that? If it were not an organ able to expand and contract, there might be some sense in what Erasistratus says. But since even he agrees that it is able to contract, what hinders it now from contracting by just so much as it is emptied by the heart? For among other things, Erasistratus says the thorax is moved by the muscles by the animal's / volition. And now, what difficulty is there in squeezing it with K478 the muscles on all sides and at the same time blocking the way for it to empty itself upwards—as happens in so-called stoppages of breath and in straining at the stool? For in actions of this kind the thorax is pressed and compressed on all sides, the upper opening of the windpipe being forcibly closed, so that nothing can pass through it. So that, if we not only press, but

---

5 γε om. M   δή FM: om. edd.

8 συστέλλεται M

9 καὶ νῦν FM edd.: del. Kühn

11 καὶ τί νῦν Furley: κἂν ὁτιοῦν FM: et in hoc nullum N: κἀνταῦθ' οὐδὲν Noll

12 θλῖψαι: Noll: θλῖψαι in -ψη mut. F: θλίψῃ M edd.: comprimere N   post μυσὶ add. κινεῖσθαι Cornarius

13 ἄνωθεν FM edd.: corr. Noll   ἐν ταῖς] fort. ἐν <τε> ταῖς

17 ὡς om. FM: add. Aldus   δὲ FM: δι' Aldus   κενοῦσθαι] κτείνεσθαι FM: corr. Aldus   μὴ μόνον <μὴ> θλίψαιμεν Cornarius

18 ἀθρόως Noll (cf. v. 21 et Gal. II 689. 883 K. De usu partium tom. I p. 475,15 sqq. He.): λάθρους F: λαῦρος M edd. λάβρος Kühn: multus repente N

ἀλλὰ καὶ τοῦτον ἀνοίξαιμεν, ἀθρόως ἐκτὸς ὁ ἀὴρ μετά τινος
φέρεται ψόφου· καὶ καλεῖται τὸ τοιοῦτον ἐκφύσησις τῆς ἀψό-
20 φου μόνον ἐκπνοῆς διαφέρουσα πλήθει καὶ τάχει <τῆς> κινήσεως. ἵνα γὰρ ὁ εἰσπνευσθεὶς ἀὴρ ἀθρόως αὖθις ἀντεκπνευσθῇ, /
N7 τάσεως πολλῆς πανταχόθεν ἐδέησε τῷ θώρακι. τὸ μὲν δὴ τῆς
τάσεως κοινὸν <ταῖς> τρισὶν ἐνεργείαις, τὸ δὲ ἠνεῶχθαι τὸν
ἄνω πόρον ἴδιον τῆς ἐκφυσήσεως. οὐδὲν μὲν οὖν χαλεπόν, οὐδ'
ὅταν ἐπέχωμεν τὴν ἀναπνοήν, θλίβειν πανταχόθεν τὸν θώρακα
K479 / 5 κλείσαντας τὸν ἄνω πόρον· οὕτως / γὰρ οὐχ ὅπως ἀντιπράττειν,
ἀλλὰ καὶ συνεργεῖν ἑλκούσῃ τῇ καρδίᾳ δυνήσεται.

7. καὶ φανερῶς ἐξελήλεγκται ψεῦδος ὂν τὸ πρὸς Ἐρασιστράτου λεγόμενον, ὡς οὐχ οἷόν τέ ἐστι τὴν καρδίαν μετα-
λαβεῖν ἐκ πνεύμονος ἀέρα κατὰ τὰς ἐπισχέσεις τῆς ἀναπνοῆς.
10 ἔστι γὰρ ἑκάστῳ τὴν πεῖραν ἐφ' ἑαυτοῦ λαβεῖν, μυριάκις εἰσπνεύσαντα πλεῖστον θλίβειν πανταχόθεν τὸν θώρακα καὶ μηδὲν
ἀντεκπνέοντα. φανήσεται <γὰρ> σφύζουσα μὲν ἐν τούτῳ ἡ καρδία,
πνιγόμενος δ' ὁ ἄνθρωπος, καὶ τοσοῦτόν γε μᾶλλον καὶ θᾶττον
πνιγόμενος, ὅσον πλεῖον εἰσέπνευσεν. ὅπερ οὐδ' αὐτὸ μετρίως
15 ἐνδείκνυται τὸ μή τι τῆς οὐσίας, ἀλλὰ τῆς ποιότητος τοῦ πνεύματος δεῖσθαι τὴν καρδίαν· εἰ γὰρ ἡ καρδία τῆς οὐσίας ἐδεῖτο,
μείζονες ἂν ἐκ τῆς ἀπορίας αὐτῆς ἤπερ ἐκ τῆς [αὐτῆς] εὐπορίας
αἱ βλάβαι συνέπιπτον. οὐ μὴν φαίνεταί γε τοῦτο γιγνόμενον,
ἀλλ' ὅταν εὐπορῇ πλείστου πνεύματος, ἀνιᾶται τηνικαῦτα μάλιστα.
20 τρίτον <δ'> ἐπὶ τούτοις οὐ τὸ τυχὸν γνώρισμα τὸ τὴν ἴασιν τοῖς
οὕτω πνιγομένοις ἐκπνοὴν εἶναι· χρῆν γὰρ μᾶλλον εἰσπνοὴν
εἶναι, <εἰ δι'> ἔνδειαν οὐσίας ἀέρος ἐπνιγόμεθα. /

---

19 τῆς *Noll:* τις FM *edd.*

20 ἀψόφου μόνον ἐκπνοῆς *Noll:* αὐτοῦ τὸ μὲν ἐκπνοεῖν FM: ἀπὸ τῆς ἀψόφου
μόνον ἐκπνοῆς *edd.:* ab insonituosa solum expiratione N τῆς *add. Noll*
κινήσεως *Cornarius:* κενώσεως FM *edd.:* motus N

21 ὁ εἰσπνευθεὶς F: ὁ εἰσπνευσθεὶς M *Aldus:* ὁ om. a *Basil. edd.* ἀντιπνευσθῇ
FM *Chartier:* ἀντεκπνευσθῇ *recte Aldus Kühn:* ἀντεπνευσθῇ *Basil.*

N7

1 πολλῶν FM: *corr. Aldus*

2 ταῖς *add. Noll*

4 ἐπέχωμεν M *edd.:* ἐπέχομεν F

5 κλείσαντες FM: *corr. Aldus*

10 εἰσπνεύσαντα *et* 12 ἀντεκπνέοντα ιn -τι *mut. Cornarius*

12 γὰρ *add. Aldus:* enim N

14 οὐδ' FM: καὶ *edd.:* etiam non mensurate N: non *om. ed. Veneta a. 1490*

also open the windpipe, the air rushes out all at once with a certain sound; and this is called blowing,[11] differing from the soundless expiration only by its copious and rapid motion. So that the inspired air may be expired again all at once, / a con- N7 siderable force is needed, acting on the thorax from all sides. Now the force is common to these three activities; but the act of opening the upper passage, peculiar to blowing. There is, then, no difficulty, even when we hold our breath, in constricting the thorax on all sides, while we close the upper passage: thus / it will be possible not only not to resist, but even to K479 assist the heart drawing in air.

7. And clearly Erasistratus' doctrine has been shown to be false, that it is impossible for the heart to take over air from the lung during the holding of the breath. For everyone can do the experiment on himself a thousand times:[12] breathe in very deeply and compress the thorax on all sides without breathing out in turn. It will be perceived that the heart indeed beats during that time, but the subject stifles; and stifles the more, and the more quickly, the more deeply he breathed in. Which itself goes a good way toward proving that the heart needs not the substance but the quality of the pneuma; because if it required the substance, greater ill effects would accrue from the lack of it than from overabundance. But that is evidently not the case but, on the contrary, whenever there is the greatest abundance of pneuma, precisely then is the greatest distress. Third, it is no small indication that the remedy for those who are stifling in this way is breathing out; it would rather have to be breathing in, if we were to stifle through lack of the substance of air. /

---

15 τὸ μὴ τι Noll: τῷ μήκει FM: μὴ edd.

16 εἰ Kühn: ἤδη FM: ἦν edd.

17 μείζονες Noll: μείζονας FP: μειζόνως M edd.: maiora ... nocumenta N ἐκ τῆς ἀπορίας] ἐκτήσατο πορείας FM: ἐκ τῆς ἀπορείας Aldus Basil.: corr. Chartier ἤπερ Kühn: εἴπερ FM edd. αὐτῆς del. Noll: om. N εὐπορίας Kühn: πορείας FM edd.

18 βλάβαι] φλέβες FM Aldus Basil.: corr. Cornarius Chartier

19 πλείστου] fort. πλεῖστον

20 δ' add. Noll

21 ἐκπνοήν] εἰσπνοήν FM: corr. Aldus χρὴ γὰρ FM: χρὴ δὲ edd.: χρῆν δὲ Kühn

22 ἦν δι' add. Aldus Basil. Chartier: εἰ δι' Kühn

K480   8. τρία δὴ ταῦτα φανερῶς καταβάλλει τὸν Ἐρασιστράτου
λόγον, ἓν μὲν δὴ καὶ πρῶτον τὸ δύνασθαι τὴν καρδίαν ἕλκειν /
N8 ἀέρα κατὰ τὰς τῆς <ἀνα>πνοῆς ἐπισχέσεις (οὐδὲν γὰρ ἐφάνη
πρὸς τοῦτο ἀντιπράττων ὁ θώραξ), ἕτερον δὲ δεύτερον τὸ τηνικαῦτα πνίγεσθαι μᾶλλον, ἡνίκ' ἂν <εἰσ>πνεύσωμεν πλέον, καὶ
τρίτον τὸ μηδ' εἰ πάνυ σφόδρα θλίβομεν τὸν θώρακα παντα-
5 χόθεν ἐν ταῖς ἐπισχέσεσι τῆς ἀναπνοῆς, δαπανᾶσθαι τὸν ἀέρα
πρὸς τῆς καρδίας, ἀλλ' ὀρέγεσθαι τὸ ζῷον ἐκπνεῦσαι, καὶ τοῦτ'
εἶναι τὸ τῆς πνίξεως ἄκος. ἐκ τούτων μὲν δὴ φανερῶς περαίνεται
τὸ μὴ <δι'> ἔνδειαν οὐσίας ἀέρος, ἀλλὰ δι' ἄλλο τι πνίγεσθαι
τὰ ζῷα.

10 9. πρὸς δὲ τὰς ὑπολοίπους τῶν εἰρημένων ἀμφισβητήσεων
αὖθις μεταβάντες ἐπισκεψώμεθα, πότεροι λέγουσιν ἀληθέστερα.
καὶ πρώτην γε πάλιν ἐξ αὐτῶν μεταχειρισώμεθα τὴν περὶ τῆς
κινήσεως τῶν ἀρτηριῶν. οἱ γὰρ [τοι] τοῖς Ἐρασιστρατείοις
ἀμφισβητοῦντες ἀλλοιοῦσθαί φασι χρῆναι τὴν κίνησιν τῶν ἀρτη-
15 ριῶν παρὰ τὸν τῆς ἐπισχέσεως καιρόν, ἄν τε κραδαίνεσθαι τὴν
K481 καρδίαν μόνον ἄν τε καὶ καταστέλλεσθαί τις ὑποθῆ/ται· κρα-
δαινομένης μὲν γὰρ παντάπασιν ἀκινήτους χρῆν γίνεσθαι μηδὲν
λαμβανούσας παρ' αὐτῆς, διαστελλομένης δὲ καὶ συστελλομένης
διπλοῦν φαίνεσθαι [δεῖ] τὸν σφυγμόν. ἐν μὲν γὰρ δὴ τῷ κατὰ
20 φύσιν ἔχειν τὸ ζῷον συστελλομένη μὲν τὸ πνεῦμα ταῖς ἀρτηρίαις
ἔπεμπεν, αἱ δὲ πληρούμεναι διεστέλλοντο, διαστελλομένη δὲ [ἤδ']
εἷλκεν ἐκ τοῦ πνεύμονος, αἱ δὲ τηνικαῦτα κενούμεναι συνεστέλ- /
N9 λοντο· κατὰ δὲ τὸν τῆς ἐπισχέσεως καιρόν, ἐπειδὴ διαστελλομένη
παρὰ τῶν ἀρτηριῶν ἕλκει, παντί που δῆλον ὅτι παλινδρομήσει

N8

1 ἀναπνοῆς] πνοῆς FM: corr. Aldus
3 ἡνίκ' ἄν Noll: ἡνίκα FM edd.   εἰσπνεύσωμεν Kühn: πνεύσομεν FM: εἰσ-
πνεύσομεν Aldus Basil. Chartier
4 μηδ' εἰ] μηδὲν FM: μηδέ Aldus Basil.: corr. Chartier: μηδ' εἰ καὶ Cornarius
5 δαπανᾶσθαι] δύνασθαι FM: corr. Aldus
6 ἐκπνεῦσαι] ἐμπνεῦσαι FM: corr. Aldus
8 δι' add. Cornarius Basil.
11 πότεροι Noll: πρότερον, εἰ FM Aldus Basil.: πρότερον, οἱ Cornarius Chartier
Kühn: qui N   ἀληθέστατα FM: corr. Aldus: veriora N
12 μεταχειρισώμεθα FM: μεταχειρισόμεθα edd.
13 τοι del. Noll
15 ἄν τε] τῷ FM: corr. Aldus
16 τις hab. F.: om. M edd.

8. These three arguments clearly overthrow Erasistratus' doc- K480
trine: first and foremost, the ability of the heart to draw in / air N8
during the suspension of breathing (for it has been shown that
the thorax offers no resistance to this); then, second, the fact
that stifling is more marked just when we have breathed in
more deeply; and third, that even if we compress the thorax as
much as we possibly can on all sides, during the suspension of
breathing, the air is not expended upon the heart, but the
animal desires to breathe out, and that is the cure of the stifling.[18] From the above it is clearly concluded that it is not from
lack of the substance of air, but from something else, that the
animal stifles.

9. Now about the remaining grounds of disputation already
mentioned, let us turn our attention to them again and see
which of the two groups speaks the truer words.[14] And first of
these let us deal again with what has been said about the movements of the arteries. Those who differ from the disciples of
Erasistratus say that the motion of the arteries must be altered
during the suspension of breathing, whether it is suggested that
the heart only oscillates, or that its motion is reduced. / For if it K481
merely oscillates, they [the arteries] must stop altogether, since
they get nothing from it; if, however, it expands and contracts,
the pulse should be perceptible as double. For when the animal
was in its natural state, the heart, contracting, sent pneuma into
the arteries, and they, in their turn being filled, expanded; and
then the heart, expanding, drew from the lung, while they, at
the same time emptying, / contracted. But during the time of N9
suspension of breathing, since the heart, expanding, draws from

---

17 γὰρ] γε FM: corr. Aldus   ἀκινήτου FM: corr. Aldus   χρήν γίνεσθαι Noll:
χρὴ ἐγγίνεσθαι FM edd.: oportere fieri N
18 λαμβανούσης FM: corr. Aldus
19 δεῖ del. Noll: om. N
21 ἥδ' del. Noll: om. N
22 πνεύμονος] πνευ ... , reliqua descissa in F: verisim. πνεύμονος, cum ita
legitur in P: πνεύματος Medd.: corr. Cornarius: ex pulmone N   κενούμεναι]
ἐνούμεναι FM: corr. Aldus   συνεστέλλοντο] συστέλλονται FM Aldus: corr.
Basil.
N9
1 τῆς hab. FM: om. edd.
2 παρὰ FM Kühn: περὶ Aldus Basil. Chartier

τὸ δι' αὐτῶν πρότερον ἐκ τῆς καρδίας ἐνηνεγμένον πνεῦμα. καὶ
οὕτως εἰ μὲν ἴσον εἴη τῷ πρόσθεν, ἴσην καὶ ποιήσεται τὴν διαστο-
5 λὴν τῶν ἀρτηριῶν, εἰ δὲ ἔλαττον, ἐλάττονα πάντως τοῦ <πρόσθεν>
ποιήσεται τὴν διαστολήν· καὶ αὕτη δῆλον ὅτι κατὰ τὸν καιρὸν
ἐκεῖνον ποιη<θή>σεται, καθ' ὃν συνεστέλλοντο πρότερον, τοῦτο
δὲ οὐδέν ἐστιν <ἄλλο> ἢ διπλασιασθῆναι τὰς κινήσεις τῶν ἀρτηριῶν. οὐ μὴν φαίνεται τοῦτο γιγνόμενον· ᾧ δῆλον ὅτι ψευδεῖς
10 αἱ ὑποθέσεις εἰσίν.

10. ἔτι δὲ καὶ τοῦτο ἐπανερωτῶσιν, εἰ μηδὲν ἐκ τῶν ἀρτη-
K482 ριῶν / κενοῦται παρὰ τὸν τῆς ἐπισχέσεως καιρόν. ἔμπροσθεν μὲν
γάρ, ἡνίκ' ἀνέπνει κατὰ φύσιν τὸ ζῷον, αὐτὸς ὁ Ἐρασίστρατος
οἴεται πᾶν ἐκκενοῦσθαι τὸ παρὰ τῆς καρδίας ἐκπεμπόμενον αὐταῖς
15 δῆλον ὡς ἐκτὸς τοῦ σώματος ἐκκρινόμενον ἤ πως ἄλλως κενούμενον. νυνὶ δὲ τί ποτε φήσουσιν; ἆρα διεξέρχεσθαι μὲν οὕτως
ὠκέως αὐτὸν διὰ τῶν ἀρτηριῶν ὥσπερ καὶ πρόσθεν, οὐ μὴν
ἐκκενοῦσθαι οὐδὲ τὸ βραχύτατον αὐτοῦ; καὶ πῶς ἐνδέχεται;
ἀλλὰ κενοῦσθαι μέν, ὅλως δ' ἕλκεσθαι αὖθις ἐκ τοῦ περιέχοντος,
20 ὅταν ἡ καρδία παρὰ τῶν ἀρτηριῶν ἀνθέλκῃ διαστελλομένη; οὐδὲ /
N10 τοῦτο εἰπεῖν ἐγχωρεῖ. καὶ μὴν εἴπερ ὅλως ἐστὶ[ν ἀ]δύνατον ἐν
τῷ διαστέλλεσθαι τὴν καρδίαν ἕλκεσθαί τι παρὰ τῶν ἀρτηριῶν
ἔξωθεν, ἐκ τοῦ περιττοῦ θώραξ καὶ πνεύμων ἐγένετο. οὐδὲ γὰρ
τοῦτο ἔστιν εἰπεῖν, ὡς ἔλαττον ἂν εἷλκεν ἐκ τῶν ἀρτηριῶν ἢ τοῦ
5 πνεύμονος, ὅθεν τῶν ὑμένων [ὑποκειμένων] ἐπικειμένων ἕλκειν
· [οὐδὲν] ἧττον δύναται· δηλοῦται δὲ τοῦτ' ἐκ τοῦ μεγέθους τῶν

---

5 τῶν ἀρτηριῶν ... τὴν διαστολήν hab. F: om. M   τῶν ἀρτηριῶν F: τῶν om.
edd.   ἔλαττον F: μεῖον edd.   τοῦ πρόσθεν Noll: γοῦν F: ἢ πρόσθεν edd.:
quam prius N

6 τὴν διαστολήν F: τὴν om. edd.   αὕτη FM: αὐτήν edd.

7 ἐκεῖνον] ἔκτινων FM: corr. Aldus   ποιηθήσεται Noll: ποιήσεται FM edd.:
hoc ... fiet N   καθ' ὃν] καθὸ FM: corr. Aldus   συνεστέλλοντο Cornarius:
συνεστέλλετο FM edd.

8 ἄλλο add. Aldus: aliud N   διπλασιασθῆναι] διαπλασθῆναι FM: corr. Aldus

9 τοῦτο Noll, cf. p. 7,18: οὕτως FM edd.: hoc N

12 παρά FM: περί edd.: circa N, sed cf. p. 8,15; Galenus plerumque κατὰ scribit,
cf. v. 1 huius pag. et saep.

13 ἡνίκα ἔπνει FM edd.: corr. Noll

15 ἐκκρινόμενον Noll: ἐκκρινον FM: ἐκρίνατο Aldus Basil.: ἐκεκρίνατο Cornarius: ἐκρίνετο Chartier Kühn: excretum N   κενούμενον Noll: κενῶτο FM:
ἐκενοῦτο edd.: evacuatum N

17 μὴν F Cornarius Kühn: μὲν M Aldus Basil. Chartier

the arteries, it is clear to all that the pneuma which previously was carried into them from the heart will flow back. And thus, if it is equal to what it was before, it will make an equal expansion of the arteries, and if less, of course it will make an expansion less than before; and clearly this expansion will occur at the same time as they were contracting before. And that amounts to the same thing as doubling the movements of the arteries. But the thing is not perceived to happen thus; hence it is clear that the hypotheses are false.[15]

10. Then again they [the Erasistrateans' opponents] raise the question whether nothing is / emptied out from the arteries K482 during the suspension of breathing. For before, when the animal was breathing naturally, Erasistratus himself believes that everything that was sent out from the heart to them [the arteries] was emptied out—clearly, as being extruded from the body, or otherwise emptied out.[16] But now, whatever are they [the Erasistrateans] going to say? Surely not that it goes just as quickly as before through the arteries, but not even the least part of it is emptied out? How is that possible? Or that it is indeed emptied, but then entirely drawn in again from the surroundings when the heart, expanding, draws in from the arteries?[17] That / cannot be conceded either. Indeed, if it is N10 perfectly possible for the heart in expanding to draw something through the arteries from outside, then thorax and lung are to no purpose.[18] For this cannot be said either, that it would draw less from the arteries than from the lung because when the valves are closed it is able to draw less.[19] That is proved from

---

18 οὐδὲ *Noll:* τοῦδε F: *om.* M *edd.:* etiam N

19 ὅλως δ᾿ *Furley:* οὐ μὴν δὲ FM

20 ὅταν] ὅτι γὰρ *Cornarius* ἀνθέλκῃ FM: ἀνέλκῃ *edd.*

N10

1 ἐστι δυνατὸν *corr.* P *et Cornarius:* ἐστὶν ἀδύνατον FM *edd.:* est possibile N

2 παρὰ FM *Chartier Kühn:* περὶ *Aldus Basil.*

3 οὐδὲ] οὐδὲν FM *Aldus: corr. Basil.:* nec N

4 ἀνθεῖλκεν *Noll:* ἂν εἶλκεν FM *edd.:* attraheret N

5 ὅθεν *Noll:* ὅπου FM *edd.:* ex quo enim N ὑποκειμένων *del. Aldus* ἕλκειν] ἐκείνου δὲ FM

6 οὐδὲν *secl. Furley* δύναται *Kühn:* δύνηται FM *edd.* δηλοῦται *Noll:* δηλοῦνται FM *edd.* τοῦτ᾿ F: ταῦτ᾿ M *edd.:* patet autem hoc N

95

σφυγμῶν· <καὶ> παντί που δῆλον, ὡς πολὺ μᾶλλον εἷλκεν ἄν,
K483 εἰ μηδ' <ἐπ>επε/φύκεσαν ὑμένες ἐν τῷ στόματι τῆς μεγάλης
ἀρτηρίας.

11. τὸ δ' ὅλον, εἰ μήθ' ἡ καρδία μήτε <τις> τῶν κατὰ
10 μέρος ἀρτηριῶν ἀποροίη πνεύματος ἐν ταῖς τῆς ἀναπνοῆς ἐπισχέσεσιν, ὡς δηλοῦσιν αὐτῶν αἱ διαστολαὶ τὸν ἴσον ὄγκον ὂν
πρόσθεν διασώζουσαι, τῷ πνίγεσθαι δεδειγμένον <ἂν εἴη> σαφῶς,
<ὡς> οὐχὶ τῆς οὐσίας αὐτῆς τοῦ ἀέρος ἔνδεια πνίγει τὰ ζῷα.
δήλη μὲν ἤδη καὶ ἡ Ἀσκληπιάδου ἐξεληλεγμένη
15 δόξα μετὰ τῆς Ἐρασιστράτου, δήλη δὲ καὶ ἡ Πραξαγόρου
καὶ Φιλοτίμου καὶ εἴ τις ἕτερος ἕνεκα θρέψεως μόνης τοῦ
ψυχικοῦ πνεύματος ἀναπνεῖν ἡμᾶς φησιν. πρόσκειται δ' ἐν τῷ
λόγῳ τὸ 'μόνης' εὐλόγως· οὐδὲ γὰρ ὡς <οὐκ> ἐνδέχεται τρέφεσθαι
τὸ ψυχικὸν πνεῦμα πρὸς τῆς ἀναπνοῆς, ἀπέδειξεν ὁ λόγος, ἀλλ' /
N11 ὡς τὸ πνίγεσθαι τοῖς ζῴοις ἐπεχομένης τῆς ἀναπνοῆς οὐ διὰ τὴν
ἀτροφίαν τοῦ ψυχικοῦ πνεύματος γίνεται. πάρεστι γὰρ αὐτοῖς
δαψιλὲς ἐν τῷ πνεύμονι τὸ πνεῦμα, καὶ ἄλλως χρόνου μακροτέρου δεῖται τὸ δι' ἔνδειαν τοῦ τρέφοντος πνεύματος ἀπόλλυσθαι
K484 / 5 μέλλον. Ἀσκληπιάδῃ δὲ / οὐ[δὲ] ταῦτα μόνον, ἀλλὰ καὶ τὰ
δι' ἑτέρων ἡμῖν εἰρημένα πρὸς τοὺς Περὶ ψυχῆς αὐτοῦ λόγους
μάχεται. δείκνυται γὰρ ἐν ἐκείνοις, ὡς ἡ τῆς ψυχῆς οὐσία,
κἂν μὴ μία ᾖ διὰ παντὸς τοῦ βίου, μέχρι χρόνου συχνοῦ
διαμένει. κατὰ δὲ τὸν Ἀσκληπιάδην οὐδὲ ἀριθμῆσαι δυνατὸν
10 ὅσας ἔχει· ἡ μὲν γὰρ ὀλίγον πρόσθεν οὖσα νῦν οἴχεται τελέως,
ἄλλη δέ ἐστιν ἡ νῦν οὖσα, μικρὸν δ' ὕστερον οἰχήσεται μὲν αὕτη,

---

7 καὶ add. Noll εἷλκεν] ἕλκειν FM Aldus: corr. Basil.
8 μηδ' ὅλως ἐπεπεφύκεσαν Noll: μὴ δὲ πεφύκεσαν F: μὴ δὲ πεφύκεισαν M:
μηδὲ πεφύκεισαν Aldus: μηδ' ἐπεφύκεισαν a Basil. edd.: non superimplan-
tatae fuissent N
9 τις add. Aldus
11 ὂν Noll: τὸν FM edd.
12 τῷ Noll: τὸ FM edd. δεδειγμένον ἂν εἴη Noll: διδαγμένους F: δεδιδαγ-
μένους M: δέ δέχεται edd.
13 ὡς add. Noll: δῆλον ὡς Aldus Basil.: δηλοῦν ὡς Chartier Kühn: suffocari
autem contingit, patet manifeste quod non N
14 Ἀσκληπιάδου Noll: ἀσκληπιάδος F: Ἀσκληπιάδειος M edd.: Asclepiadis N
ἐξεληλεγμένη Noll: ἐληλεγμένη ἢ ἐξηλαγμένη F: ἐληλεγμένη ἢ ἐξηλεγμένη
M: ἐξηλεγμένη edd.
15 δὲ Noll: τε FM edd.

the size of the pulses. It is quite clear to all that it would draw much more, if there were / no membranous outgrowth [valves] K483 in the mouth of the great artery.[20]

11. Altogether, if neither the heart nor any of the arteries in turn were to lack pneuma during the cessation of breathing, as their expansions show, since they preserve the same bulk as before, then from the fact of suffocation it would have been shown clearly that it is not the lack of the substance itself of the air that stifles animals. Obviously the opinion of Asclepiades has been refuted along with that of Erasistratus, and clearly also that of Praxagoras and Philotimus and of anyone else who says we breathe only to nourish the psychic pneuma.[21] The "only" in the proposition is added advisedly. For the argument does not prove that it is impossible for the psychic pneuma to receive nourishment from breathing, but / only that suffocation does N11 not afflict animals upon the suspension of breathing because of the starving of the psychic pneuma. For there is plenty of pneuma for them in the lung, and, further, something about to die through lack of nourishing pneuma needs a longer time. Not only these [arguments] / but also what we have said elsewhere K484 against his work *On Soul* tell against Asclepiades. For there it is shown that the substance of the soul, even if it does not remain one and the same through the whole life, nevertheless persists for a considerable time. But according to Asclepiades there is no counting how many souls one has: for even the one existing a moment ago is now totally gone, and that which exists now is another, and a moment later that will go too and another will

18 οὐκ add corr. P et Cornarius: μὴ add. a Basil. edd.   ἐνδέχεται F et a Basil. edd.: ἐνδέχεσθαι M Aldus

N11

3 ἄλλως] fort. δῆλον ὡς   μακτοτέρου FM Aldus: μικροτέρου a Basil. edd.
5 Ἀσκληπιάδης FM Aldus: corr. Cornarius Basil.   οὐδὲ FM edd.: οὐ Noll: non hec solum N
8 μὴ μία ᾖ] ἡμῖν FM: corr. Aldus: etsi non una esset N   comma post ᾖ hab. edd.: post βίου transpos. Mewaldt: usque tamen tempus multum N
9 διαμένει] -νει in -νη mut. F: διαμένη M Aldus Basil.: corr. Chartier: permaneret N   Ἀσκληπιάδην] -δη F
10 ἡ Noll: κᾶν FM edd.: que N: καὶ ἡ M. Wellmann, N. Jahrbb. 21 (1908) 699 n. 3   οὖσα] ὅσα FM: corr. Aldus

γενήσεται δ' ἑτέρα. <ὅπερ> ὡς ἔστιν ἀδύνατον καὶ ἄτοπον, δι' ἐκείνων ἀποδέδεικται.

3. Εἰ τοίνυν ἤτοι τῆς οὐσίας αὐτῆς τοῦ ἀέρος ἢ <ἦσ>τινοσοῦν
15 ἐνδείᾳ ποιότητος ἀποθνῄσκει τὰ ζῷα πνιγόμενα, δέδεικται <δὲ>
θάτερον ἀδύνατον, ἀπολείπεται θάτερον, ἐνδείᾳ ποιότητός τινος
ἐν ταῖς ἐπισχέσεσι τῆς ἀναπνοῆς πνίγεσθαι τὰ ζῷα. τίς οὖν
ἐστιν αὕτη, σκεπτέον.

2. ἐπεὶ τοίνυν, ὅταν ἐν τοῖς κατὰ τὴν καρδίαν καὶ τὸν
20 θώρακα τόποις ἀθροισθῇ θερμασία πλείων τῆς κατὰ φύσιν, ὡς /
N12 ἐν τοῖς καυσώδεσι πᾶσι συμπίπτει νοσήμασιν, εὐθὺς καὶ πλέον /
K485 τοῦ συνήθους ἀναπνεῖν ὀρεγόμεθα, δόξειεν ἂν ἐμψύξεως ἕνεκεν
ἡ ἀναπνοὴ γίγνεσθαι. ἀλλὰ πάλιν εἰ κατεψυγμένων τῶν αὐτῶν
τούτων ὀργάνων, ὡς ἔν τε τοῖς βουλίμοις καλουμένοις κἀπειδὰν
5 ἰσχυρῷ τις ὁμιλήσῃ κρύει, μὴ ὅτι ψύχειν τὴν ἐν ἡμῖν θερμασίαν,
ἀλλὰ καὶ θερμαίνειν δεῖ ὀλίγου δεῖν ἅπασαν ἐψυγμένην,
ὅμως εἰσπνεῖν ὀρεγόμεθα, δόξει ἐναντιοῦσθαι <τοῦτο τῷ>
τὴν ἀναπνοὴν ἐμψύξεως ἕνεκα γίνεσθαι.

3. καίτοι τινὲς ἀντιλαμ-
βανόμενοι δεῖσθαι μὲν ἀεί φασιν ἐμψύξεως τὴν ἐν τοῖς ζῴοις
10 θερμασίαν, ἀλλ' ὅταν μὲν αὐξηθῇ, πλείονος, ἐλάττονος δέ, ὅταν
ἀρρωστοτέρα γένηται· καὶ τὰς τοιαύτας διαθέσεις οὐχ ὅπως ἐναντιοῦσθαι τῷ δόγματί φασιν, ἀλλὰ καὶ μαρτυρεῖν οἴονται. χαλεπὸν
τοίνυν αὐτὸ τοῦτο πρότερον ὂν γίγνεται καὶ δυσδιαίτητον, ὅταν ἀπὸ
τῶν αὐτῶν φαινομένων ἐπ' ἐναντίας ἐνδείξεις ἔρχωνται· μετα-
15 στῆσαι γὰρ οὐδετέρους οἷόν τε, τοὺς μὲν ὡς ἐμψυξίς ἐστιν ἡ

---

12 ὅπερ om. FM edd.: ὃ Kühn: corr. Mewaldt: que quoniam sunt N
14 εἰ τοίνυν] εἴποι νῦν FM: corr. Aldus   ἦστινος οὖν Kühn: τινοσοῦν FM edd.
15 δὲ add. Noll: autem N
17 τίς οὖν Noll: τί γοῦν FM edd.
18 αὕτη Kühn: αὐτῆς FM: αὐτὴ edd.
N12
  2 ἕνεκεν Noll: ἕνεκα FM edd.
  3 γίγνεσθαι FM: γενέσθαι edd. κατεψυγμένον FM: corr. Aldus
  4 ὀργάνων] ἀρτηριῶν FM: corr. Aldus
  5 ἰσχυρῷ τις Mewaldt: τις ἰσχυρῶς FM: τις ἰσχυρῷ edd.   ψύχειν Cornarius:
    ψύχει FM edd.: infrigidare N   ἐν ἡμῖν FM Chartier Kühn: ἐν om. Aldus
    Basil. ἐφ' ἡμῖν Cornarius

come into being. That this is impossible and ridiculous has been proved in that place.

Chapter 3

If animals die suffocating either from lack of the substance itself of air, or from the lack of some quality or other, and one alternative has been proved impossible, the other remains:[22] animals, during suspensions of breathing, stifle from lack of some quality. So we must inquire what this is.

2. Since, then, whenever there is gathered together in the places about the heart and the thorax a warmth greater than the natural one, as is the case / in all febrile illnesses, we immediately want to breathe more fully / than usual, it would seem that breathing occurs for the sake of cooling. But then again, if, those same organs being chilled, as in the case of what is called *bulimus*[23] and when we meet sharp cold, it is necessary not only not to chill the heat in us but actually to warm it up because it is pretty well entirely chilled, and yet we feel a desire to breathe in, this will seem to contradict that breathing happens for the sake of cooling. K485 N12

3. However, some attack this and say that the heat in animals always requires cooling, but more when it waxes, less when it wanes. And they say such conditions do not go against the theory but even confirm it. Now this was hard in itself in the first place, but it becomes even impossible to decide, when from the same appearances they proceed to opposing proofs.[24] For it is impossible to shake either those, on the one hand, who

---

6 θερμαίνειν δεῖ Cornarius: θερμαίνειν δ' FM: calefacere oportet N: θερμαίνειν <ἐχρῆν> Noll

7 εἰσπνεῖν Noll: εἰσπνέειν FM edd. δόξει FM edd.: videbitur utique N: δοξειεν ἄν Noll τοῦτο τῷ add. Noll: hoc huic N

9 μὲν om. edd. ἐν om. Basil.

11 ἀρρωστέρα] ἐρεστότερον FM: corr. Aldus οὐχ ὅπως Cornarius: οὐ γὰρ οὕτως FM edd.

13 <ὂν> add. DeLacy

14 ἐπ' ἐναντίας Noll: ὑπεναντίας FM edd.: ad contrarias N ἔρχωνται Noll: ἔχωνται FM edd.: veniunt N μεταστῆσαι Noll: μεταστῆναι FM edd.: transponere N

15 οἷόν τε Cornarius: οἴονται FM edd.: possibile est N

K486   χρεία τῆς ἀναπνοῆς, εἰ θερμαινομένων <μὲν> τῶν ἀνα/πνευστικῶν
       ὀργάνων <πλέον, ἐμψυχομένων δ'> ἔλαττον ἀναπνέομεν, τοὺς /
N13   δ' <ὡς> οὐδαμῶς, ὅσον ἐπὶ τούτοις, ἐμψύχεσθαι δεόμεθα <λέ-
       γοντας.> λέγοντος γοῦν, φασιν, Ἱπποκράτους ἐν Προγνω-
       στικῷ "ψυχρὸν δ' ἐκπνεόμενον ἔκ τε τῶν ῥινῶν καὶ τοῦ στόματος
       ὀλέθριον κάρτα ἤδη γίγνεται", τὴν τοιαύτην τις ἐννοησάτω
    5 διάθεσιν, οἵα τίς ποτ' ἐστίν· εὑρήσει γάρ, οἶμαι, κατεψυγμένων
       ἱκανῶς τῶν ἀναπνευστικῶν ὀργάνων γινομένην αὐτήν. ἐχρῆν οὖν,
       φασί, μηδ' ὅλως ἀναπνεῖν τοὺς οὕτω διακειμένους, ὡς ἂν τὸ
       τῆς ἐμψύξεως δεόμενον οὐκ ἔχοντας. ὡς γάρ, εἰ μηδ' ὅλως εὐθὺς
       ἐξ ἀρχῆς ἐγένετό τι τὸ δεησόμενον ἐμψύξεως, οὐκ ἂν ἦν οὐδεμία
   10 χρεία τῆς ἀναπνοῆς, οὕτως, εἰ πρόσθεν <μὲν> ἦν, οἴχεται δὲ
       νῦν, οὐ δεησόμεθα.
             4. πρὸς δὴ ταῦτά φασιν, <ὡς> ἡ διὰ τῆς ἀνα-
       πνοῆς κίνησις ἐξάπτει ῥιπίζουσα. τοῦτο δὲ ὡς μὴ ταὐτόν ἐστιν
       ὃ πρόσθεν, οὐ μακροῦ μοι δοκεῖ δεῖσθαι λόγου. πρόσθεν μὲν
       γὰρ ἔλεγον ἐμψύχεσθαι, νῦν δὲ ἐξάπτεσθαι. ἐναντίον δὲ δήπου
   15 τὸ ἐμψύχεσθαι τῷ ἐξάπτεσθαι· τὸ μὲν γὰρ σβέννυσι, τὸ δὲ
K487   ἐξάπτει τὴν θερμό/τητα, καὶ τὸ μὲν ἵνα μὴ καυθῇ τὸ δεδεγμένον
       αὐτὴν σῶμα, τὸ δὲ ἵνα μὴ καταψυχθῇ γίνεται· πλὴν εἰ κατὰ
       συμβεβηκὸς καὶ τὸ ψυχρὸν ἐξάπτειν λέγοιεν. οὕτως δ' οὐ τὴν
       χρείαν τῆς ἀναπνοῆς, ἀλλὰ τὴν ποιητικὴν τῆς χρείας αἰτίαν
   20 εἰρήκασιν. /
N14   5. ἐστὶ γοῦν ἄμεινον ἐπὶ τὸ κοινὸν τῶν τοιούτων αἱρέσεων

---

16 εἰ] ἦ FM *Aldus: corr. Cornarius Basil.*   μὲν *add. Noll:* quidem N
17 πλέον, ἐμψυχομένων δ' *add. Noll:* magis consueto respirare desideramus,
infrigidatis autem e converso N, *quae verba Cornarius ita vertit:* μᾶλλον τοῦ
συνήθους ἀναπνεῖν ὀρεγόμεθα, κατεψυγμένων δὲ ἀνάπαλιν: *cf. supra p.*
11,19–12,3   τοὺς δ' <ὡς> *Cornarius:* τοὺς δ' (om. ὡς) FM *edd.:* illos vero
quoniam N
N13
  1 λέγοντας *add. ac lac. stat. Noll:* dicentes *add supra p. 12,15 inter* est *et* utilitas
resp. N
  5 οἵα τίς ποτ'] οὗτοι ἀπότ F: οὗτοι ἀπότ⁰ᵘ M: *corr. Aldus*   εὑρήσεις MP
  7 ἀναπνεῖν] ἀναπτύειν F
  8 μηδ' ὅλως *Cornarius:* μηδὲν ὅλως FM *edd.*
  9 δεησόμενον F: δεόμενον M *edd.*
 10 μὲν *add. Noll*
 11 ὡς *add. Noll*   ἡ διὰ] ἰδία FM: *corr. Aldus*

say breathing is for cooling if we breath more when the organs of / respiration are heated and less when they are cooled,[25] or those, / on the other hand, who say we do not need to be cooled at all in these latter conditions. At any rate, they say, since Hippocrates says in the *Prognostic*, "cold being breathed out of the nose and mouth is fatal indeed," one should take note of the nature of this condition; for he will find, I suppose, that it occurs when the organs of breathing are chilled enough. They say, then, that those who are in this case should not be breathing at all, since they have nothing that is in need of cooling.[26] Just as there would be no need of breathing at all, if from the beginning there were nothing that needed to be cooled, so, if there were once something but it has now passed away, we shall not need it.

4. Well, to this the reply is made that the activity of breathing kindles by fanning. Now, that this is something new, I think it needs no great argument to show. For before they said "to cool," and now they are saying "to kindle," and obviously cooling and kindling are contraries, since the one quenches and the other kindles / heat, and the one happens so that the body which receives it shall not burn, the other so that it shall not grow cold; unless they would say that the cold also kindles *per accidens*. In that case, however, they would not have said anything about the use of breathing,[27] but about the productive cause of its use. /

5. In any case, it is better to pass to what these alternatives

K486
N13

K487

N14

---

12 κίνησις] κίνησιν FM *Aldus: corr. Cornarius Basil.* ῥιπίζουσα] ῥιπίζουσαν FM: *corr. Aldus:* motus ... flabellans N τοῦτο δέ φασιν FM: τὸ δὲ ὅτι *edd.*
13 ἐστιν ὁ *Noll:* ἐστι τὸ FM: ἐστι τῷ *edd.:* est ei quod N μακροῦ *Cornarius Kühn:* μικροῦ FM *edd.*
14 ἐναντίον ... ἐξάπτεσθαι] hoc loco hab. N et ab Aldo edd.: ante μὴ ταὐτὸν (12) transpos. FM
16 δεδεγμένον αὐτὴν *Mewaldt:* λελεγμένον αὐτῆς FM: δεχόμενον αὐτῆς ab Aldo edd.: δεχόμενον αὐτὴν *Kühn:* suspiciens eam N
18 οὐ] οὖν FM: *corr. Aldus*
19 τῆς χρείας F: utilitatis N: *om.* M *edd.*
20 εἰρήκασιν *Noll:* εἴρηται F: εἴρηκεν M *edd.:* εἰρήκοιεν *Cornarius:* dicent N
N14
1 ἐστὶ γοῦν] ἐνισοῦν F: ἔνι γοῦν M: *corr. Aldus*

μεταβάντας ἐκεῖνο πρότερον διασκέψασθαι. κινδυνεύουσι γὰρ
ἅπαντες, ὅσοι περὶ τῆς ἐμφύτου θερμασίας εἰρήκασί τι, τὴν μὲν
σωτηρίαν αὐτῆς ὀνειρώττειν, οὐ δύνασθαι δὲ ἀκριβῶς καὶ διηρ-
5 θρωμένως ἐξηγήσασθαι τὸ σφέτερον νόημα· καὶ διὰ τοῦτο οἱ
μὲν ἔμψυξιν, οἱ δὲ ῥίπισιν, οἱ δὲ ῥῶσιν γράφουσι. μάλιστα δὲ
αὐτοὺς οἶμαι προτρέπειν τὰ περὶ τὰς φλόγας φαινόμενα. ταύτας
γὰρ ἐναργῶς ὁρῶμεν οὕτως ταχέως ἀπολλυμένας, ὅταν ἀποστερη-
θῶσιν ἀέρος, ὥσπερ τὰ ζῷα, καθάπερ δηλοῦσιν αἱ τῶν ἰατρῶν
10 σικύαι καὶ πάνθ' ὅσα στεγανὰ καὶ κοῖλα περιτεθέντα τῆς <τε>
διαπνοῆς αὐτὰς εἴρξαντα ῥᾳδίως κατασβέννυσιν. ἂν τοίνυν
εὑρεθῇ, τί ποτε φλόγες ἐν ταῖς τοιαύταις διαθέσεσι πάσχουσαι
K488 σβέννυνται, τάχα ἂν εὑρεθείη, / τί ποτέ ἐστιν ὃ παρὰ τῆς ἀναπνοῆς ἀπολαύει χρηστὸν ἡ ἐν τοῖς ζῴοις θερμασία. πρὸς δὴ
15 τὴν εὕρεσιν αὐτοῦ πάντας ἐπέλθωμεν τοὺς τρόπους, καθ' οὓς
αἱ φλόγες ὁρῶνται σβεννύμεναί τε καὶ αὐξανόμεναι. οὐ γὰρ μόνον
εἰ περι<τε>θείη τι στεγανὸν αὐταῖς, ἀλλὰ καὶ τοῖς βαλανείοις τε
καὶ τοῖς ἡλίοις τοῖς διακαέσι καὶ τοῖς ψύχεσι τοῖς ὑπερβάλλουσι
καὶ σφοδρῶς ῥιπιζόμεναι καὶ πλήθει ὕλης ἐπ' αὐτῶν σωρευθείσης
20 καὶ τοὐναντίον ἐνδείᾳ τροφῆς ὁρῶνται σβεννύμεναι, ῥωννύμεναι /
N15 δὲ καὶ αὐξανόμεναι πρός τε τοῦ μετρίου ψυχροῦ κἂν εἰ μετρίως
ῥιπίσῃς καὶ τροφῆς εὐπορούσαι συμμέτρου.

6. ἐπὶ τοίνυν τούτοις ἔτι κἀκεῖνο προσκείσθω τὸ φαίνεσθαι
πάσας τὰς φλόγας διττὴν κίνησιν κινουμένας, ἑτέραν μὲν ἀπὸ
5 τῆς ὕλης ὅθεν ἐξάπτονται μάλιστα μὲν ἄνω φερομένας ἤδη καὶ
πάντη σκιδναμένας, ἑτέραν δὲ ἐναντίαν ταύτῃ πρὸς τὴν ἀρχὴν
ἑαυτῶν καὶ οἷον ῥίζαν συστελλομένας τε καὶ συνιζούσας. καὶ

---

2 μεταβάντες F
3 εἰρήκασί Cornarius: παρήκασί FM edd.: dixerunt N
5 οἶμαι ante οἱ μὲν add. M. edd.: om FN
6 ἔμψυξιν ... ῥίπισιν ... ῥῶσιν M edd. ἔμψυξις ... ῥίπισις ... ῥῶσις F γράφουσι M edd.: scribunt N: γράφει F
7 αὐτοὺς] αὐτὸν F: αυτος M: corr. Aldus: eos N
10 στεγανὰ Noll: στεγνὰ F: στενὰ MP edd.: constricta N περιτεθέντα Noll:
περιτιθέμενα FM edd. τε add. Noll
11 αὐτὰς Cornarius: αὐτὰ FM edd. κατασβέννυσιν Noll: κατασβεννύουσιν
FM edd.
12 φλόγες] φλ' ... reliqua oblitterata (infra versum ἤ ε) in F: φλογὸς M Aldus
Basil.: corr. Cornarius Chartier πάσχουσαι σβέννυνται F Cornarius Chartier
Kühn: πασχούσαις σβέννυται M Aldus Basil.

have in common and to consider that first.[28] For all those who have spoken of the innate heat seem to have a vague idea about its preservation, but to be unable to expound their own meaning precisely and articulately; and on this account some write "cooling," some "fanning," and others "strengthening." What encourages them most, I suppose, are the phenomena associated with flames. For these we clearly see perishing when they are deprived of air, just as quickly as animals; as is shown by the cupping instruments of medical men, and by all closed and hollow vessels, which readily extinguish the flames when, placed about them, they cut them off from the draught. If it could be discovered what happens to flames in these circumstances to quench them, it would perhaps be discovered / what that useful K488 something is in breathing, from which the natural heat in animals profits.[29] To find this out, let us run over all those ways in which flames are seen to be quenched or to be increased.[30] They are seen to be quenched not only if some cover is put over them, but also by baths and by scorching sunbeams, and by excessive colds, and by too violent fanning, and by too much stuff heaped upon them, and, on the contrary, by lack of sustenance; but they are strengthened / and increased with moderate N15 cold, and if you fan them moderately, and when they enjoy a due proportion of sustenance.[31]

6. Now to all this let it also be added that all flames are seen to move with a double motion, one being away from the matter from which they are kindled, mostly going upward and dispersing in all directions, and the other being opposed to the first, gathering themselves together toward their own source and

---

15 εὕρησιν F   αὐτοῦ Cornarius: αὐτῶν FM edd.

17 περιτεθείη Noll: περιθείη FM edd.: superponatur N   τι στεγανὸν Noll: τίς τίτανον FM edd.: τι κοῖλον Cornarius: quid constrictivum N

18 fort. διαρκέσι, cf. Gal. VII 621 K. (ἰσχυροτέρα γὰρ ἡ τῶν ἡλιακῶν ἀκτίνων ῥώμη καὶ διαρκεστέρα τοῦ πυρός): et sole adurentibus N

19 πληθ’, postea " add. F: πλήθεσιν M edd.: et multitudine materie super eas acervata N

N15

4 ἑτέραν μέν] ἑτέραν δὲ FM: corr. Aldus

7 ῥίζαν F: ῥίζας M edd.: radicem N

γὰρ ἐὰν λαμπάδος μεγίστης τὸ ἄνω πέρας ἐξάψῃς, ἐπὶ τὸ κάτω
ταχέως ἀφίξεται τὸ πῦρ· κἂν εἰ τὴν λυχνιαίαν φλόγα σβέσας
K489 / 10 τῷ πέρατι τῆς / ἄνω φερομένης αἰθαλώδους λιγνύος προσενέγκῃς
ἕτερον πῦρ, εἶτ᾽ αὖ καιομένην ὄψει τοῦ λύχνου τὴν θρυαλλίδα,
οὐδενὸς τῶν τοιούτων γίγνεσθαι δυναμένου, εἰ μόνην τὸ πῦρ
ἔσχε τὴν ἐπὶ τὰ ἄνω κίνησιν. ἐπὶ δὴ τούτοις ἅπασι τοῖς φαινομένοις τῷ λόγῳ σκεψώμεθα πρῶτον μὲν τὸ πάντων ὕστατον
15 ῥηθέν, τὸ διττὸν τῆς κινήσεως, ὑπὸ τίνος ἀνάγκης γίνεται, μετὰ
δὲ τοῦτο καὶ τῶν ἄλλων ἕκαστον.

7. ἐπεὶ τοίνυν ἅπασα φλὸξ ὠκυ-
τάτην ἔχει τὴν διαφθοράν (ἀεὶ γὰρ εἰς τὸ περιέχον σκίδναται),
διὰ τοῦτο ἀναγκαῖον αὐτῇ καὶ τὴν γένεσιν ταχίστην ὑπάρχειν·
<ἄλλως γὰρ> οὐκ ἂν οὐδ᾽ ἐπ᾽ ἐλάχιστον <χρόνον> διήρκεσεν.
20 ἀλλ᾽ ἐστὶν ἑκάστῃ φλογὶ γένεσις ἐκ τῆς ὑποκειμένης ὕλης ἐξά-
πτεσθαι· εἰκότως ἄρα κίνησιν οὐ τὴν ἔξω μόνον ἀπὸ τῆς ἰδίας
ἀρχῆς, ἀλλὰ καὶ τὴν ἐναντίαν αὐτῇ τὴν εἴσω σύμφυτον ἔχει.
καὶ τοίνυν καὶ φθείρεσθαι πᾶσαν φλόγα ἀναγκαῖόν ἐστι
τῆς ὕλης στερηθεῖσαν ἢ τῶν κινήσεων τῆς ἑτέρας. καθόλου γὰρ /
K490 / N16 εἰπεῖν, ὡς πολλάκις ἐν ἑτέ/ροις δέδεικται, τῶν <δια>δεχομένων ἀλ-
λήλας κινήσεων [μὲν] ἐναντίων τὴν ἑτέραν χωρὶς τῆς ἑτέρας <ἀδύ-
νατόν ἐστι> διασῴζεσθαι. ταῦτ᾽ ἄρα δεῖται συμμέτρως ψυχροῦ τοῦ
περιέχοντος ἀέρος πᾶσα φλόξ. ὁ μὲν <γὰρ> ὑπερβαλλόντως ἔκ-
5 θερμος τὴν ἔξω κίνησιν αὐτῆς ἀμέτρως ἐργαζόμενος, ὁ δὲ ψυχρὸς
τὴν ἔσω[θεν], σβεννύ<ου>σιν ἀμφότεροι. τὸ μὲν οὖν ῥιπίζεσθαι
ἀσυμμέτρως ἀναστέλλει τὴν φλόγα πρὸς τὴν ὕλην ὥσπερ καὶ
τὸ ψυχρόν, τὸ δὲ ὑπερβαλλόντως κινεῖσθαι σκεδάννυσιν ὥσπερ
καὶ τὸ θερμόν. τῶν δὲ τὴν ἔσω κίνησιν ἄμετρον ἐργαζομένων

---

8 ἐάν coll. v. 9 sq. Mewaldt: εἰ FM edd.   ἐξάψοις Aldus: ἐξάψοιας F: ἐξάψοιεν
M: ἐξάψαις Kühn: ἐξάψῃς Mewaldt
10 λιγνύος] λιχνύος FM Aldus Basil.: corr. Cornarius Chartier   προσενέγκῇς
Noll: -καις FM edd.
12 εἰ μόνην Noll: εἰ μὴ μόνον FM: εἰ μόνον edd.: si solum (... motum) N
14 σκεψώμεθα M edd.: σκεψόμεθα F
18 αὐτῇ] αὐτὴν F: αὐτῆς M: corr. Aldus
19 ἄλλως γὰρ add. Aldus: aliter enim N   οὐκ ἄν] που· κἂν FM: corr. Aldus
χρόνον add. Noll: nec paucissimo tempore N: cf. supra p. 1.2
21 ἀπό FM: om. edd.
22 αὐτῇ] αὐτὴν FM: corr. Aldus
23 ἐστι FM: est N: ἐστι<ν ἤτοι> Noll

root, so to speak. For if you light the upper end of a long torch, the fire will speedily reach the lower end, and if, when you have put out the flame in a lamp, you bring to the top of the / upward-streaming smoky soot another light, you will see the   K489 wick of the lamp burning again; things like this could not happen at all if fire had only the upward motion. Well, with all these phenomena in mind, let us consider first of all in our discussion what was last mentioned, the duality of motion and what necessarily brings it about; and after that, each of the other topics.

7. Since every flame has a most swift destruction, as it is always being scattered abroad, on this account it is necessary that its generation must also be very swift; otherwise it would not endure even for the shortest time. But the genesis of each flame is its kindling from the matter that supports it. So it is reasonable, then, that it has by nature not only the outward motion from its proper source, but the contrary to this, the inward. And furthermore, every flame must be destroyed when deprived either of matter or of one of its motions. For to speak / generally, as has been proved many times / elsewhere, when   N16 / K490 opposing motions succeed each other, one cannot persist without the other.[32] Every flame, therefore, requires the surrounding air to be cold in due proportion, for the excessively hot, by making its outward motion out of proportion, and the excessively cold its inward motion, both quench it. Immoderate fanning presses the flame against the matter, just as the cold does; but excessive motion scatters it, just as the hot does. Now

---

N16

1 <δια> add. Noll

2 μὲν del. Noll: om. N   ἀδύνατον ἐστι add. Noll: om., postea οὐ add. F: οὐ hab. M edd.: del. et post διασῴζεσθαι add. οὐχ οἶόν τε Cornarius: impossibile est salvari N

3 δεῖται] hoc loco hab. FN: post ἀέρος hab. M edd.

4 γὰρ add. Aldus: enim N

6 ἔσω Noll: ἔσωθεν FM edd.   σβεννύουσιν ἀμφότεροι Noll: σβέννυσιν. ἀμφότεροι FM edd.: extingunt alteruter. N   τὸ μὲν οὖν ῥιπίζεσθαι Noll: τοίνυν ῥιπίζεσθαι F: τοίνυν ῥιπιζόμενοι M edd.: nam flabellari quidem N

7 ἀσυμμέτρως] fort. ἀμέτρως   ἀναστέλλει Noll: ἀναστέλλεις F: ἀναστέλλουσι M edd.: remittit N

9 ἔσω Cornarius: ἔξω FM edd.: ıntus N

105

10 ἐστὶ καὶ σικύα καὶ πᾶν ὅτιπερ ἂν τὸν ὑπὸ τῆς ἐντὸς φλογὸς
διακεκαυμένον ἀέρα εἴρξῃ τῆς πρὸς τὸν ἔξω [πυρός], τὸν ψυχρόν,
ὁμιλίας.

8. εἴδομεν <οὖν ὡς> πάντη συμμετρία σωτηρία τῆς φλογός
ἐστιν. οὕτως οὖν οὐκ ἀπεικὸς ἔχειν κἀπὶ τῆς ἐν τοῖς ζῴοις θερ- /
N17 μασίας. [εἰς] ὕλην μὲν <γάρ>, ὅθεν ἀνάπτεται, τὸ αἷμα, σύμφυτον δὲ ἔχουσα κινήσεως ἀρχὴν ἐφ' ἑκάτερα, τῆς ἑτέρας στερη-
θεῖσα καὶ τῆς λοιπῆς ἐξ ἀνάγκης στερίσκεται· καὶ διὰ τοῦτ'
K491 αὐτό, ἐάν τε ἀναπνοῆς / εἴρξῃς ἐάν θ' αἵματος, εὐθέως διαφθερεῖς.
5 καὶ γὰρ καὶ τὴν τοῦ λύχνου φλόγα διαφθερεῖς ἢ καταπνίξας
[ὀργάνῳ τὸν πνεύμονα] ἢ παντάπασιν ἐλαίου στερήσας. ἀνάλογον
οὖν <τίθεσο> τῇ μὲν θρυαλλίδι τὴν καρδίαν, τῷ δὲ ἐλαίῳ τὸ
αἷμα, τῷ δὲ στεγανῷ τὸν πνεύμονα· περίκειται γὰρ δή τοι ἔξωθεν
τῇ καρδίᾳ δίκην σικύας. ἀλλὰ παρ' ὃν μὲν ἀναπνεῖ τὸ ζῷον
10 χρόνον, εἰκάσαις ἂν αὐτόν, οἶμαι, τετρημένῃ σικύᾳ, κατὰ δὲ τὸν
τῆς ἐπισχέσεως καιρὸν ἀτρήτῳ τε καὶ πανταχόθεν στεγούσῃ.
ὡς οὖν ἡ μὲν τετρημένη σικύα σβεννύειν οὐ δύναται τὴν ἐντὸς
φλόγα διὰ τοῦ τρήματος ἀναπνέουσαν, ἡ δὲ τοὐναντίον <στεγανὴ>
παραχρῆμα σβέννυσιν καταπνίγουσα, τὸν αὐτὸν ὁ πνεύμων τρόπον
15 ὁ μὲν στεγανός, οἷος ὁ κατὰ τὰς ἐπισχέσεις, σβέννυσιν, ὁ τετρη-
μένος δέ, οἷος ὁ κατὰ τὰς ἀναπνοάς, διασῴζει τὴν ἔμφυτον θερμασίαν. ἐγὼ δέ ποτε καὶ κάμινον ἰδὼν σβεννυμένην ὑπὸ τοῦ μὴ

---

10 ἐστὶ καὶ σικύα] fort. εἰσι σικύαι: sunt ventosa N   τὸν Noll: τῶν FM edd.:
τὸν τῶν Cornarius
11 ἀέρα] ἄρα FM: corr. Aldus: post διακεκαυμ. transpos. Cornarius   διακεκαυμένον Noll: διακεκαυμένων FM edd.: acrem combustum N   εἴρξῃ τῆς ...
ὁμιλίας· εἴδομεν οὖν ὡς πάντη Noll (πυρὸς del. ut ex πρὸς iterato corruptum):
εἴρξητί πρὸς τῶν ἔξω πυρὸς τῶν ψυχρῶν ὁμ᾽ εἰδέναι. πάση F: εἴρξητί πρὸς
τὴν ἔξω τοῦ πυρὸς τῶν ψυχρῶν εἰδέναι. πάση M edd. εἴρξῃ (τι del.) Chartier
Kühn: εἴρξῃ (τι del.) Cornarius: pro εἰδέναι coni. ἰέναι Basil. in mg., quod in
text. recep. Chartier Kühn: pro εἰδέναι, πάση coni. ἡ δὲ ἐπὶ πάντων, sed
deinde ἰέναι. πᾶσα δὲ praetul. Cornarius: pro πάση hab. ἡ δὲ Chartier Kühn:
prohibet ab ea quae extra et versus frigidum conversatione. commensuratio
vero in omnibus salus flammae est N
13 φλογός] πάσης φλογός Chartier Kühn
N17
1 εἰς ὕλην FM edd.: εἰς del. Kühn: ἢ τὴν ὕλην Cornarius   γὰρ add. Noll: enim
N

106

among things that make the inward motion excessive are the cupping instrument and everything whatever that prevents the air, overheated by the flame within, from going to meet the cold air outside.[33]

8. So we see that it is always due proportion that keeps flame going. And so it is not unreasonable that it is thus with the warmth in / animals too. For as its matter, whence it is kindled,   N17 it has the blood, and it has by nature a principle of motion in either direction, so that of necessity if the one fails so does the other. And for this same reason, if you cut if off / from breath-   K491 ing or from blood, you will at once destroy it. For you will stop the flame of the lamp also, if you either stifle it or deprive it totally of oil. Consider the heart as the analogue of the wick, the blood of the oil,[34] and the lung of the lamp cover (for it lies around the outside of the heart like a cupping vessel); during the time the animal is breathing you might liken it, I suppose, to a pierced vessel, whereas during the time of stoppage, to one that is closed and shut in on all sides.[35] As, therefore the pierced vessel cannot quench the fire within, because it breathes at the hole, but on the contrary when shut up it quenches it immediately by stifling it, in the same way the lung when closed quenches, as in suspensions of breathing, but when open, and in breathing, maintains the innate heat. I have sometimes seen

---

2 ἔχουσα] -σαν FM Aldus Basil.: corr. Cornarius Chartier στερηθεῖσα] στε-
ρη θ -F: στερηθεὶς M Aldus Basil.: corr. Cornarius Chartier

4 εἴρξης Kühn: ἔξει FM: εἴρξεις edd.   διαφθερεῖς Noll: διαφθείρεται FM edd.:
corrumpes N

5 διαφθερεῖς ἤ Noll: ἅμα ἀφαιρήσει FM: ἅμα ἀφαιρήσεις edd.: corrumpes vel
N

6 ὀργάνῳ τὸν πνεύμονα (cf. v. 8) FM: del. Aldus   ἐλαίῳ FM Aldus Basil.: corr
Chartier   ἀνάλογον οὖν <τίθεσο>/ ἀναλογοῦν⁷ F: ἀναλογοῦν M: corr
Aldus: proportionale igitur pone N

8 αἷμα. τῷ δὲ στεγανῷ Noll coll. p. 14,17: αἱματῶδες, ὀργάνω FM: αἱματῶδες,
τῷ δὲ ὀργάνῳ edd.: sanguinem, organo autem N

9 ἀναπνεῖ] ἀνάπτει⁻¹ᵉⁱ F: ἀνάπτει, πνεῖ M.: corr. Aldus

13 στέγανὴ add. Noll: constricta vero N

16 θερμασίαν F: θερμότητα M edd.

17 ποτε F: om. M edd.   ἰδών] εἰδῶν FM: corr. Aldus: videns N

διαπνεῖσθαι, κἄπειτ' αὐτὴν παρανοιχθεῖσαν <καὶ> πολὺ μὲν αἰθα-
λῶδες ἐκπνεύσασαν, πολὺν δ' ἔξωθεν εἰσπνεύσασαν τὸν ἀέρα
20 καθαρὸν ἐπ' ἀμφοτέροις ἀναλάμψασαν, οὐ μικρὰν οὐδὲ τῆς ἐκ- /
K492 / N18 πνοῆς / ἐλογισάμην εἶναι τὴν χρείαν εἰς τὸ κενοῦν τὴν οἷον
λιγνὺν τοῦ αἵματος· αἴθαλος γὰρ καὶ καπνὸς καὶ λιγνὺς καὶ
πᾶν τὸ τοιοῦτον περίττωμα τῆς καιομένης ὕλης οὐδὲν ἧττον
ὕδατος ἀποσβεννύναι πέφυκε τὸ πῦρ.

                           9. ἐξ ἁπάντων οὖν τούτων
5 ἐστὶν ἀποδέξασθαι τῶν λεγόντων τῆς ἐμφύτου θερμασίας ἕνεκεν
ἀναπνεῖν τὰ ζῷα. καὶ γὰρ τό <τε> ῥιπίζεσθαι συμμέτρως χρήσιμον καὶ τὸ μετρίως ψύχεσθαι (ἄμφω γὰρ ταῦτα φαίνεται ῥων-
νύντα τὴν εἴσω θερμασίαν), κίνησίν <τε> ἀναγκαῖον † ἔχει
κάτω † τὸ καπνῶδες, <ὡς> ἂν εἴποι τις, ἐκκενοῦν τῆς τοῦ
10 αἵματος συγκαύσεως.

        10. ταῦτ' ἐπιστημονικὴν μὲν οὐκ ἔχει τὴν πίστιν οὐδ' ἀναγκαίαν
τὴν ἀπόδειξιν, οἵαν ἐν τοῖς ἄλλοις λόγοις ἀεὶ μεταχειρίζεσθαι
σπεύδομεν, οὐ μὴν ἐστέρηται τοῦ πιθανοῦ. τὸ γὰρ τάχος τῆς
ἀπωλείας τοῦ ζῴου τοιαύτην ἐπιζητεῖ τὴν αἰτίαν, τῆς <μὲν> τροφῆς,
15 ἣν οἱ θρέψεως ἕνεκα ψυχῆς ἀναπνεῖν ἡμᾶς λέγοντες αἰτιῶνται,
χρόνου μακροτέρου δεομένης, τῆς δὲ [τῆς] γενέσεως τῆς ψυχῆς,
K493 <ἣν> Ἀσκληπιάδης φησίν, / ὁμολογουμένης μὲν τῷ τάχει, μαχο-
μένης δὲ ἄλλοις μυρίοις καὶ τοῖς κατ' ἀρχὰς εἰρημένοις ἐν τῷδε
τῷ λόγῳ κοινῇ πρὸς ἁπάσας τὰς αἱρέσεις, ὅσαι δι' ἔνδειαν ἀέρος
20 ἀπόλλυσθαι τὰ ζῷα νομίζουσι στερηθέντα τῆς ἀναπνοῆς. εἰ /
N19 τοίνυν τὸ τάχος τῆς ἀπωλείας τοῦ ζῴου διὰ μὲν ἀτροφίαν τῆς

---

18 sq. αὐτὴν παρανοιχθεῖσαν ... ἐκπνεύσασαν ... εισπνεύσασαν] αὐτὴ ...
    -σα ter FM Aldus Basil.: corr. Cornarius Chartier: accusativos hab. N καὶ add.
    Noll: et N
19 πολὺν Noll: πολὺ FM edd.
20 ἀναλάμψασαν Cornarius: ἀναλάμψαι FM edd. refulgentem N οὐδὲ FM:
    om. N edd. τῆς ἐκπνοῆς] τὴν ἔκτινος FM: corr. Aldus
N18
1 ἐλογισάμην M: ἐλογησάμην F: εὐλογηνσάμην Aldus: εὐλογισάμην Basil.:
    recte Chartier
2 καπνὸς] κάμινος FM: corr. Aldus
4 ἀποσβεννύναι F: ἀποσβέννυσθαι M edd.
6 τε add. Noll: etenim et flabellari N σύμμετρον FM: corr. Aldus
8 κίνησιν ἀναγκαῖον (ἀναγκείαν sic F) ἔχει κάτω τὸ καπνῶδες ἂν εἴποι τις
    ἐκκενοῦν τῆς τοῦ αἵματος συγκαύσεως FM: motumque necessarium est

an oven quenched through lack of draught, and after it has been opened at the side, belching forth black smoke in abundance and drawing in from outside much pure air; and on these two conditions flaming up again; and I have reckoned that // even breathing out must be of no small use, in that it purges K 492 / N18 the smoky vapor, as it were, of the blood.[36] For soot and smoke and murk and every such waste product of the burning material naturally quench fire just as much as water does.

9. From all these things, therefore, it is possible to accept the view that animals breathe for the sake of the innate heat. For both the right amount of fanning and moderate cooling are needed, as they are both seen to strengthen the inner heat, and motion is necessary for emptying out the smokiness, as one might say, from the combustion of the blood.[37]

10. This is not to be received as science, nor is the demonstration a necessary one, such as we always strive to achieve in our other discussions; but it is not devoid of persuasiveness.[38] For the rapidity of the death of the animal requires some such cause; nourishment, the cause given by those who say we breathe to nourish the soul, would require a longer time; while the generation of the soul, which is Asclepiades' view, / is K493 consistent with the speed, but in conflict with very many other facts, particularly with those points raised at the beginning of this treatise against all the schools that think it is from lack of the substance of air that animals die when breathing is stopped. If, / then, the rapidity of the animal's death does not allow its N19

---

habere quod fumosum ut utique dicat quis evacuans de sanguinis adustione
N: τε et ὡς add., ἔχειν vult Aldus: pro κάτω mavult ἔξω Cornarius: pro ἔχει κάτω proposuit ὑπάρχειν κὰν τῷ Mewaldt
12 οἴαν] οἶαν F: οἶον M: corr. Aldus λόγοις FM: sermonibus N: om. edd.
14 μὲν add. Cornarius: quidem N
15 ἦν οἱ] φθίνοιεν F: φθίνοῖ M: corr. Aldus
16 δεομένης Cornarius: ἀεὶ ὁ μὲν εἰς FM: δεῖν edd.: indigente N τῆς δὲ γενέσεως Noll: τῆσδε τῆς γενέσεως FM: γενέσεως δὲ edd.
17 ἦν add. Cornarius: quam N φησὶν FM: φυσιν Aldus: φύσιν Basil.: recte Chartier
N19
1 ἀπωλείας F edd.: ἀπολείας M

ψυχικῆς οὐσίας οὐκ ἐγχωρεῖ γίγνεσθαι, διὰ δὲ τὴν γένεσιν ἐγχωρεῖ
μέν, ἀλλ' ἐπὶ ψευδέσι ταῖς ὑποθέσεσιν, ἡ δὲ τῆς ἐμφύτου θερμασίας ἀπωλεία μηδὲν ἔχει τῶν φαινομένων ἐναντιούμενον, εὐλο-
5 γώτερον ἐκείνων προελέσθαι.

4. Πάλιν τοίνυν αὐτὴν ἀναλαβόντες βασανίσωμεν, ἐπεὶ τῶν
ἄλλων ἀληθεστέρα φαίνεται. οὐκοῦν ἔκ τε τοῦ ῥιπίζεσθαι τὴν
ἀρχὴν τῆς ἐμφύτου θερμασίας κὰκ τοῦ συμμέτρως ἐμψύχεσθαι
κὰκ τοῦ τὸ οἷον καπνῶδες αὐτῆς ἅπαν ἀπορρεῖν ἓν ἠθροίζετο
10 κεφάλαιον, ἡ σωτηρία τῆς κατὰ φύσιν θερμασίας. εἰς ταύτας
οὖν τὰς ἀρχὰς ἴδωμεν εἰ δυνατὸν ἀναγαγεῖν τὰ κατὰ μέρος
ἅπαντα.

K494   **2.** καὶ πρῶτόν γε προχειρισθήτω τὸ κατὰ τὰ / βαλανεῖα
συμβαῖνον, ἐν οἷς ἐπὶ πλέον διατρίψαντες ἐκλυόμεθα, τελευτῶντες
15 δὲ καὶ ἀποθνήσκομεν. εἰ γὰρ διότι θερμὸν ἀναπνέομεν, ἐχρῆν,
φασί, καὶ τοὺς ὑπὲρ λέβητος [θ'] ὕδατος θερμοῦ στάντας, εἶτα
ἀναπνέοντας τὸν ἀναφερόμενον ἀτμὸν ὁμοίως ἀδικεῖσθαι· οὐ μὴν
φαίνεσθαι ἀδικουμένους· ᾧ δῆλον, ὅτι μὴ διὰ τὴν ἀναπνεομένην
θερμασίαν, ἀλλὰ διὰ τὴν ἐξ ὅλου τοῦ σώματος κένωσιν τοῦ
20 πνεύματος ἐν τοῖς βαλανείοις ἐκλυόμεθα. πῶς οὖν καὶ ταύτην
τὴν ἀμφισβήτησιν διαιτῶμεν; ἣν τὸ μὲν συνημμένον ἀληθὲς
εἶναι φήσωμεν, ὡς "δεῖ πνίγεσθαι τοὺς τὸν ἐκ λέβητος ἀτμὸν /
N20   εἰσπνέοντας, εἴπερ ὅλως ἐμψύξεως ἕνεκεν ἀναπνέομεν," οὐ μὴν τήν
γε πρόσληψιν αὐτῶν· "ἀλλὰ μὴν οὐ πνίγονται" πνίγονται γὰρ οὐδὲν
ἧττον <τῶν> ἐν τοῖς βαλανείοις οἱ τὸν ἐκ τῶν λεβήτων ἀτμὸν ἀνα-

---

2 ψυχικῆς FM: ψυχῆς *edd.*: anime N: <τῆς> τῆς ψυχῆς *Wifstrand (Eikota
VIII 42)*

3 ὑποθέσεσιν *Cornarius:* ὑποσχέσεσιν FM *edd.*: suppositionibus N

5 ἐκεινων προελέσθαι *Cornarius:* ἐκείνην προέσθαι FM: ἐκείνου προέσθαι
edd.: illam suscipere N

6 πάλιν *Noll:* πασαν F: πᾶσαν M *edd.*: rursus N   ἐπεὶ] ἐπὶ F

9 τὸ οἷον] τοῖον FM: *corr. Aldus*   ἓν ἠθροίζετο *Noll:* ἐν οἷς ἠθροίζετο FM: ἐν
οἷς ἠθροίζεται *Aldus Basil.*: ἓν ἀθροίζεται *Chartier Kühn:* ἐν συναθροίζεται
Cornarius: unum acervatur N

11 εἰ *edd.*: οὐ F: οὐ *in* εἰ *corr.* M

13 πρῶτον γε F: πρότερον M *edd.*: primum N

14 τελευτῶντες] τελευταῖον *Cornarius*

16 τούς] τοῦ FM *Aldus Basil.: corr. Cornarius Chartier*   θ' *del. Aldus*   στάντας
Kühn: συστάντος FM *Aldus Basil.:* συστάντας *Cornarius Chartier:* stantes N:
ad εἶτα *asynd. cf. Gal. XV 24 K. (I CMG V 9,1 p. 14,28) et 83 K. (ib. 44,16)*

happening through lack of nourishment of the substance of the soul, and does allow its happening on account of generation [of soul], but only on false suppositions, whereas the loss of the innate heat has nothing contrary to the appearance, it is more reasonable to prefer the latter to the two former opinions.

Chapter 4

Now let us take it [this theory] up and examine it again, since it seems nearer to the truth than the others. From the fanning of the source of the innate heat, and from the cooling in due proportion, and from the expulsion of the smoke, so to speak, of that heat, we put together a single item: the preservation of the natural heat. So let us see whether all the particulars can be brought under these principles.

2. First let what happens at / the baths be considered: if we K494 spend too long in the baths we become faint, and at last even die. If it is because we are breathing what is hot, then, they say, those also who stand over a cauldron of hot water and then breathe the rising vapors should likewise suffer; but there is no appearance that they do suffer, whence it is clear that we grow faint in the baths, not from the heat breathed in, but from the loss of pneuma from the whole body. How then are we to decide this disputed matter? By allowing the conditional proposition to be true: "those who breathe the vapor of / cauldrons N20 must stifle, if we breathe only for the sake of cooling," but not their second premiss: "but they do not stifle."[39] For the breathers of vapor from cauldrons stifle no less than those in the

---

21 διαιτῶμεν; ἦν Noll: διαιτωμένην FM: διαλύσομεν; ἦν edd.

22 φήσωμεν, ὡς δεῖ Noll: φήσομεν· ἐν ᾧ δὴ FM: φήσωμεν, ὅτι δεῖ edd.

N20

1 ἀναπνέομεν FM: ἀναπνεύμεν Aldus: ἀναπνεύομεν Basil ἀναπνεύσαιεν Chartier Kühn: respirant N

2 οὐδὲν ἧττον τῶν Chartier Kühn: οὐδὲν ἧττον FM Aldus Basil.: οὐδὲν ἧττον τοῖς Cornarius: οὐθ᾽ οἱ τὸν Noll

3 οἱ edd : ἢ FM: οὐθ᾽ οἱ Noll: suffocantur enim non minus his qui in balneis, qui ex lebetibus ipsum inspirant N τῶν λεβήτων F: τῶν om. M edd.

πνέοντες. εἰ δὲ καὶ μὴ πνιγόμεθα, θαυμαστὸν οὐδέν ἂν ἦν ἴσως·
5 ἡ γὰρ καθ᾽ ὅλον τὸ σῶμα διαπνοὴ κατὰ τὰ βαλανεῖα τῇ διὰ
K495 τοῦ στόματος ὁμοίως βέβλαπται. οὐκ ἔστι δὲ ταὐτὸν τὸ / κατὰ τὸ
στόμα μόνον ἀναπνεῖν τινα κακῶς τῷ καὶ κατὰ τοῦτο καὶ καθ᾽
ὅλον τὸ σῶμα. μεγίστη δ᾽ ἀπόδειξις ἐπὶ πολλῶν ἀρρώστων γίγνεται
δι᾽ ὅλης μὲν ἡμέρας ἱδρούντων κρισίμως πολλῷ μᾶλλον <τῶν> ἐν
10 τοῖς βαλανείοις, οὐ μὴν ἐκλυομένων ὁμοίως ἐκείνοις οὐδὲ πνιγο-
μένων ὅλως, ἔστ᾽ ἂν ἀναπνέωσι τὸν ἔξωθεν ἀέρα τὸν ψυχρόν·
εἰ δὲ καὶ συνείρξας αὐτοὺς ἱματίοις τι θερμὸν ἀναπνεῖν ἀναγκάσαις,
ἀποπνίξαις αὐτίκα. τοὺς μέντοι κατεψυγμένους καὶ ῥιγοῦντας
οὕτω συνείρξας οὐχ ὅπως οὐκ ἀποπνίξεις, ἀλλ᾽ οὐδ᾽ ἀδικήσεις
15 οὐδέν, ἄχρις ἂν ἐκθερμανθέντες τύχωσι· τηνικαῦτα δ᾽ οὐκέθ᾽
ὑπομένουσιν <ὡς μὴ> σύνηθες. ἐξ ὧν ἁπάντων δῆλον, ὡς οὐ διὰ
τὸ κενούμενον ἐξ ὅλου τοῦ σώματος ἐν τοῖς βαλανείοις πνεῦμα
καταλυόμεθά τε καὶ τελευτῶμεν τὸν βίον, ἀλλὰ διὰ τὴν θερμασίαν. θαυμάσαι δὲ ἔστιν οὐ τῶν ἄλλων τοσοῦτον <ὅσον> Ἐρα-
20 σιστράτου τῶν τοιούτων φαινομένων ἀποτολμῶντος κατα- /
N21 ψεύσασθαι, ὃν οὐκ εἰκὸς ἄπειρον εἶναι τῆς διὰ τοῦ πίθου πυρίας
τῶν ὑδερικῶν, εὐδοκιμησάσης οὐχ ἥκιστα τῶν ἄλλων παλαιῶν
K496 παρὰ Χρυσίππῳ τῷ Κνιδίῳ. / κενοῦνται γὰρ οὗτοι τὸ πᾶν σῶμα
πολὺ θᾶττόν τε καὶ μᾶλλον ἢ ἐν τοῖς βαλανείοις, οὐ μὴν πνί-
5 γονται δὲ διὰ τὸ ψυχρὸν εἰσπνεῖν ἀέρα. τούτου δ᾽ εἴ τις αὐτοὺς
στερήσειεν, ἀποθνήσκουσιν ἐν τάχει.

3. πῶς οὖν, φασίν, ἔν τε τοῖς Χαρωνίοις βαράθροις καὶ τοῖς
νεωστὶ κεχρισμένοις οἴκοις τιτάνῳ καὶ πρὸς τῆς τῶν ἐσβεσμένων
ἀνθράκων ὀσμῆς πνιγόμεθα; κατὰ μὲν τὸν Ἐρασίστρατον,

---

4 οὐδὲν ἂν ἦν ἴσως M edd. ἂν ἦν ἴσως del. Noll: ἂν ἴσως οὐδὲν ἂν ἦν F:
mirabile nullum esset N
5 κατὰ] καὶ FM: corr. Aldus
6 στόματος] σώματος FM: corr. corrector Parisini Suppl. 35 et Aldus βέβλαπ-
ται] βέβληνται FM: corr. Aldus τὸ στόμα] τὸ om. F
7 καὶ κατὰ F: καὶ om. M. edd.
9 τῶν add. Noll: τοῖς add. Cornarius: ἢ add. Kühn
12 αὐτοὺς] αὐτοῖς FM: corr. Aldus
14 οὐκ ἀποπνίξῃ FM edd.: pro οὐκ vult ἂν Cornarius: οὐκ ἀποπνίξεις Noll:
nedum non suffocabis N
16 ὡς μὴ add. Aldus: ut non consuetum N
19 ὅσον add. Noll Ἐρασιστράτου Noll: Ἐρασίστρατ F: Ἐρασίστρατον M
edd.: tantum ut de Erasistrato N

baths. But even if we do not stifle, there would perhaps be nothing surprising in that. For at the baths the breathing throughout the whole body has been affected in the same way as the breathing by the mouth; that someone breathes badly / by the mouth only, however, is not the same as breathing badly K495 both by the mouth and throughout the whole body.[40] But the greatest proof comes from many sick people who sweat acutely through a whole day, much more than those at the baths, and yet do not faint as the latter do, nor stifle at all, so long as they breathe the cool air from outside; but if by confining them with clothes you compel them to breathe something hot, you will stifle them at once.[41] However, if you confine in the same way those who are chilled through and shivering, you will not only not stifle them, you will not even do them any hurt, until it comes about that they are warmed through and through; but then they no longer endure it, as not being normal. From all of which it is clear that it is not through the loss of pneuma from the whole body in the baths that we become faint or even lose our lives, but through the heat. The others are not to be wondered at so much as Erasistratus, who dared to fly in the face of / such appearances, though he could hardly be in ignorance of N21 the vapor-baths in a wine-cask, for the dropsical, made famous not least among the ancients by Chrysippus of Cnidos.[42] / For K496 these patients have their whole body emptied much more rapidly and completely than in the baths, yet they do not stifle, because they breathe cold air. If anyone deprives them of this, then they quickly die.

3. How, then, they say, are we stifled in Charonion pits,[43] and in newly whitewashed houses, and from the smell of quenched coal? According to Erasistratus,[44] because the air,

---

20 ἀποτολμῶντος Noll: coll. Εἰ κατὰ φύσιν ἐν αρτηρίαις p. 16,12 Albr. et saep.: κατατολμῶντα FM edd.: [κατα]τολῶντα Rob. Fuchs Philolog. LVI (1897), 375
N21

1 ἄπειρον] πειρατὸν FM: corr. Aldus

2 τῶν ὑδερικῶν edd. et e corr. F: τὸν ὑδερικόν M et ante corr. F

5 δὲ διὰ τὸ Cornarius: δὲ διὰ τὸ FM: δὲ διὰ τὸν edd.: γε διὰ τὸ Kühn εἴ Mewaldt: ἄν FM edd.

7 Χαρωνίοις Noll: βαρωνίοις F: βαροδμείοις M edd.: βαρυόδμοις Kühn: in charoniis · s · letabilibus cavernis N

10 ὅτι λεπτὸς ὢν ἐν ταῖς τοιαύταις καταστάσεσιν ὁ ἀὴρ οὐ στέγεται
πρὸς τῶν ἀρτηριῶν, ἀλλ' ἐκκενοῦται ῥαδίως, καὶ ἐνδείᾳ πνεύματος
ἀπόλλυται τὸ ζῷον. ἡμεῖς δέ φαμεν, ὡς οὐδὲν ἐξετέλεσεν Ἐρασίστρατος, οὐ δείξας ἢ λεπτὸν ἐν τοῖς τοιούτοις τὸν ἀέρα
γιγνόμενον ἢ μὴ στεγόμενον τοῖς ζῴων σώμασιν ἢ μὴ τῆς ἀλη-
15 θοῦς αἰτίας ἑτέρας οὔσης ἢ χαλεπῆς ὑπαρχούσης εὑρεθῆναι.
μακρότερα μὲν οὖν ἀναγκαζόμεθα λέγειν πρὸς τὰ † μακρω * * †,
χρὴ δέ, ὅσον οἷόν τε, πειρᾶσθαι συντεμεῖν αὐτὰ συντομώτερον.
ἄλλο δ' οὐδὲν ἔχω φάναι, τὰς πολλὰς ἀντιλογίας περικόψας, ἢ
K497 τὸ φαίνεσθαι τὰς κινήσεις τῶν ἀρτηριῶν / ἐν ταῖς τοιαύταις
20 διαθέσεσι μηδὲν ἀπολειπομένας μεγέθει τε καὶ χρόνῳ τῶν ἔμ- /
N22 προσθεν, ὡς ἂν πλήρεις οὔσας δηλονότι τοῦ δι' αὐτῶν φερομένου
πνεύματος. ἐχρῆν δ' αὐτὰς μηδ' ὅτι θᾶττον ἢ μικρότερον φαίνεσθαι [τε] σφυζομένας, ἀλλ' ἀσφύκτους γίνεσθαι παντάπασιν, ὡς
ἂν ἐστερημένας τελέως τοῦ πληροῦντος αὐτῶν τὰς κοιλίας ἀέρος.
5 4. ἀλλ' εἰ τὴν Ἐρασιστράτου, φασίν, διαβάλλεις αἰτίαν,
ἑτέραν εἰπέ.

<ἐρῶ δή>, ἐὰν πρότερον ὑμεῖς εἴπητέ μοι, διὰ ποίαν
αἰτίαν θαλαττίου ζῴου νάρκης ἀψάμενοι ναρκῶμεν. εἰ δὲ
οὐδὲν λέγειν ἔχετε, τοσοῦτον ἴσως ἡμῖν εἰπεῖν συγχωρήσετε τὸ
τὴν δύναμιν εἶναι τοῦ ζῴου ναρκωτικὴν τῶν ἀψαμένων οὕτως
10 ἰσχυράν, ὥστε καὶ διὰ τοῦ πεπηγότος <ἐν> αὐτῷ τριόδοντος εἰς
τὰς χεῖρας τῶν ἁλιέων ῥαδίως ἀνατρέχειν τὸ πάθος. οὐκοῦν

---

12 ὡς post ἐξετέλεσεν hab. FM et edd.: huc transpos. Noll: ὅτι huc edd.   Ἐρασίστρατος οὐ δείξας Noll: Ἐρασιστράτου δείξαντος FM edd.: οὐ interponi
voluit iam Cornarius: quod nihil profecit quemadmodum Erasistrato non pre-
monstrante N
13 τοιούτοις M edd.: τοιούτης F
14 ἢ μὴ στεγόμενον] εἰ μὴ στ. Cornarius
15 χαλεπῆς M edd.: χαλεπούς F
16 μακρω cum spat. 5 litt. FM: εἰρημένα (om. μακρῶ) edd.: longe dicat N: longe
om. Veneta a. 1490: fort. μακρολογούμενα sive μακρηγορούμενα
17 συντεμεῖν Noll: οὖν τεμεῖν F: τεμεῖν M edd.: incidere N
18 ἄλλο Furley: εἰ FM edd.   ἔχω] ἔχων F   περικόψας, ἢ τὸ Furley: περικόψας
τοῦ FM edd.:   περικόψω <ἀρχόμενος ἀπὸ> τοῦ sugg. Noll: abscidam in
apparendo N
N22
1 ὡς ἂν τὸ μὲν, deinde spat. 3 vel 4 litt., tum ἦν FM: ὡς ἂν πλῆρας (sic) οὔσας
Aldus Basil.: πλήρας in πλήρει (sic) mut. Chartier: in πλήρεις Cornarius
Kühn: ut utique plenas entes N: fort. πεπληρωμένας legendum

being thin under those conditions, is not contained by the arteries but is easily emptied out, and the animals die for want of pneuma. But we say that Erasistratus has accomplished nothing, because he has not proved either that the air becomes thin in such conditions, or that it is not contained by the bodies of animals, or that the true cause is not different or hard to discover.[45] Now, we are forced to speak at greater length in answer to longer disquisitions, but we must try to be as brief as may be. Having cut out the many counterarguments, I have nothing else to say except that the motions of the arteries / in these condi- K497 tions are seen to be deficient neither in magnitude nor in time compared with what they were / before, clearly as though they N22 were full of the pneuma coursing through them. But they should not only appear with either more rapid or smaller pulse, but become altogether pulseless, as being totally deprived of air to fill their cavities.

4. "But," they say, "if you find fault with Erasistratus' explanation, tell us another."

I reply: "If you will first tell me how it is to be explained that we are numbed when we touch the sea-animal, the numbing fish.[46] If you are unable to say anything, perhaps you will agree to my saying so much, that the numbing power of the animal upon those that touch it is so strong that the effect easily passes right through the fisherman's trident implanted in the fish into

---

2 μηδ' ὅτι FM: μὴ ὅτι edd.

3 τε del. Aldus σφυζομένης FM Aldus: corr. Cornarius Basil. ὡς ἂν FM: ἂν om. edd.

4 ἀέρος] ἀνέμου FM: corr. Aldus

6 ἑτέραν om. a Basil. edd. ἐρῶ δὴ add. Mewaldt: λέξω δὲ add. Aldus: dicam
autem eam N ὑμεῖς] ὑμεῖς F εἴποιτέ FM edd.: corr. Kühn

7 θαλαττίου ζώου ... ναρκῶμεν Furley: θαλάττιοι (θ. οἱ F) ζωγρεῖς νάρκης ἀψάμενοι ναρκῶσι (ναρκῶμα ut vid. F) FM edd.: torpiginem marinum animal (i.e. θαλαττίου ζώου) tangentes torpemus (i.e. ναρκώμεν) N· θαλαττίας νάρκης ἀψάμενοι ναρκῶμεν Noll

8 τοσοῦτον ἴσως Noll: τούτων ἴσως FM; τοῦτο ὅμως edd.

9 τοῦ ζώου M edd.: τὸ ζῷον F

10 <ἐν> αὐτῷ Noll: αὐτοῦ FM edd.: ei N

συγχωρήσετε εἶναί τινας μὲν ποιότητας καὶ δυνάμεις, <ὧν> ἡ μὲν νάρκην, ἡ δὲ κάρον, ἡ δὲ ψύξιν, ἡ δὲ σῆψιν, αἱ δὲ ἄλλο τι φέρουσι κακόν, ἀέρος δὲ οὐδεμίαν συγχωρήσετε εἶναι τοιαύτην

K498 / 15 δύναμιν;

   ἀλλ᾽ οὐκ / ἔχομεν, φασίν, ἐναργῶς δεῖξαι, τίς ἡ ποιότης αὕτη καὶ τίς ἡ δύναμις αὕτη.

   τί οὖν τοῦτο πρὸς τὰ παρόντα; διὰ γὰρ τῶν ἀδήλων οὔτε ἀνατρέπεσθαί τι δίκαιον οὔτε κατασκευάσασθαι. /

N23   5. μεταβαίνωμεν οὖν ἀπὸ τῶν τοιούτων ἐπὶ τὸ κατασκευάζειν ἐναργῶς, ὁποτερανοῦν τῶν αἱρέσεων ἀνατρέπειν δυνάμεθα. τὰ μὲν οὖν ἐξ ἀνάγκης ἀνατρέποντα τὴν Ἐρασιστράτου δόξαν εὐθὺς κατ᾽ ἀρχὰς ἡμῖν ἐρρήθη, τὰ δὲ τὴν ἡμετέραν κατασκευά-

5 ζοντα τοιαῦτα μὲν οὖν οὐχ εὕρομεν ὡς ἐξ ἀνάγκης περαίνειν, ἁπάντων μέντοι τῶν ἄλλων πιθανώτατα πρὸς τῷ μηδ᾽ ἀνατρέπεσθαι πρός τινος τῶν φαινομένων ταύτην τὴν δόξαν. ὥστε τὴν μὲν Ἐρασιστράτου περὶ χρείας ἀναπνοῆς ὑπόληψιν ἤδη καταλιπεῖν δίκαιον, ἐπειδὴ κἂν τοῖς Περὶ σφυγμῶν λόγοις ἐξελέγχεται

10 πολυειδῶς σφαλλομένη, αὐτοὺς δὲ διὰ βραχέων ἐπιδραμεῖν τῶν ἄλλων φαινομένων τὰς αἰτίας εἰς τὴν προκειμένην ἀναφέροντας ὑπόθεσιν· ὥσπερ κατά γε τὴν γυμνασίαν μεῖζόν τε καὶ πυκνότερον ἡμᾶς ἀναπνεῖν· οὐ γὰρ ἀπεικὸς οὐδὲ τοῦτο γίνεσθαι διὰ τὴν ἐν

K499   τοῖς σφοδρῶς κινουμένοις / αὐξανομένην θερμασίαν· ὅτι γὰρ οὐδ᾽

15 ἐνταῦθα διὰ τὴν τῶν ἀρτηριῶν ἐπιπλήρωσιν, ἐναργές ἐστιν ἐκ τοῦ κινεῖσθαι μὲν ἐξ ἀρχῆς εὐθὺς πολλάκις σφοδρῶς, οὐ μὴν ἀλλοιοῦσθαι τὴν ἀναπνοήν, πρὶν ἱκανῶς θερμανθῆναι, ἐκθερμανθέντων δέ, κἂν παυσώμεθα κινούμενοι,

---

12 συγχωρήσεις FM: corr. Aldus   μὲν Furley: ἀέρων F: ἀέρος M: ἰχθύων edd.: del. Noll: piscium quidem concedetis esse quasdam qualitates N   ἡ μὲν FM: <ὧν> αἱ μὲν Aldus: <ὧν> ἡ μὲν Noll

14 φέρουσαι FM: φέρουσι Aldus: quarum hec quidem ... hec vero (quater) ... infert N   συγχωρήσομεν FM: corr. Aldus

15 φασίν] φάναι FM: corr. Aldus

17 ἀδήλων] ἀλλήλων FM: corr. Aldus

N23

1 μεταβαίνομεν FM Aldus Basil.: corr. Chartier   Ἐρασιστράτειον MP

4 ἡμετέραν] ἑτέραν FM: corr. Aldus: nostram N

5 ante τοιαῦτα hab. spat. 6 litt. F: nullum spat. M   post οὖν add. ὡς edd.   περαίνειν] παραινεῖν FM: παραίνειν Aldus Basil.: corr. Cornarius Chartier

116

his hands. Now, will you agree that there are certain qualities and powers, of which one brings numbness, another torpor, another chilling, another putrefaction, and others some other ill, and will you nevertheless deny that there is any such power in air?"

They answer: / "We cannot clearly show what this quality K498 and this power are."

Well, what is this to the present case? It is wrong to argue for or against anything from things that are unclear.[47] /

5. Let us pass on, then, from such things, to show clearly N23 which of the two schools we are able to refute.[48] Well, what necessarily refutes the opinion of Erasistratus was set down by us right at the beginning;[49] but as to what establishes our own opinion, we have not found such [arguments] as prove it by necessity, but only what is more persuasive than all the others, in addition to the fact that this opinion is not refuted by any of the phenomena. So it is proper now to leave Erasistratus' theory about the use of breathing, since it is shown to be erroneous in many ways also in my work *On Pulse*,[50] and for our own part to run over briefly the causes of other phenomena, relating them to our present thesis. For example, that we breathe more deeply and more frequently when at exercise. For it is not unreasonable that this should happen, because of / the increased heat in K499 those who move vigorously.[51] That here too the reason is not the filling of the arteries[52] is clear from the fact that often the movement is vigorous[53] right from the beginning, though the breathing is not changed until there is sufficient warming up, whereas when we are warmed thoroughly, even though we

---

6 πιθανώτατον FM *edd.:* πιθανώτατα *Cornarius:* probabilissima N   πρὸς τῷ
   Furley: προς τὸ FM *edd.:* cum hoc quod N (*i.e.* πρὸς τῷ)   ἀνατρέπεσθαι M
   edd.: ἀντιτρέπεσθαι F
11 τὸ προκείμενον FM: *corr. Aldus*
12 γυμνασίαν] ἀσίαν FM: *corr. Aldus*
13 ἐν *om. Chartier Kühn*
15 ἐκ] οὐ FM: *corr. Aldus*
16 κινεῖσθαι *Furley:* γίγνεσθαι FM *edd.*   σφοδροὺς FM: σφοδρῶς *edd.:* fortiter
   N   *post* σφοδρῶς, τοὺς σφυγμούς *add. Noll*
18 κἂν *Aldus:* καὶ FM   παυσώμεθα *Mewaldt:* ἐπαυσάμεθα FM *edd.*

μέχρι πολλοῦ διασῳζομένην ὁρᾶσθαι τὴν αὐτὴν ἰδέαν τῆς ἀνα-
20 πνοῆς. ἀλλὰ κἂν τοῖς καυσώδεσι πυρετοῖς ὁμοίως ἀναπνεῖν ὀρεγόμεθα διὰ τὴν αὐτὴν αἰτίαν· ὅπου γὰρ ἂν ᾖ μέγιστον τὸ τῆς
χρείας δεόμενον, ἐνταῦθα εἰκὸς αὐξάνεσθαι καὶ τὴν χρείαν αὐτήν· /
N24 ἡ μὲν γὰρ μείζων φλὸξ μείζονος ἀέρος, ἡ δὲ ἐλάττων ἐλάττονος
δεῖται· πᾶσα δ' οὖν δεῖται δι' ἣν ἔμπροσθεν εἴπομεν ἀνάγκην.
οὔκουν ἐστὶ θαυμαστόν, εἰ κατεψυγμένοι τὰ περὶ τὴν καρδίαν
καὶ τὸν πνεύμονα τὸν ἔξωθεν ἀέρα ποθοῦσί τε καὶ δέονται διὰ
5 τῆς εἰσπνοῆς ἐπισπᾶσθαι. ἐπισπῶνται μὲν γάρ, ἀλλ' ὀλίγον καὶ
διὰ πολλοῦ· μεγάλως γὰρ καὶ πυκνῶς οὐκ ἐγχωρεῖ ῥιπίζειν τὴν
βραχεῖαν θερμασίαν.
K500 6. διὰ τί τοίνυν οἱ μὲν παῖδες πλεῖόν τε καὶ / πυκνότερον,
οἱ δ' ἀκμάζοντες ἔλαττόν τε καὶ ἀραιότερον ἀναπνέουσιν; ἤ, ὅτι
10 "τὰ αὐξανόμενα πλεῖστον ἔχει τὸ ἔμφυτον θερμόν," ἕπεται ἐξ
ἀνάγκης πλήθει θερμασίας μέγεθός τε καὶ πυκνότης ἀναπνοῆς;
εἰ δὲ καὶ τρέφεται τὸ ψυχικὸν πνεῦμα πρὸς τῆς ἀναπνοῆς, καὶ
διὰ τοῦτ' ἀναπνέουσι πλεῖστόν τε καὶ πυκνότατον οἱ παῖδες, ὅτι
καὶ τροφῆς πλείονος ὡς ἂν αὐξανόμενοι δέονται. εἰ δὲ τὸ λιγνυῶδες
15 ἀποχεῖται πλεῖστον ἐν ταῖς ἐκπνοαῖς, καὶ διὰ τοῦτο ἀναπνέουσι
πλεῖστόν τε καὶ πυκνότατον· ἔνθα γὰρ ἡ τῆς τροφῆς ἐργασία
πλείων, ἐκεῖ καὶ τὸ περίττωμα πλέον. <οἷς μὲν οὖν οἱ παῖδες
θερμότεροι τῶν νεανίσκων εἶναι δοκοῦσιν, οὗτοι τοιαύτην ἐροῦσι
τὴν αἰτίαν> τοῦ τοὺς παῖδας <οὕτως> ἀναπνεῖν· οἷς δ' οἱ
20 νεανίσκοι θερμότεροι τῶν παίδων εἶναι δοκοῦσιν, οὗτοι τὴν μὲν
προειρημένην αἰτίαν οὐ προσοίσονται. περὶ μέντοι τῶν γερόντων
οὐδεὶς ἀμφισβητεῖ τὸ μὴ οὐκ εἶναι πολὺ ψυχροτέρους αὐτοὺς τῶν /

---

19 διασῳζόμενοι FM *Aldus Basil.: corr. Cornarius Chartier* ἰδέαν F *et a Basil.
edd.:* ἰδίως M: ἰδίαν *Aldus*
21 ὅπου γὰρ ἂν ἦν *edd.* (ἦν *in* ᾖ *corr. Kühn):* ὅπερ ἂν ἦν FM
22 εἰκὸς *Noll:* ἱκανῶς FM: <οὐκ ἀπεικὸς> ἱκανῶς *edd.:* decens est N
N24
2 δ' οὖν *Noll:* δ' οὐ FM: οὖν *edd.*
3 ἐστὶ *Noll:* ἔτι FM *edd.:* est mirabile N κατεψυγμένον FM *Aldus Basil.:*
-μένα *Cornarius, corr. Chartier* τὰ] τὸ M
5 ἐπισπῶνται F: ἐπισπᾶται M *edd.:* attrahunt N καὶ διὰ πολλοῦ *Noll coll. p.*
23,19: ἐρκεαία (*sic*) πολλ⁻ FM: καὶ διὰ καιροῦ πολλοῦ *edd.:* et per multum
tempus attrahunt non multum N
10 ἔχει τὸ ἔμφυτον M *edd.:* τὸ ἔμφυτον ἔχει F
12 τρέφεται FM *edd.:* θρέψεται *Cornarius: corr. Kühn*

cease moving, the same pattern of breathing is seen to be preserved for a long time. In burning fevers too we desire to breathe similarly, for the same reason; for wherever there is the greatest lack of the use, there it is reasonable that the use itself should be increased. / For the greater flame requires more air, N24 and the lesser flame less—though every flame requires it, because of the necessity we have described before;[54] so there is nothing surprising if when chilled in the regions round the heart and the lung they desire the outside air and need to draw it in through breathing. For they do draw it in, but only a little in a long time, as it is not permissible to fan their diminished heat either greatly or frequently.

6. Now, why is it that children breathe much and / rapidly, K500 while those of full growth breathe both less and less quickly? Unless it is that, since "growing things have innate heat in abundance,"[55] abundance and rapidity of breathing follow of necessity upon abundance of heat? And if the psychic pneuma draws nourishment from the breathing,[56] on this account also children breathe most deeply and most often, because, as growing things, they need more nourishment. Then, if most smoky stuff is shed in breathing out, for this reason also they breathe most and most rapidly. For the more nourishment is worked up, the greater is the surplus.[57] Now, those who think children to be warmer than young people will offer such an explanation of children's breathing in this way; those, however, to whom young people appear warmer than children will not proffer the explanation just mentioned. On the other hand, regarding the old, no one will wish to say otherwise than that they are much

---

13 ὅτι Cornarius: ἔτι FM edd.: ἐπεὶ Kühn

15 ἐκπνοαῖς Noll: ἀναπνοαῖς FM edd.: in expirationibus N   διὰ ταῦτα FM: corr. Aldus

17 πλείων M edd.: πλεῖον F

18 οἷς μὲν ... αἰτίαν om. FM edd.: add. Cornarius: quibus igitur infantes calidiores iuvenibus esse videntur, hii talem causem dicent infantes ita respirandi N

19 τοῦ τοὺς παῖδας ἀναπνεῖν FM: om. edd.: οὕτως ex N add. Noll: τῆς αὐτῶν πυκνοτέρας ἀναπνοῆς Cornarius

N25 παίδων καὶ νεανίσκων· ὁμολογεῖ δὲ τῇ ψύξει καὶ ἡ τῆς ἀναπνοῆς ἰδέα μικροτέρα τε ἅμα καὶ ἀραιοτέρα γιγνομένη.

7. παραπλήσια δὲ τοῖς ἐπὶ τῶν ἡλικιῶν φαινομένοις

K501 κἂν ὥραις καὶ χώραις καὶ φύσεσι συμ/βέβηκε·

5 καὶ ὁμολογεῖ γὰρ ἀεὶ τοῖς μὲν θερμοῖς ἡ μείζων τε καὶ πυκνοτέρα, τοῖς δὲ ψυχροῖς ἡ ἐλάττων τε καὶ ἀραιοτέρα. μικρόν τε καὶ πυκνὸν ἀναπνέουσιν οἵ τε ἐδηδοκότες καὶ οἱ πεπωκότες στενοχωρίᾳ τοῦ διαφράγματος, οὕτω δὲ καὶ αἱ κυοῦσαι· κἂν τοῖς ὑδέροις τε καὶ ταῖς φλεγμοναῖς τοῦ ἥπατος καὶ τῆς γαστρὸς καὶ

10 τοῦ σπληνὸς ὁμοίως ἀναπνέουσι διὰ τὴν αὐτὴν αἰτίαν. ἀλλὰ περὶ μὲν τῆς οἰκείας <τούτων> ἀναπνοῆς ἐν τοῖς Περὶ δυσπνοίας εἰρήσεται. νῦν δὲ ἀρκεῖ καὶ ταῦτα αὖθις <εἰς> ἔνδειξιν τοῦ πάνθ' ὁμολογεῖν τὰ φαινόμενα τῷ προειρημένῳ δόγματι περὶ χρείας ἀναπνοῆς.

15 **5.** Ἴδωμεν δ' ἐφεξῆς, εἰ δύναται τρέφεσθαι τὸ ψυχικὸν πνεῦμα πρὸς τῆς ἀναπνοῆς. εἴπωμεν δὲ πρότερον, πῶς καλοῦμέν τι ψυχικὸν πνεῦμα, ἀγνοεῖν ὁμολογοῦντες οὐσίαν ψυχῆς. ἐπεὶ τοίνυν αἱ κατὰ τὸν ἐγκέφαλον κοιλίαι <στερηθεῖσαι> τοῦ πνεύματος, ἐπειδὰν τρωθῇ, εὐθὺς ἀκινήτους τε καὶ ἀναισθητοῦντας ἐργάζονται, χρὴ

K502 / 20 τοῦτο τὸ πνεῦμα / πάντως ἤτοι τὴν οὐσίαν αὐτὴν εἶναι τῆς ψυχῆς ἢ τὸ πρῶτόν γε αὐτῆς ὄργανον. εἴρηται δὲ ἑτέρωθι περὶ αὐτοῦ διὰ πλειόνων ἀκριβέστερον, ἐν οἷς καὶ τοῦτ' εὐθὺς εὕρηται δῆλον /

N26 ὡς ἀναγκαῖόν ἐστι τοῦτο τὸ πνεῦμα τρέφεσθαι. πόθεν οὖν ἄλλοθεν ἕξει τὴν τροφήν, εἰ μὴ παρὰ τοῦ διὰ τῆς εἰσπνοῆς ἑλκομένου; καίτοι κἀκ τῆς τοῦ αἵματος ἀναθυμιάσεως οὐκ ἀπεικὸς αὐτὸ τρέφεσθαι, καθάπερ καὶ πολλοῖς τῶν ἐλλογίμων ἰατρῶν τε καὶ

N25

3 ταῖς ... φαινομέναις FM *edd.:* τοῖς ... φαινομένοις *Kühn*

4 κἂν] ἐν FM

11 τούτων *add. Aldus:* de propria his respiratione N

12 ταῦτα] τοῦτο *Cornarius* <εἰς> ἔνδειξιν τοῦ *Noll:* ἐνδείξειν τὸ FM *edd.*

16 πρὸς] πρ° *(i.e. πρὸς)* F: πρὸ M: *recte ab Aldo edd.*

18 < > *Furley*

19 *post* ἀναισθητοῦντας *add.* ἡμᾶς *ab Aldo edd.*

20 τῆς οὐσίας αὐτῆς FM: *corr. Aldus*

21 ἑτέρωθεν FM *Aldus Basil.: corr. Chartier* αὐτοῦ *Noll:* αὐτῶν FM *edd.:* de eo N

colder than / children or young people, and the form of breath- N25
ing in them suits their coldness by becoming both less and
sparser.

7. Similar to these phenomena which depend on various ages
are the accompaniments of seasons, places, and / characters; for K501
the greater and more frequent breathing corresponds always
with hot conditions, lesser and less frequent with cold. Both
those who have eaten and those who have drunk breathe little
and fast, because of the constrained condition of the diaphragm,
and so too, pregnant women; and those who suffer from water
or phlegm in the liver or in the stomach or in the spleen
breathe similarly, from the same cause. But the peculiar breathing of these will be treated of in the tract on *Difficulty in Breathing*.[58] For the present, this will suffice to show again how all the
appearances are agreeable to the doctrine already stated about
the use of breathing.

Chapter 5

Let us consider next whether it is possible for the psychic
pneuma to draw sustenance from the breathing. Let us first say
how we give something the name "psychic pneuma," ignorant
as we confessedly are of the substance of the soul.[59] Since the
emptying of the pneuma from the hollows in the brain, when it
is wounded,[60] at once makes men both motionless and without
feeling, it must surely be that this pneuma / is either the very K502
substance of the soul or its primary organ. This has been treated
of elsewhere[61] at more length and more exactly, and there it
was immediately found clear / that this pneuma must of neces- N26
sity be nourished. From what other source, therefore, will it get
nourishment unless from that which is drawn in while breathing
in? But it is not improbable that it may be nourished also from
the vapor rising from the blood, as has seemed true to many

---

22 εἴρηται δῆλον ὡς οὐκ FM: οὐκ *postea del.* F: δῆλον *et* οὐκ *del Aldus:* dictum
   est quoniam necessarium est N: εἴρηται δῆλον <ὄν> *placet Mewaldtio,*
   εὕρηται δῆλον Noll (*coll. p. 29,8 sq.* ἐδείχθη γὰρ ἀδύνατος)
N26
   1 φασιν *ante* ἄλλοθεν *add. edd.: del.* Mewaldt: aiunt aliunde N, *fort. per ditto-
   graphium* (aliunt aliunde p)

5 φιλοσόφων ἔδοξεν. ἀλλ' οὐδ' ἐκ τῆς εἰσπνοῆς ὁμοίως οἱ περὶ τὸν
Ἐρασίστρατον τοῖς <περὶ τὸν> Ἱπποκράτην τρέφεσθαί φασι
τὸ ψυχικὸν πνεῦμα· τοῖς μὲν γὰρ ἐκ τῆς καρδίας διὰ τῶν ἀρτηριῶν ἐπὶ τὰς μήνιγγας, τοῖς δὲ εὐθὺς διὰ τῶν ῥινῶν εἰς τὰς
κατὰ τὸν ἐγκέφαλον κοιλίας ἔρχεσθαι τὸ πνεῦμα δοκεῖ.

10 2. τὴν μὲν οὖν Ἐρασιστράτου περὶ τούτων δόξαν κἀνταῦθα καταλίπωμεν, ἐξελεγχομένην πολυειδῶς <ἐν τοῖς> Περὶ
τῶν ἐν σφυγμοῖς αἰτίων. ἐπὶ <δὲ> τὴν ἀληθῆ μεταβάντες τὴν
καὶ ταῖς ἀρτηρίαις αἵματος μεταδιδοῦσαν ἐπισκεψώμεθα τουτὶ
τὸ φαινόμενον, οὗ πολλάκις ἐπειράθημεν. ἐν γὰρ τῷ βρόχοις
K503 / 15 διαλαμ/βάνεσθαι τὰς κατὰ τὸν τράχηλον ἀρτηρίας οὐδὲν πάσχει
τὸ ζῷον οὔτ' εὐθὺς οὔθ' ὕστερον, ὡς ἡμεῖς ἐνίοτε πειρώμενοι ἐν
βρόχοις αὐτὰς διελαμβάνομεν. ὅλην δὲ ἡμέραν τὸ ζῷον εἰσπνέον
τε καὶ ἐκπνέον καὶ κινούμενον ἀκωλύτως ἰδόντες νυκτὸς ἤδη
βαθείας ἐσφάξαμεν, οὐκέθ' ἡγούμενοι τὴν ἐπὶ πλέον πεῖραν
20 πιστὴν ὑπάρχειν· δύνασθαι γὰρ ἐν τοσούτῳ χρόνῳ διὰ τοὺς περι- /
N27 κειμένους βρόχους συμπαθῆσαί τι τῶν κυριωτάτων μορίων. ἐθαυ-
μάζομεν οὖν τὰς ἐκ τοῦ κυριωτάτου τῶν ζωτικῶν ὀργάνων, [τῶν]
τῆς καρδίας, εἰς τὸ κυριώτατον τῶν ψυχικῶν, τὸν ἐγκέφαλον,
τεταμένας ἀρτηρίας οὕτως ἄλυπον τῷ παντὶ βίῳ τὴν βλάβην
5 ἐχούσας εὑρίσκοντες. ἀλλὰ περὶ μὲν τούτων κἀν τῷ Περὶ χρείας
σφυγμῶν ἐπὶ πλέον ζητήσομεν· ὅπερ δ' ἐξ αὐτῶν ἐστιν εἰς τὰ
παρόντα χρήσιμον, οὗ χάριν ἐμνημόνευσα τῶν καρωτίδων ἀρτηριῶν, τοῦτ' αὖθις λεγέσθω, τὸ μὴ πάνυ τι δεῖσθαι τοῦ παρὰ
τῆς καρδίας πνεύματος τὸν ἐγκέφαλον. ἀπολείπεται γοῦν ἤτοι
K504 / 10 τὴν ἀναθυμίασιν / αὐτῷ τὴν ἐκ τοῦ αἵματος ἱκανὴν ὑπάρχειν
<ἢ τὴν> διὰ τῶν ῥινῶν εἰσπνοήν. ἀλλ' οὐδὲ τὴν ἀναθυμίασιν

5 οὐδ' ἐκ] οὐδεὶς ἐκ FM: corr. Aldus
6 τοῖς <περὶ τὸν> Aldus: καὶ FM: hiis qui ab N
7 τοῖς μὲν edd.: τοὺς μὲν FM
8 ἐπὶ τὰς Chartier: ἐπὶ τοὺς FM Aldus Basil.
10 οὖν F: om. M edd.
11 ἐν τοῖς add. Noll: in libro N
12 δὲ add. Aldus   τὴν ... μεταδιδοῦσαν FM edd. (αἵματος FM: αἷμα edd.):
om. N: del. Cornarius
16 ὡς ὑμῶν ἔνιοι περὶ μὲν οὖν τὴν ἐν βρόχοις αὐτὰς διαλαμβάνομεν FM: ὡς
ἡμεῖς (ὑμεῖς Aldus Basil.: corr. Chartier) ἐνίοτε πειρώμενοι ἐν βρ. αὐτὰς
διελαμβάνομεν edd.: quarum (sic p d Ven. 1502 in mg.: quantum Ven. 1490.
1502 in textu) nos aliquando experientiam sumentes ... assumebamus N
20 πιστὴν Cornarius: πίστιν FM edd.: experientiam esse fidem N

distinguished physicians and philosophers. But Erasistratus and his school do not say that the psychic pneuma is nourished by what is breathed in, in the same way as does the school of Hippocrates. For to the former the pneuma appears to come from the heart through the arteries to the membranes of the brain, to the latter, to come directly through the nostrils into the hollows in the brain.[62]

2. And here too let us leave alone the opinion of Erasistratus on this matter, for it was refuted in many ways in the treatise *On the Causes of the Pulse*.[63] But passing to the truth, which is that blood is distributed to the arteries also, let us consider this fact, of which we have often made experiment. When the arteries that run through / the neck are ligatured, the animal suffers K503 nothing, either at once or later on; we have more than once so ligatured them in our experiments, and having seen the animal all day long breathing in and out and moving without hindrance, when night was already advanced we killed it, no longer supposing the experiment, continued longer, to be reliable: for it was possible / the principal organs might suffer indirectly N27 from the ligatures applied over so long a time. We were astonished, then, finding the arteries that stretch from the most important of the vital organs, the heart, to the most important of the psychic organs, the brain, bearing the damage thus without harm to vitality as a whole. This, however, we shall examine more fully in *The Use of the Pulse*.[64] But one thing may be repeated from that work, as being serviceable to the present discourse, for which purpose I have called to mind the carotid arteries: that the brain does not at all need the pneuma from the heart. It is accepted that either the vapor / rising to it from K504 the blood is sufficient, or what is inhaled through the nostrils;

N27

1 συμπαθῆναι FM *edd.: corr. Kühn*

2 τῶν κυρωτάτων FM: *edd.: corr. Noll:* a principalissimo N   τῶν *del. Noll*

3 τὰ κυρώτατα FM *edd.: corr. Noll:* ad principalissimum N

4 βίῳ· ᾧ τὴν FM

8 τὸ *Cornarius:* τοῦ FM *edd.*   παρὰ τὴν καρδίαν FM: *corr. Aldus*

10 αὐτῶν FM: *corr. Aldus*

11 ἢ τὴν *add. Aldus*   εἰσπνοῆ FM: *corr. Aldus*

εἰκὸς γίνεσθαι δαψιλῆ βρόχῳ διαληφθεισῶν τῶν ἀρτηριῶν·
δείκνυται <δὲ καὶ> τοῦτ' ἐν τῷ Περὶ χρείας σφυγμῶν. ἀναγκαῖον
<οὖν> ἐκ τῆς διὰ τῶν ῥινῶν εἰσπνοῆς τὴν πλείστην εἶναι τροφὴν
15 τῷ ψυχικῷ πνεύματι. τοῦτ' ἐστι τὸ παρ' Ἱπποκράτους λεγό-
μενον· "ἀρχὴ τροφῆς πνεύματος στόμα ῥῖνες βρόγχος πνεύμων
καὶ ἡ ἄλλη ἀναπνοή." ἐξ ἁπάντων [ἢ] γὰρ τούτων τρέφεται
μηδαμῆ παρεμποδιζόμενον· εἰ δὲ καὶ [μὴ] παρεμποδίζοιτο καθ'
ἓν ὁτιοῦν αὐτῶν, ἀλλ' ἔτι διά γε τῶν λοιπῶν ὑπηρετεῖται. μαθεῖν
20 δ' ἐναργῶς ἔστιν ἐξ οὗ μέλλομεν εἰπεῖν φαινομένου περὶ τῆς ἐκ /
N28 τοῦ πνεύμονος εἰς τὰς καθ' ὅλον <τὸ ζῷον> ἀρτηρίας μεταλήψεως
τοῦ πνεύματος, ὡς ἤτοι βραχυτάτη παντελῶς ἢ οὐδ' ὅλως γίγνεται.
περι[τι]θέντες γὰρ παιδὸς τῷ στόματι καὶ ταῖς ῥισὶ μεγάλην κύστιν
βοείαν ἤ τι τοιοῦτον ἕτερον ἀγγεῖον, ὡς μηδαμῇ παραπνεῖσθαι μηδὲν
K505 / 5 τῆς ἀναπνοῆς, δι' ὅλης ἡμέρας εἴδομεν / ἀκωλύτως <ἀνα>πνέοντ'
αὐτόν. ἐξ οὗ δῆλον ὡς ἕλκουσι μικρὸν παντελῶς ἢ οὐδὲν ὅλως
αἱ κατὰ τὸ ζῷον ἀρτηρίαι [οὐδ' ὁμοίου] τῶν ἔξωθεν ἀέρα.
    3. . . . . . τῶν ποιοτήτων ἀναγκαῖα καὶ μάλιστα
τῆς [τὴν οὐσίαν] θερμότητος. τὸ μὲν γὰρ ψυχρότερον οὐχ
10 ὁμοίως εὔπορον ἁπάντη (χρὴ δ' ἑτοίμως ἰέναι διὰ πάντων τῶν
ὀργάνων τὸ τῆς·ψυχῆς πνεῦμα), τὸ δ' αὖ θερμότερον ἁπάντη
μὲν πόριμον, ἀλλὰ πρῶτον μὲν κατακαίει τε καὶ συντήκει τὸ
σῶμα, τελευτῶν δὲ καὶ αὐτὸ συναπόλλυται καὶ ἀποσβέννυται.
καὶ [συνει] ἐν μὲν ταῖς ἀποπληξίαις ψυχρότερον, ἐν δὲ τοῖς

---

12 διαληφθεισῶν FM: διαλειφθεισῶν edd.: corr. Cornarius
13 δὲ καὶ τοῦτ' ἐν Noll: οὔτ' ἐν FM: δὲ τοῦτο ἐν edd.: demonstratum autem est
    et hoc in libro N: et om. Veneta a. 1490
14 οὖν add. Aldus εἰσπνοῆς Noll: ἐστιν ὡς FM edd. ἐστιν uncis inclus. Basil.
    inspiratione N
15 τὸ] τῷ FM: corr. Aldus λεγόμενον] λεγομεν F: λέγομεν M: corr. Aldus
17 ἀναπνοή] διαπνοῇ Hipp. ἢ del. Aldus τρέφονται FM: corr. Aldus
18 παραποδιζόμενον FM edd.: corr. Kühn μὴ del. Aldus
19 ἔτι] εἴτι FM: corr. Aldus μαθεῖν] μέθην FM: corr. Aldus
20 τῆς ἐκ τοῦ πνεύμονος Cornarius: τοῦ οἰκείου πνεύματος FM: τῆς οἰκείας
    πνεύμονος edd.: de ea que ex pulmone N
N28
1 τὸ ζῷον add. Noll: animal N: cf. infra v. 7
2 βραχυτάτη Noll: βραχὺ ἔτι FM edd.: βραχύ τι Cornarius: breve quid N
3 περιτιθέντες FM edd.: corr. Noll σώματι πλὴν τῷ add. Noll (cf. K VII 15
    sq., ubi Galenus ad hunc locum respicere videtur): om. N
4 ἤ τι] ἤτοι FM: corr. Aldus

but it is probable that the rising vapor too becomes scarce, when the arteries are ligatured (this too is shown in *The Use of the Pulse*).[65] So it must be that it is for the most part[66] from breathing in through the nostrils that the nourishment comes for the psychic pneuma. This is what Hippocrates says: "the source of the food of the pneuma is the mouth, the nostrils, the windpipe, the lung, and the other breathing."[67] For from all these it is nourished, if nothing prevents; and if there is impediment to any one of these, yet it is still served through the others. But it can be learned clearly from the following observation, about the [supposed] distribution of pneuma from / the   N28
lung into the arteries of the whole creature, that this occurs little or not at all. For, covering the mouth and nostrils of a boy with a large ox-bladder, or any such vessel, so that he was unable to draw any breath at all outside it, we saw him / breath-   K505
ing unhindered through a whole day.[68] Hence it is clear that the arteries all through the animal < draw in the outer air very little or not at all.

3. If the psychic pneuma has no need of the substance of the outer air, however, attraction> of its qualities is necessary, and especially of heat. For if it [the pneuma] is too cold, it has not the same facility of moving everywhere (yet the psychic pneuma must move readily through all the members), whereas if it is too hot it is able to move everywhere but first burns and consumes the body, and finally also perishes and is quenched itself.

---

5 εἴδομεν] εἰ μὲν FM *Aldus Basil.*: ἴδομεν *Chartier: corr. Cornarius Kühn: om.* N ἀναπνέοντ᾽ αὐτόν *Noll:* πνέομεν ταυτόν FM *Aldus Basil.*: πνέοντα ταυτόν *Chartier:* πνέοντα αὐτόν *Kühn:* respiramus N

6 ὡς ἕλκουσι *Furley:* ἕνωσίν τε FM: ὡς ἤτοι *Kühn*

7 αἱ *Kühn:* ἢ FM   οὐδ᾽ ὁμοίου *om. Kühn*   τὸν ἔξωθεν ἀέρα *Noll:* τὸν ἔξωθεν ἠρεμία FM

8 *lacunam stat. Noll*

9 τὴν οὐσίαν *om. edd.*

10 *et* 11 ἁπάντη *Noll:* ἅπαντι FM *edd.:* πάντη *Cornarius, fort. recte, cf.* 16 *et* 17: undecumque et undique N

12 κατακαίει τε] κατακαίεται FM *edd.: corr. Cornarius Kühn*

13 τελευτῶν FM *(cf. p. 19,14):* τελευταῖον *edd.*   αὐτό] αὐτ᾽ F   αὐτά M: *recte Aldus*

14 συνεῖεν FM: ἐν *edd.*

15 πυρετοῖς θερμότερον τοῦ μέτρου γιγνόμενον, ἐν μὲν ταῖς ἀποπληξίαις ἴσχεται τοῦ πάντη ῥαδίως ἰέναι, καὶ διὰ τοῦτο εἰς ἀκινησίαν
τελευτᾷ τὸ πάθος, ἐν δὲ τοῖς πυρετοῖς εὔπορον μὲν ὂν πάντη, /

N29 καύσιμον δὲ καθάπερ πῦρ, οὔτε τρέφειν οὔτ᾽ αὐξάνειν τὰ σώματα
δύναται. μὴ τοίνυν εἶναι μικρὰν νομίζωμεν τὴν χρείαν τοῖς ζῴοις
τῆς συμμέτρου θερμασίας, ἀλλ᾽ ἐν τοῖς ἀναγκαιοτάτοις, μάλιστα
μὲν οὖν τῷ πνεύματι τῷ ψυχικῷ καὶ τοῖς κυριωτάτοις ὀργάνοις,
5 ἤδη δὲ καὶ καθ᾽ ὅλον τὸ σῶμα. /

K506 4. εἰκότως ἄρα τὴν ἀρχὴν τῆς φυσικῆς θερμασίας, τὴν
καρδίαν, εἰς τοσοῦτον χρῄζουσαν <ἀναπνοῆς> ἔχομεν, εἰς ὅσονπερ
καὶ συμμέτρου θερμασίας αὐτοὶ χρῄζομεν. ἐδείχθη γὰρ ἀδύνατος
ἡ σωτηρία τῆς θερμασίας χωρὶς τῆς ἀναπνοῆς. "ἔκπνουν μὲν
10 δὴ καὶ εἴσπνουν ἐστὶν ὅλον τὸ σῶμα" κατὰ τὸν <Ἱπποκράτους>
λόγον· ἀλλὰ καὶ πρὸς ἡμῶν ἑτέρωθι δέδεικται. σύμμετρος δὲ
ἀναπνοὴ τοῖς μὲν ἄλλοις ἅπασι μορίοις ἡ διὰ τῶν ἀρτηριῶν
ἐστιν, ἐγκεφάλῳ δὲ καὶ καρδίᾳ δύο ἐξαίρετα πρόσκειται τῆς
ἀναπνοῆς ὄργανα, τῷ μὲν ῥῖνες, τῇ δὲ πνεύμων. ὅπως δὲ ὁ
15 πνεύμων κινοῖτο, θώρακος ἐδεήθη· καὶ διὰ τοῦθ᾽ ὡς μὲν τῇ
καρδίᾳ συνημμένος ὁ πνεύμων τὸ πρῶτόν ἐστι<ν ἀνα>πνευστικὸν
ὄργανον, ὡς δὲ <πρὸς> τοῦ θώρακος κινούμενος τὸ δεύτερον.

5. <εἰ> δὲ καὶ τῆς τοῦ αἵματος ἀναθυμάσεως εἰς θρέψιν
δέοιτο τὸ ψυχικὸν πνεῦμα (πιθανὸν γὰρ καὶ τοῦτο), μεγίστην ἂν
20 ἔχοι καὶ ταύτην συμμέτρου θερμασίας τὴν χρείαν τὰ ζῷα. τὸ /

N30 μὲν γὰρ ψυχρὸν αἷμα πῶς ἂν εἰς ἀτμοὺς λύοιτο; <τὸ> δ᾽ ἀμέτρως
K507 θερμὸν εὐσκέδαστον μὲν εἰς ἀτμούς, ἀλλ᾽ εἰς θο/λεροὺς τούτους

---

16 ἰέναι Noll: εἶναι FM: εἰσιέναι edd.

17 μὲν ὂν Noll: μέντοι FM: μέν τοι edd.: quidem est (i.e. μέν ἐστι) N
N29

1 καύσιμον δὲ Noll: κασσίβην δὴ FM: κατακαίειν δὴ edd.: comburere vero N
πῦρ, οὔτε Noll: πυροῦ FM: πῦρ, ἀλλὰ μήτε edd.   οὔτε τρέφειν οὔτ᾽ Noll: οὐ
τροφείου δὲ FM: οὔτε τρέφειν μήτε edd.

3 συμμέτρου] συμμετρίας FM: corr. Aldus

7 ἀναπνοῆς ante χρῄζουσαν add. Aldus: post χρ. add. Noll: egens respiratione
N

8 ἀδύνατον FM: corr. Aldus

9 μὲν bis F

10 ἐστίν] εἰς FM: om. Hipp.: ἐστὶ add. Aldus   κατὰ] καὶ FM: corr. Aldus
Ἱπποκράτους add. Aldus: Hippocratis N

13 ἐγκεφάλου τε καὶ καρδίας FM edd. (τε in δὲ corr. Aldus): corr. Noll: cerebro
vero et cordi N

And being cooler than the norm in apoplexies, and hotter in fevers, it is prevented in apoplexies from moving everywhere easily, and therefore this affliction ends in immobility, whereas in fevers, being mobile everywhere / but tending to burn like N29 fire, it can neither nourish bodies nor cause them to grow. So let us not imagine that there is small use for animals in moderate heat, but rather that it is among the most essential things, particularly for the psychic pneuma and the most essential organs, but at the same time for the whole body. /

4. So it is understandable that we possess a source of natural K506 heat, the heart, which has need of breathing to the same extent that we ourselves need regulation of heat. For it has been shown that the preservation of the heat is impossible without breathing. "Indeed, the whole body breathes in and out," as Hippocrates says; and it has been proved elsewhere by ourselves too.[69] The breathing through the arteries is enough for all other members, but for the brain and the heart two special organs of breathing are provided; for the first, the nostrils; for the second, the lung. But that the lung might move, the chest was needed; and so, considered as the companion of the heart, the lung is the first organ of breathing; but insofar as it is moved by the chest, it is the second.

5. Now, if the psychic pneuma should also need the vapor arising from the blood as nourishment[70] (for this too is plausible), then animals would have this very great use for heat in due proportion. For how could / the blood that is cold be re- N30 solved into vapor? On the other hand, that which is unduly hot easily disperses into vapor, only / it is a dark and smoky vapor. K507

---

14 τῷ μὲν ... τῇ δὲ *Noll:* τὸ μὲν ... τὸ δὲ FM: τῷ μὲν ... τῷ δὲ *edd.*

15 διὰ τοῦθ᾽ *Noll:* δι᾽ αὐτοῦ FM: δι᾽ αὐτὸ *edd.*   τὴν καρδίαν F

16 ἐστι πνευστικόν FM *edd: corr. Noll*

17 πρὸς *add Cornarius:* ὑπὸ *add. Chartier Kühn*   κινούμενον FM *edd.: corr. Kühn*

18 <εἰ> δὲ καὶ *Noll:* δὲ ἐκ FM: <εἰ> δὲ *edd.*

19 δέοιτο *Noll:* διὰ FM: χρῄζει *edd.*

20 post ταύτην *add. τῆς edd.*   συμμέτρου] συμμετρίαν F: *om.* M: *corr. Aldus* N30

1 δ᾽ ἀμέτρως FM: τὸ *add. Noll:* ἀμέτρως δὲ *edd.*   ἀτμούς] ἀναίμους F: ἀνατμούς M

127

καὶ καπνώδεις. οὐ μὴν τοιούτῳ γε εἶναι πρέπει τῷ ψυχικῷ πνεύματι, ἀλλ' εἴπερ τῳ ἄλλῳ καθαρωτάτῳ τε καὶ χρηστοτάτῳ.
5 ταῦτ' ἄρα [τῷ τὸ μέλαν χρηστοτάτῳ· ταῦτ' ἄρα] τὸ μελαγχολικὸν
αἷμα καὶ τὸ πικρόχολον εἰς ἀτμοὺς μοχθηροὺς λυόμενον τὸ μὲν
εἰς μελαγχολίαν, τὸ δὲ εἰς φρενῖτιν ἄγει. διὰ τοῦτο δὲ κἂν τοῖς
καυσώδεσι πυρετοῖς ἑτοίμως παραφρονοῦσιν. ἢν γὰρ καὶ χρηστὸν
ᾖ τηνικαῦτα τὸ αἷμα, διὰ γοῦν τὸ πλῆθος τῆς θερμασίας ἀτμίζει
10 καπνωδῶς. εἴη δ' ἂν καὶ τοῦτο τῆς κατὰ φύσιν θερμασίας ὄφελος
οὐ σμικρόν, ἀτμίζειν σύμμετρόν τε καὶ καθαρὸν καὶ χρηστόν.

6. οὐ μὴν οὐδ' εἰ τῆς οἰκείας κατασκευῆς δεῖ<ν> ὅτῳ τῶν
μορίων ὑπόθοιτό τις, οὐδ' ἂν οὕτως εἰς τὴν φυλακὴν τῆς κατασκευῆς ὠφελοίη μικρὸν ἡ σύμμετρος θερμασία. ξηρὸν μὲν γὰρ
15 ἀμέτρως ἢ ὑγρὸν οὐκ ἂν <ἐν> ἀκαρεῖ χρόνῳ γίγνοιτο τῶν μορίων
οὐδέν, ψυχρὸν <δ'> ἐσχάτως ἢ θερμὸν δύναιτ' ἂν ἐμφανῶς
γενέσθαι. καὶ μὴν ἰδίως ἑκάστου τῶν μορίων οὐσία ψυχροῦ καὶ
θερμοῦ καὶ ξηροῦ καὶ ὑγροῦ ποία τις κρᾶσίς ἐστιν· ὥστε καὶ
K508 διαφθείρεσθαι ταύτην ὑπ' οὐδενὸς οὕτω ταχέως / εἰκὸς ὡς ὑπὸ
20 τῆς κατὰ τὴν θερμασίαν ἀμετρίας. εἰ δὲ καὶ τοῦτο, καὶ τὴν
ἐνέργειαν ὑπ' οὐδενὸς ἑτοιμότερον ἐγχωρεῖ βλαβῆναι. τῶν μὲν
οὖν ἄλλων ὀργάνων αἱ βλάβαι τῶν ἐνεργειῶν μικραί, τῶν δ' εἰς
αὐτὴν τὴν ζωὴν διαφερόντων μεγάλαι, τῶν δ' οὐ μόνον εἰς /
N31 αὐτὴν τὴν ζωὴν διαφερόντων, ἀλλὰ καὶ πρὸς τὰ ἄλλα λόγον
ἀρχῆς ἐχόντων μέγισται. τοιαῦτα δ' ἐστὶν ἐγκέφαλός τε καὶ
καρδία. ὥσθ' ἡ τούτων τῆς κατασκευῆς βλάβη παραχρῆμα
βλάψει τὴν ζωήν. ἀλλ' οὐδὲν ὑπαλλάττειν αὐτὴν οἷόν τέ ἐστιν
5 ἑτοιμότερον ἀμέτρου θερμασίας. ὥστε ἄμφω δέδεικται διὰ τοῦ
λόγου τοῦδε, τὸ χρήσιμον τῆς συμμέτρου θερμασίας <καὶ> τὸ ἐν τῇ
ἀναπνοῇ εἰς αὐτήν.

7. ἀναγκαῖον οὖν μὴ πιθανὸν μόνον, ἀλλὰ καὶ τὸ

---

4 τῷ ἄλλῳ M edd.: τῳ καὶ ἄλλῳ F

5 τῷ τὸ μέλαν χρ. ταῦτ' ἄρα FM: del. Aldus: om. N

7 φρενίτιν F: φρενίτην M: recte Aldus

8 ἢν γὰρ καὶ χρηστὸν ᾖ Noll: ἢ γὰρ ἢ χρηστὸν ἢ FM: εἰ γὰρ χρηστὸν ἢ
edd.: καὶ post γὰρ add. Cornarius: nam etsi benignus fuerit N

12 οὐδ' εἰ Cornarius: οὐδὲ FM edd. τῆς οἰκείας κατασκευῆς Noll: ταῖς οἰκείαις
κατασκευαῖς FM edd. δεῖν Noll: δεῖ FM: δεῖσθαι edd. at etiam si propriis
constitutionibus singulam particulam egere N

13 οὐδ' ἂν Noll: οὐδὲν FM: οὐδὲ edd.

14 ὠφελοίη Noll: ἀφέλοι FM: ὠφέλοι Aldus Basil.: ὠφελοῖ Chartier: ὠφελεῖ Kühn

15 ἂν <ἐν> Noll: ἂν FM: ἐν edd.

Such a character, of course, cannot suit the psychic pneuma: it above all other things must be most pure and excellent. After all, when the blood is carrying either black or yellow bile, being resolved into nasty vapors it leads in the former case to melancholy, in the latter, to phrenitis. On this account also, in burning fevers, the sufferers become easily distraught. For though the blood is wholesome at this time, yet, because of the excess heat, it gives off a smoke. But to give off a vapor that is temperate, clean, and good: this too would be no small benefit of natural warmth.

6. But even if someone were to suggest that every part requires its own peculiar composition, still a moderate warmth would be of no small service in preserving this composition. For whereas none of the parts could become immoderately dry or wet in a short time, they could manifestly become extremely hot or cold. And indeed the proper being of each of the parts is a certain blend of cold and hot, and dry and wet:[71] hence it / stands to reason that this is ruined by nothing so swiftly as by K508 disproportion in the heat. And if so, the activity too can be injured by nothing more readily. Injuries to the activities of other organs are minor; injuries to those essential to life are great; but injuries to those that not only / are essential to life N31 but also have the status of principles with respect to the others are the greatest: and such are the brain and the heart. So injury to the composition of these will immediately injure life. But nothing is able to change it more readily than immoderate heat. So both the value of heat in moderation and of breathing in regard to this have been shown by the argument.

7. It must now be readily apparent that we have found not

---

16 οὐδέν] οὐδὲ FM: corr. Aldus   δ' add. Aldus
18 κρᾶσις] τάσις FM: corr. Aldus
23 αὐτήν] ταύτην F: ταύτην in αὐτήν corr. M   μεγάλαι ... διαφερόντων (31,1) hab. F edd.: om. M
N31
1 αὐτὴν τὴν ζωὴν F: ζωὴν αὐτὴν edd.
2 τοιαῦται FM Aldus Basil.: corr. Chartier   ἐγκέφαλός τε F: τε om. M edd.
6 τοῦδε τὸ Furley: τόδε τὸ FM: τό τε Basil. Noll   καὶ τὸ] τοῦ FM: corr. Aldus
8 ἀναγκαῖον οὖν edd.: ἀναγκαίου δρᾶν FM: ἀναγκαῖον δ' ἅμα Noll: necessarium autem erit N

ἀληθὲς εὑρηκέναι ἑτοίμως [μὲν] ἀποφαίνεσθαι. καὶ χρείαν εἶναι
10 τῆς ἀναπνοῆς λέγομεν ἐμφύτου θερμασίας φυλακήν. ἔνεστι δ᾽,
εἰ καὶ τὴν οὐσίαν τῆς ψυχῆς ἀγνοοῦμεν, ἀλλ᾽ ἐκ διαιρέσεως
οὐδὲν ἧττον συλλογίσασθαι, λήμμασι τῶν ἀποδείξεων τοῖς ἐναργῶς
K509 γινωσκομένοις / χρησαμένους· ὧν καὶ τοῦτό ἐστι, τὸ περιεχόμενον
ἐν ταῖς κατὰ τὸν ἐγκέφαλον κοιλίαις πνεῦμα δυοῖν θάτερον ἀναγ-
15 καῖον εἶναι, ἤτοι τὴν οὐσίαν τῆς ψυχῆς ἢ τὸ πρῶτον αὐτῆς
ὄργανον. † οὐ τούτου πρῶτον ὄντως δὲ ἀναγκαῖον ὁ ἐγκέφαλος
ἐν ἑαυτῷ τὴν οὐσίαν τῆς ψυχῆς ἔχειν καὶ ταύτην † ἤτοι τὴν
ἔμφυτον εἶναι θερμασίαν ἢ τὸ πνεῦμα ἢ τὸ σύμπαν αὐτῆς τῆς
κατασκευῆς εἶδος ἢ παρ᾽ αὐτὴν εἴ τις δύναμις ἀσώματος. ἀλλ᾽
20 ἀναγκαῖον τοῦτο, πρῶτον εἰς τὰς κινήσεις ὄργανον ἕν τι τῶν /
N32 εἰρημένων ἔχειν αὐτὴν ἀπαθῆ μὲν παντελῶς ὑπάρχουσαν, ἐν δὲ
τοῖς θανάτοις, τῶν πρώτων αὐτῆς ὀργάνων πασχόντων, λυομένην.
ὥστ᾽ ἐξ ἀνάγκης ἤτοι τῆς κατασκευῆς τοῦ ἐγκεφάλου βλαπτομένης ἢ ὁμοῦ τοῦ κατ᾽ αὐτὸν πνεύματος ἢ τῆς θερμασίας μόνης,
5 ὁ θάνατός ἐστι τοῖς ζῴοις. ἀλλ᾽ οὔτε τὴν κατασκευὴν ἐν τάχει
βλαβῆναι δυνατὸν ἑτέρως ἀλλ᾽ ἢ διὰ τὴν τῆς θερμασίας ἀμετρίαν,
ὡς ἐδείξαμεν, οὔτ᾽ αὐτὴν πολὺ μᾶλλον τὴν θερμασίαν· ἀλλ᾽ οὐδὲ
K510 τὸ λοιπὸν ἔτι καὶ τρίτον ἔχειν τινὰ τὸ πνεῦμα δύναται / πρόφασιν
ἑτέρας φθορᾶς ἐξαιφνιδίου παρὰ τὰς ἔμπροσθεν εἰρημένας, τήν
10 τε τῆς οὐσίας ὅλης αὐτοῦ κένωσιν καὶ τὴν τῆς θερμασίας ἀμετρίαν.
ἀλλ᾽ ἐν ταῖς τῆς ἀναπνοῆς ἐπισχέσεσιν οὐκ ἔχομεν αἰτιᾶσθαι
τὴν κένωσιν ὅλης τῆς οὐσίας, ὡς [ἐπὶ τῶν εἰς τὰς κοιλίας τρώ-
σεων] ἐπὶ ταῖς εἰς τὰς κοιλίας τρώσεσιν.

---

9 μὲν del. Mewaldt   invenire parate autem non emicare N
10 φυλακήν Cornarius: ἀναπνοήν FM edd.: custodiam N
12 συλλογίσασθαι Noll: οὖν λογίσασθαι FM: οὖν del. Aldus: sillogizare N
λήμμασι Cornarius: λήμμα^a F: λήμματα M edd.: assumptionibus — utentes
N
16 locus desperatus: verba οὐ τούτου ... ταύτην descripsit Noll ad codicum fidem
additis crucibus: verba οὐ τούτου πρῶτον et ἀναγκαῖον ex v. 20 huc trans-
posita; verba τὴν οὐσίαν τῆς ψυχῆς fort. ex v. 15; verba ἔχειν καὶ ταύτην ex
32,1 (ἔχειν αὐτήν): ἀλλ᾽ εἰ πρῶτον, ὁ ἐγκέφαλος ἐν ἑαυτῷ τὴν οὐσιάν τῆς
ψυχῆς ἔχει, ἀνακαῖόν ἐστι καὶ ταύτην edd.: . . ἔχειν ἀνακαῖόν ἐστι, καὶ
ταύτην Cornarius: sed si hoc primum, cerebrum in se ipso substantiam
anime habere necessarium est, et hanc N
17 ἤτοι τὴν FM: om. edd.: vel N
18 τῆς om. F
19 εἴ τις] ἤτις FM: corr. Aldus: si qua N

merely what is plausible, but the truth itself.[72] And we say: the use of breathing is the conservation of the innate heat. However, it is possible, even though we are ignorant of the substance of the soul, nevertheless to make inferences by a disjunction, using as premises of our demonstrations things / clearly K509 known[73]—among which is this: the pneuma contained in the cavities of the brain is necessarily one of these two: either the substance of the soul, or the soul's first organ. But if it is the *first* organ, then the brain necessarily contains within itself the substance of the soul, and this must be either the natural heat, or the pneuma, or the form of the composition taken as a whole, or some incorporeal power beyond it.[74] And it is necessary that this, one of the / aforementioned, as the primary N32 organ for motion, must keep it [the soul] absolutely unaffected, though dissolved in death when its primary organs suffer.[75] So necessarily animals die, either because the composition of the brain is damaged, or by the same act the pneuma in it, or only the heat. But the composition cannot be damaged rapidly except through the excess of heat, as we have shown, and much less the [natural] heat itself; but the third and remaining alternative, the pneuma, cannot / have any cause of sudden destruction K510 other than those formerly mentioned, namely, the emptying out of its substance or the excess of heat. But in the stoppage of breathing, we have no reason to allege the emptying of the whole substance, as we have when the cavities [of the brain] are wounded.

N32

1 αὐτὴν ἀπαθῆ μὲν *Noll:* αὐτὴν μὲν ἀπαθῆ FM *edd.:* ipsam quidem impassibilem N

2 αὐτῆς *Cornarius:* αὐτῶν FM *edd.:* eius N

3 βλαπτομένης F *edd.* -νην M

7 οὔτ᾽ αὐτήν] οὐ ταῦτ᾽ F: οὐ ταῦτα M: *corr. Aldus*   οὐδὲ] οὐ δὲ FM: οὐ διὰ *edd.* οὔτε *Cornarius:* nec propter N

8 τινὰ F: *om.* M *edd.*

9 ἐξαιφνιδίου] ἐξαίφνης δι᾽ οὗ FM: *corr. Aldus*

10 αὐτοῦ *Cornarius:* αὐτῶν FM *edd.:* ipsius N   κένωσιν] ἔνωσιν FM: *corr. Aldus*

11 αἰτᾶσθαι *Noll:* αἰτίας αἱρεῖσθαι FM: causam dicere N: αἰτίας ἐρεῖσθαι *Aldus Basil.:* αἰτίας εἰρῆσθαι *Chartier Kühn*

12 ὅλης] ἀλλ᾽ οὐδὲ FM: *corr. Aldus*   ἐπὶ τῶν εἰς τὰς κοινὰς τρώσεων FM: *del. Noll:* ἐπὶ ταῖς εἰς τὰς κοιλίας τρώσεσιν *del. edd.*

8. ἀπολείπεται δή, <ὅτι διὰ> θερμασίας συμμετρίαν ἀνα-
15 πνέομεν. αὕτη μὲν οὖν ἡ μεγίστη χρεία τῆς ἀναπνοῆς· δευτέρα
δ' ἡ θρέψις τοῦ ψυχικοῦ πνεύματος. γίγνεται δὲ ἡ μὲν προτέρα
δι' ἀμφοτέρων τῆς ἀναπνοῆς τῶν μερῶν, εἰσπνοῆς τε καὶ ἐκπνοῆς,
τῆς μὲν οὖν ἀναψυχούσης τε καὶ ῥιπιζούσης, τῆς δὲ τὸ αἰθα-
λῶδες ἀποχεούσης, ἡ δευτέρα δὲ διὰ τῆς εἰσπνοῆς μόνης. ὅτι
20 μὲν οὖν εἰς τὴν καρδίαν ἕλκεταί τις ἀέρος μοῖρα κατὰ τὰς /
N33 διαστολὰς αὐτῆς ἀναπληροῦσα τὴν γενομένην κενότητα, τὸ μέγεθος
αὐτῆς τῆς διαστάσεως [ὡς] ἱκανὸν ἐνδείξασθαι. ὅτι δὲ καὶ εἰς τὸν
ἐγκέφαλον εἰσπνεῖται, δι' ἑτέρας ἐπιδέδεικται πραγματείας, ἐν ᾗ
Περὶ τῶν Ἱπποκράτους καὶ Πλάτωνος δογμάτων διαλεγόμεθα. /
K511 / 5 9. διὰ τί δέ, τῆς καρδίας εἰς ἑαυτήν τέ τι παρὰ τοῦ πνεύμονος ἑλκούσης ἀέρος ἐπιπεμπούσης τε ταῖς πλησίον ἀρτηρίαις,
ὅμως γε ὁ ἐκπνεόμενος οὐδὲν ἐλάττων φαίνεται τοῦ κατὰ τὴν
εἰσπνοὴν ἑλχθέντος, εἰρήσεται μὲν καὶ δι' ἑτέρων ἐπὶ πλέον,
ἀποχρήσει δὲ καὶ νῦν εἰπεῖν τοσοῦτον, ὡς ἀτμός τις ἐκπνεῖται
10 τοὐπίπαν ἴσος τῷ πλήθει τῆς μεταληφθείσης μοίρας τοῦ πνεύματος εἴς τε τὴν καρδίαν καὶ τὰς ἀρτηρίας. αἵτινες <δ'> εἰσὶν αἱ διαθέσεις τοῦ σώματος, ἐν αἷς ἤτοι βραχεῖ πλείων ὁ ἀτμὸς τοῦ μεταληφθέντος ἀέρος ἢ ἐλάττων ἢ ἴσος, ἐν τοῖς <Περὶ δυσπνοίας εἰρήσεται.
10. ἀρκεῖν μοι δοκεῖ ταῦτα> περὶ χρείας ἀναπνοῆς. ὃ γὰρ ὑπὲρ
15 αὐτῆς τισιν εἰρήσεται μοχθηρῶς, ῥᾷστα φωραθῆναι δύναιτ' ἂν μὴ
παρέργως ἕκαστον τῶν ἐνταυθοῖ γεγραμμένων ἀναλεξαμένοις.

---

14 ἀπολίποιτο δὴ θερμασία (sic M: θερμ^α F) συμμετρίας ἀναπνέομεν FM:
ἀπολείπεται ὅτι θερμασίας συμμετρίᾳ ἀποθνήσκομεν Aldus: δὴ om. edd.:
γοῦν eodem loco add. Cornarius: διὰ add. Cornarius Basil.: ἀσυμμετρίαν
Cornarius: ἀμετρίαν a Basil. edd.: relinquitur itaque caliditatis immensuritate
mori nos N
16 δ' ἡ Noll: δὲ FM edd.
17 δι' ἀμφοτέρων] διαφέρον FM: corr. Aldus
19 ὅτι … ἕλκεται] ἔστι … ἕλκει τέ FM: ἐπεὶ — ἕλκηται Aldus Basil.: corr.
Chartier
N33
1 κενότητα Noll: ἐγγύτατα FM: κένωσιν edd.
2 αὐτῆς Noll: αὐτοῦ τὲ FM: αὐτό γε edd. magnitudo ipsa N ὡς del. Aldus
4 διαλεγόμεθα F edd.: διελεγόμεθα M: disputamus N
5 ἑαυτήν τέ τί F: τε om. M edd.
6 ἐπιπεμπούσης] ἐπιπνεούσης FM: corr. Aldus
8 ἑλχθέντος] ἔχοντος FM: corr. Aldus

8. It remains, then, that we breathe for regulation of heat. This, then, is the principal use of breathing, and the second is to nourish the psychic pneuma.[76] And the first is brought about by both parts of breathing, both in-breathing and out; to the one belong cooling and fanning, and to the other, evacuation of the smoky vapor; the second is brought about by in-breathing only. That some portion of air is drawn into the heart at its / swelling, filling the space produced, the size of the swelling N33 proves sufficiently.[77] And that there is breathing into the brain has been shown in another work of ours, in which we discuss *The Doctrines of Hippocrates and Plato*.[78] /

9. But why it is that, though the heart both draws some air K511 from the lung into itself, and sends some on to the nearby arteries, what is breathed out nevertheless appears no less in quantity than what is drawn in, will be told elsewhere in full;[79] it is enough to say here only this, that some vapor is breathed out, equal as a whole to the volume of the pneuma taken over into the heart and arteries. Which are the states of the body in which the vapor is somewhat more than the air taken over, or less, or the same—this will be spoken of in *Difficulties in Breathing*.[80]

10. This, I think, is enough on the use of breathing. For whatever has been badly said by some on this subject will easily be faulted by those who read with consequence everything of what is here written.

---

9 τοσοῦτον *Noll:* τόν τε σῖτον FM τὸ τε μόνον *edd.:* τόδε μόνον *Kühn:* tantum N   ἐκπνεῖται *Kühn:* ἀναπνεῖν τὲ FM: ἐκπνοεῖται τε *Aldus:* ἐκπνεῖταί τε *Basil. Chartier*

10 ἴσος τῷ πλήθει] ἴσως τῷ πάθει FM: *corr. Aldus*

11 δ' *add. Chartier:* autem N   εἰσὶν αἱ *Mewaldt:* εἰσὶ καὶ FM *edd.*

13 τοις] ταῖς FM *Aldus Basil.: corr. Chartier*   Περι δυσπνοίας ... δοκεῖ ταῦτα *om.* FM: *add. Aldus:* in hiis qui de dispnia dicetur. sufficere mihi videntur hec N

14 μὲν *ante* μοι *edd.: del. Noll*   ὃ γὰρ FM: ὅσα δ' *edd.* quaecumque autem N

15 εἰρήσεται] εἴρηται *Cornarius, fort. recte:* dicta sunt N   μοχθηρῶς F *edd.:* μοχθηρᾶς M

16 ἀναλεξαμένοις *Noll:* ἐνδειξαμένοις FM: ἐκλεξαμένοις *edd.* relegerint N: elegerint *ed. Veneta a. 1490*

AN IN ARTERIIS NATURA
SANGUIS CONTINEATUR

INTRODUCTION

Title

Galen refers to this work in his *De usu partium* IV 17 (K III 329): "The fact that blood is naturally contained in the arteries has been shown separately in another treatise" (αὐτο μέντοι τοῦθ᾽ ὅτι κατὰ φύσιν ἐν ἀρτηρίαις αἷμα περιέχεται, καθ᾽ ἕτερον λόγον ἰδίᾳ δέδεικται). He says something very similar in *De usu pulsuum* 5.

The word "naturally" is an essential element in the title, because Erasistratus did not deny that blood could be in the arteries, but asserted that it was not present in the normal state of the body. In their natural state, "only pneuma is contained in them" (*An in arteriis* 1). From many passages in Galen we learn that Erasistratus asserted that fevers were due to the presence of blood in the arteries (see especially *De venae sectione adversus Erasistratum* 3, K XI 154).

The Text

There are only two Greek manuscripts extant: Laurentianus 74,3 of the twelfth century (f. 91ʳ–98ᵛ), designated "L," and Marcianus append. cl. V 4 of the fifteenth century (f. 229ᵛ–233ᵛ), designated "V." For an account of these, see F. Albrecht's edition (Marburg, 1911). That edition was based on a new collation of these manuscripts, which I have checked, with the assistance of Mr. David Blank, and found sufficiently accurate.

The Aldine edition of 1525, designated "a," may have been based on some third source, now lost. Albrecht reports that it cannot be based on L, because it shares with V 30 errors that are not found in L. But it has one complete line that is missing from V. Differences in a are recorded fully in the apparatus criticus.

Other editions occasionally cited in the apparatus criticus are the Basel edition (b) of 1538, and the editions of Charterius (c) of 1679 and Kühn (k) of 1821–1833.

Extant Latin translations are by Winter (w) in 1536, Rota in the first Juntine edition (i) in 1541, Trincavellius (t) in 1541, and Rasarius (r) in 1562.

Many emendations of the received text were made by Janus Cornarius, who lived in the first half of the sixteenth century and recorded his suggestions in the margin of his Aldine edition at Jena.

The Greek text published here differs from that of Albrecht in two respects. In a few cases, we have considered the same evidence that was used by Albrecht and rejected his conclusion about the correct reading:

1.18–19	omission of προκειμένου ... τρωθῆναι
2.4	insertion of δείκνυμεν
2.5 and 2.12	tense of verbs
12.24	μένει

Much more important, however, are the changes we have made as a result of J.S.W.'s study of the translation into Arabic, by Isa ibn Yahya, of Hunain's Syriac version of his single Greek manuscript. (For information about these translators, see Ullmann, *Die Medizin in Islam*, and Strohmaier, "Ḥunayn.") For a detailed account of these changes in the text, see notes 18, 22, 33, 35, 36, 38, 42, 47, 48, 57, 58, 59, and 61.

As a result of the Arabic find, Chapter 6 has been substantially altered, and the argument much improved: in addition to the notes *ad loc.*, see our article in *Classical Review* 22 (1972).

Pages and lines are numbered according to Albrecht's edition (A). The pages of Kühn's edition are also noted (K).

Summary

Chapter 1

1. Blood is observed to emerge when an artery is pierced; so either it was present in the artery before the piercing, or, if pneuma were originally present and not blood, then the pneuma should be observed emerging before the blood.

No pneuma is observed, so none was present.

2. The Erasistrateans reply: Pneuma is so fine and moves so rapidly that it could emerge before the blood without being observed.

If we accept this, we must ask whether the pneuma (a) moves of itself, or (b) is moved by something else.

Chapter 2

(a) Is the pneuma self-moving? It can only be self-moving if it is like aether [and so, apparently, hot in itself], or is heated in some way.

If it were aetherial, it could not be contained in the arteries so as to expand them when forced into them from the heart (as Erasistratus asserts that it is and does).

It is warmed by the body (assuming, as Erasistratus asserts, that it is drawn into the body through the lungs); but then it is also moistened and made vaporous, so it would have to be observable on emerging from the arteries.

Indeed, if much blood is allowed to emerge at once, we do perceive vapor emerging with it.

But Erasistratus asserts that no blood can emerge before all the pneuma has been emptied from all the arteries; so if we prick an artery with a fine needle and at once see blood emerge, it would have to follow that all the pneuma in the whole system had emerged in an instant through the fine hole made by the needle. But this is absurd.

Moreover, the pneuma is essential for life, according to Erasistratus; yet when an artery is pierced and bleeds, he must say that the whole pneuma has been emptied out; yet we see the animal still lives.

Chapter 3

(b) Is the pneuma not self-moved, but moved by pressure from the heart?

Then (i) are the arteries able to collapse utterly? If so, pneuma can escape from them without causing a vacuum that must be filled by blood.

Or (ii) do they collapse only partially? If so, like an elastic tube that expands when air is blown into it and returns to normal size when the pressure is released, when pneuma escapes from a wound the arteries will return to a position of rest, still retaining as much pneuma as they had before they were expanded by pressure from the heart. Again, there is nothing to cause a vacuum that must be filled by blood.

Chapter 4

What should happen, on Erasitratus' theory, when an artery is wounded?

Imagine the artery of the axilla pierced with a needle. Then, according to Erasistratus, all the pneuma will be emptied out of it, followed by all the pneuma in the body, since all the arteries are connected; and all the spaces in the arteries and the heart that are emptied of pneuma will be filled with blood. But according to Erasistratus' theory, filling the left ventricle of the heart with blood should have suffocated the animal (but he was not suffocated); emptying the vital pneuma should have killed him (but he was not killed); the loss of pneuma should have paralyzed him (but he could still move); the entry of blood into the arteries should have caused fever (but there was no fever).

This can be proved experimentally.

Moreover, it is not even necessary to pierce an artery. Even when the skin is pierced, the pneuma must, according to Erasistratus, be emptied out, because he thought the skin to be a fine network of arteries, veins, and nerves.

Chapter 5

In this chapter Galen answers an important objection raised by Erasistrateans (though he appears to think it a foolish one): that the blood may come from the nearest anastomoses, and by no means all the pneuma in the system needs to be emptied out before the blood appears in the wound. This, however, is not an objection that Erasistratus made or could make; for he said explicitly that the blood comes from the furthest anastomoses.

Galen shows by an *argumentum ex exemplo* that the objection will not cover all cases: if the abdominal wall of a kid is severed and the guts examined, the arteries of the guts are seen to be full of liquid; but these arteries are connected with those of the abdominal wall only through the aorta. Since it is the latter that are severed, the former can only be filled with blood by the suction required by the hypothesis if the aorta has first been emptied of pneuma.

140

Comparison of the arterial system with a tree illustrates how arteries close to each other in position may yet be remote from each other in the system.

How did the Erasistrateans come to be so foolish? They fall into the error of rejecting what is sure on grounds that are less sure.

Chapter 6

Galen sets out to show the reasons that persuaded the Erasistrateans to believe that the arteries are full of pneuma, and to show that these reasons are not cogent.

The following questions are raised by the Erasistrateans:

(i) Why should Nature have made two sorts of vessels to contain the same fluid (blood)?

(ii) How can pneuma be carried to the whole body, if the arteries are full of blood?

(iii) How, if pneuma is not so carried, are voluntary motions possible?

(iv) How can the regularity of the pulse be explained, if the arteries contain blood as well as pneuma?

Galen answers:

(i) Different organs may contain the same matter, but have different functions: for example, the four "stomachs" of ruminants. That the arteries have a function other than that of the veins, Galen promises to explain in another book (probably *De usu partium* VI).

(ii) The problem is based on a false assumption. It is not necessary that pneuma drawn in in respiration be distributed over the body by the heart.

(iii) The same applies to the problem of voluntary motions.

(iv) We show, by the experiment of tying an artery twice and cutting it between the ligatures, that it continues to pulsate regularly when full of blood. The Erasistratean position can be put in this form: If (a) the arteries contain blood, and (b) they are filled with pneuma from the heart, then (c) the regularity of the pulse will not be maintained. Having conceded (a) and the denial of (c), they must reject (b).

141

Chapter 7

Some Erasistrateans complain about "dialectical subtleties," but Galen presses them to live up to Erasistratus' own assocation with Peripatetic logicians.

Accepting this, some of them question whether Galen can prove anything more than that the conjunction "the arteries contain blood, and they are filled with pneuma from the heart" is not true. Galen continues, assuming that his opponents have accepted the conclusion of Chapters 1–5, that the arteries naturally contain blood: the arteries are not filled with pneuma from the heart, and their pulsation is not due to the pumping of pneuma by the heart; their own expansion (pulsation) causes them to be filled. They work not like wineskins but like bellows. When they expand, they draw in both through their extremities and through their pores.

Chapter 8

The heart is the source of this faculty in the coats of the arteries.

This is shown by the experiment of inserting a hollow reed or bronze tube into an incision in an artery, so that the incision is mended. So long as the coats are unconstricted, the pulse continues; but if the coat is tied tightly to the tube, the pulse stops in the part of the artery away from the heart, although the blood and pneuma continue to pass through it.

Moreover, the whole of an artery pulsates simultaneously, which could not happen if the expansion were due to the passage of pneuma through the blood-filled artery. Voluntary motions, however, illustrate that a faculty can cause instantaneous motion.

Sigla

L = Laurentianus 74₃ saec. XII

V = Marcianus app. cl. V₄ saec. XV

a = editio aldina 1525

ex his tota lectionum varietas annotatur praeter menda orthographica vel typothetica

b = editio basileensis 1538

c = — Charteriana 1679

k = — Kuehniana 1824

w = Guinterii interpretatio 1536

i = iuntinae et basileensis interpr. 1541 sq.

t = Trincavelli interpr. 1560

r = Rasarii interpr. 1562

hae ibi tantum laudantur, uti quid recte novaverunt

Corn = Cornarius

Ka = Kalbfleisch

Alb = Albrecht

(—) quae hisce uncis sunt inclusa per compendium anceps scripsit Laurentiani tantum librarius

Z = Istanbul: A.S. 3631, 83–94

Y = Istanbul: A.S. 3590, 37–50

ΓΑΛΗΝΟΥ ΕΙ ΚΑΤΑ
ΦΥΣΙΝ ΕΝ ΑΡΤΗΡΙΑΙΣ ΑΙΜΑ
ΠΕΡΙΕΧΕΤΑΙ

K703 / A1   1.   Ἐπειδὴ τιτρωσκομένης ἀρτηρίας ἡστινοσοῦν φαίνεται κενούμενον αἷμα, δυοῖν θάτερον ἀναγκαῖον ὑπάρχειν, ἢ ἐν αὐταῖς αὐτὸ περιέχεσθαι ταῖς ἀρτηρίαις ἢ ἑτέρωθεν μεταλαμβάνεσθαι. ἀλλ' εἰ μεταλαμβάνεται, παντί που δῆλον ὡς ὅτ'

5 εἶχον κατὰ φύσιν, πνεῦμα μόνον ἐν αὐταῖς περιείχετο. εἰ δὲ τοῦτο, ἐν ταῖς τρώσεσιν ἐχρῆν πρότερον τοῦ αἵματος ἐκκενού-

K704 μενον φαίνεσθαι τὸ πνεῦμα. οὐχὶ δέ / γε φαίνεται· οὔκουν οὐδὲ μόνον ἔμπροσθεν περιείχετο.

           2. καὶ διὰ βραχυτέρου δ' ἂν λόγου ταὐτὸν ἀποδειχθείη τόνδε τὸν τρόπον· "εἰ τιτρωσκομένων

10 ἀρτηριῶν αἷμα παραχρῆμα φαίνεται κενούμενον, ἦ[ε]ν ἄρα ἐν ἀρτηρίαις αἷμα καὶ πρὸ τοῦ τρωθῆναι." δῆλον γάρ, ὡς ἐν τούτῳ τῷ λόγῳ τὸ "παραχρῆμα" προ<σ>κείμενον ἀληθῆ ποιεῖ τὴν τοῦ ἑπομένου <ἐν> τῷ συνημμένῳ πρὸς τὸ ἡγούμενον ἀκολουθίαν. ἁπλῶς μὲν γὰρ ῥηθὲν χωρὶς τοῦ "παραχρῆμα"

15 τόνδε τὸν τρόπον· "εἰ τιτρωσκομένων ἀρτηριῶν αἷμα φαίνεται κενούμενον" ἑπόμενον ἕξει τὸ κατ' ἀρχὰς εὐθὺς ῥηθὲν τὸ "ἤτοι καὶ πρόσθεν ἐν αὐταῖς περιείχετο ἢ νῦν μεταλαμβάνεται." προ<σ>κειμένου δὲ τοῦ "παραχρῆμα" τὸ ἑπόμενον "ἦν ἐν ἀρτηρίαις αἷμα καὶ πρὸ τοῦ τρωθῆναι," συνθέτου δηλονότι τοῦ

20 παντὸς λόγου γιγνομένου τόνδε τὸν τρόπον· "εἰ τιτρωσκομένων ἀρτηριῶν φαίνεται κενούμενον αἷμα, ἤτοι ἐν αὐταῖς περιείχετο

A2 ταῖς ἀρτηρίαις ἢ ἑτέρωθεν μεταλαμβάνεται· ἀλλὰ μὴν τιτρωσκο-

K705 μένων τῶν ἀρτηριῶν φαίνεται κενούμενον αἷμα, οὐ μεταλαμ/βά-

---

A1

3 ἑτέρ(ω)θ(εν) L: ἑτέρας V: ἑτέροθι a

10 ἦν c: ἦεν La: ἦ ἐν V

12 προκείμ(ε)ν(ον) LVa: corr. Corn

13 ἐν add. Alb

18 προκεμ(έ)ν(ου) L: προκείμενον Va: corr. Corn   προσκειμένου ... τρωθῆναι om. Alb

19 αἷμα Corn: ἀλλὰ LVa

WHETHER BLOOD IS
NATURALLY CONTAINED IN
THE ARTERIES

Chapter 1[1]

Since, when any artery whatever is wounded, blood is ob- A1 / K703
served to be voided, one of two things must necessarily be the
case: either it is contained in the arteries themselves, or it is
transferred from elsewhere. But if it is transferred, it is clear to
everyone that when they were in their natural state, only pneuma was contained in them.[2] But if so, in the case of wounds,
pneuma should have been observed escaping before the blood.
But it is not / so observed; so neither was it previously the only K704
thing contained.

2. This same proposition could also be demonstrated more
briefly thus:[3] "If, when arteries are wounded, blood is observed
at once to be voided, then blood was in the arteries also before
the wounding." For it is clear that in this argument the addition
of "at once" makes true the logical consequence of that which
follows, in the conditional proposition, upon the antecedent. For
stated simply, without the "at once," in this way: "If, when
arteries are wounded, blood is observed to be voided," it will
have as consequent just what was said right at the beginning:
"Either it was present in them before, or it is now transferred."
But with the addition of "at once," the consequent is: "Blood
was also in the arteries before the wounding." The whole argument, clearly, can be put together like this: "If, when the arteries are wounded, blood is observed to be voided, then either it
was contained / in the arteries themselves, or it is transferred A2
from elsewhere. But, when the arteries are wounded, blood is
observed to be voided, and it is not transferred, / as we shall K705

---

21 φαίνεσθαι V

A2

1 ἐτέρωθ(εν) L: -θι Va

145

νεται <δέ>, ὡς δείξομεν. ἐν αὐταῖς ἄρα ταῖς ἀρτηρίαις περιείχετο." πῶς οὖν ὅτι μὴ μεταλαμβάνεται; "εἰ
5 μεταλαμβάνεται, φαίνεται δήπου πρὸ αὐτοῦ κενούμενον πνεῦμα·
ἀλλὰ μὴν οὐ φαίνεται· οὐκ ἄρα μεταλαμβάνεται."

3. ἀρκεῖ τοῦτο

εἰς ἀπόδειξιν τοῖς μήθ' αἱρέσει τινὶ προκατειλημμένοις μήτ'
ἀγνοοῦσιν ἀληθεῖς λόγους διακρίνειν ψευδῶν. ἐπεὶ δ' οὐ πάντες
τοιοῦτοι, πλειόνων ἴσως πρὸς ἐκείνους δεήσει λόγων. ἀντι-
10 λαμβάνονται γοῦν οἱ περὶ τὸν Ἐρασίστρατον ψεῦδος εἶναι
φάσκοντες τὸ συνημμένον. οὐ γὰρ ἀληθὲς ὑπάρχειν φασὶ τὸ
"εἰ μεταλαμβάνεται, φαίνεται πρὸ αὐτοῦ κενούμενον πνεῦμα."
δύναται γὰρ κενοῦσθαι μέν, μὴ φαίνεσθαι δέ, λεπτομερὲς ὂν
καὶ κοῦφον καὶ διὰ τοῦτο ῥᾳδίως ἐκπεμπόμενον.

4. ἀναγκαῖον

15 οὖν αὖθις ἡμῖν δεικνύειν ὡς οὐκ ἂν λάθοι. πῶς οὖν ἀπο-
δείκνυμεν; πολυειδῶς μὲν ἄν, <ἵνα δὲ> καὶ σαφεῖς γίγνωνται
οἱ λόγοι καὶ τάξει προΐωσιν, ἀναγκαῖον αὐτοὺς ἐκείνους ἐρέσθαι,
πῶς ἐκκενοῦσθαι θέλουσι τὸ πνεῦμα, πότερον ἐξ ἑαυτοῦ φερό-

K706 μενον ἢ πρὸς ἑτέρου / τινὸς ὠθούμενον. ἀποκρινοῦνται δ' οὐχ
20 ὡσαύτως ἅπαντες, ἀλλ' οἱ μὲν ἐξ ἑαυτοῦ φέρεσθαί φασιν, οἱ
δὲ ὑπὸ τῆς καρδίας ὠθεῖσθαι. καὶ τοίνυν καὶ ἡμῖν ἑκατέροις
ἐν μέρει δεικτέον ἐστὶν ὡς ἀδύνατα λέγουσιν.

2. Ἀρκτέον δ' ἀπὸ τῶν ἐξ ἑαυτοῦ φέρεσθαι
λεγόντων. ἢ γὰρ τοῦτο πάντως δήπου λεπτομερέστερον οἷον
25 τὸ αἰθερῶδες ἢ ἄλλως πως θερμότερον εἶναι φήσουσιν αὐτὸ
τοῦ περιέχοντος ἡμᾶς ἀέρος· οὐδὲ γὰρ τρίτον ἕξουσιν εἰπεῖν

A3 πνεύματος σύμπτωμα, δι' ὃ φέρεσθαι δύναιτο ἄν.

2. λεπτομερέ-

στερον μὲν οὖν οὐκ ἂν εἴη τὸ κατὰ τὰς ἀρτηρίας πνεῦμα τοῦ

---

3 δέ Corn: om. LVa
4-5 εἰ μεταλαμ.άνε (pars litt. μ et litt. β detritae) L: om. Va ἐφαίνετο LVa:
corr. Furley
8 ψεῦδος V
15-16 intra ἀπο et δείκνυμεν L perforatus
16 μὲν ἄν, <ἵνα δὲ> Alb: μέν, ὡς δ' ἄν a γίγνοντ(αι) LV: corr. a
17 οἱ λόγοι Va: ὀλίγοι L
20-21 ἀλλ' — ὠθεῖσθαι om. V
21 ὑπὸ L: ἀπὸ a
22 δεκτέον LV: corr. a

demonstrate. Therefore it was contained in the arteries themselves." Now, how shall we prove that it is not transferred? "If it is transferred, then pneuma is observed to be voided before it. But this is not observed. So it is not transferred."

3. This will serve as a sufficient proof for those who are not committed in advance to a particular school and who can distinguish truth from falsehood. But since not all are of this kind, probably further arguments will be needed to convince the others. At any rate, the followers of Erasistratus object, alleging that the conditional proposition is false. For they say the following is not true: "If it is transferred, pneuma is observed to be voided before it,"[4] since it might indeed be voided, but might not be observed, being composed of extremely fine particles, and light, and hence easily evacuated.

4. Thus it is necessary for us to demonstrate our position again, in a manner allowing of no evasion. How, then, do we prove it? Well, in several ways; but so that the arguments may be lucid and may proceed in order, we must put the question to them themselves, how they would have the pneuma to be emptied out, whether moving of itself, or / propelled by some- K706 thing else? However, they do not all give the same answer, but some say it moves of itself, others that it is propelled by the heart.[5] So it falls to us to show each in turn that they assert something impossible.

Chapter 2

Let us begin with those who say it moves of itself. They will say either that it is composed of finer parts altogether, like what is aetherial, or that it is in some other way warmer than the air around us. For they will not be able to mention any third / property belonging to pneuma, by which it might move.[6] A3

2. Now, the pneuma in the arteries could not be composed of finer parts than the air around us, as its origin teaches us.

---

23 ἑαυτοῦ Corn: ἑαυτ(οῦ) L: ἑαυτῶν Va
24 ἦ a: εἰ LV   πάντ(ως) L: πάντα V: πάντη a
26 τρίτ(ον) L: τρίτου V
A3
  2 τὰς Va: τῆς L

περιέχοντος ἡμᾶς ἀέρος, ὡς ἡ γένεσις αὐτοῦ διδάσκει. γίγνεται
γὰρ κατὰ τὸν Ἐρασίστρατον ἐκ τοῦ περιέχοντος ἡμᾶς ἀέρος
5 εἴσω τοῦ σώματος εἰς μὲν τὰς κατὰ πνεύμονα πρώτας ἀρτηρίας
ἐλθόντος, ἔπειτα δὲ εἴς τε τὴν καρδίαν καὶ τὰς ἄλλας. εἰς ὅσον
οὖν ὑγροτέροις ὁμιλεῖ σώμασιν, εἰς τοσοῦτον εἰκὸς αὐτὸ παχυ-
μερέστερόν τε καὶ ἀτμωδέστερον γίγνεσθαι. θερμότερον δὲ
K707 γίγνεται, ἀλλ’ ὡς ἀτμὸς / ἄνω φερόμενον οὔτε ἀφανῆ τὴν
10 κένωσιν οὔτε οὕτως ὠκεῖαν ἕξει. Πραξαγόρας μὲν οὖν καὶ
παχυμερέστερον αὐτὸ καὶ ἱκανῶς ἀτμῶδες εἶναί φησιν, Ἐρασίστρατος δέ, ὅπῃ μὲν ἔχει πάχους, οὐ διώρισεν, ἐξ ὧν δ’ ὑπὲρ
αὐτοῦ λέγει τεκμήραιτ’ ἄν τις οὐδαμῶς αὐτὸ προσήκειν εἶναι
λεπτόν. τάς τε γὰρ ἀρτηρίας ὑπ’ αὐτοῦ πληρουμένας διαστέλλε-
15 σθαί φησι καὶ τὰς τῶν μυῶν κοιλίας ὡσαύτως, οὐδετέρου δὴ
τούτων γίγνεσθαί ποτ’ ἂν δυνηθέντος, εἰ λεπτομερὲς ἀκριβῶς
ὑπῆρχεν· οὐ γὰρ δὴ ἴσχεσθαί γε τὸ τοιοῦτον μᾶλλον ἐν τοῖς
σώμασιν, ἀλλ’ ἐκπέμπεσθαι πρέπει. τί ποτ’ οὖν ἐκφυσώμενον
οὐ φαίνεται παραπλησίως τῷ κατὰ τὰς ἐκτὸς τοῦ θώρακός
20 τε καὶ τοῦ περιτοναίου καὶ τῆς φάρυγγος τρώσεις;

3. γελοῖον δ’
ἴσως ποιοῦμεν ἐξ ἑτέρων αὐτὸ συλλογιζόμενοι, παρὸν αὐτῶν
ὑπομνῆσαι τῶν ἀρτηριῶν, ἐξ ὧν ὅταν ἀθρόον ἐξακοντίζηται
τὸ αἷμα, σαφῶς ἐκφυσώμενον φαίνεται. ὡς γὰρ θερμότερον,
οὕτω καὶ ἀτμωδέστερον τὸ κατὰ τὰς ἀρτηρίας αἷμα. οὐ μὴν
25 αὐτός γε καθ’ ἑαυτὸν ἀτμὸς ἢ ἀὴρ ἢ αἰθὴρ ἢ ὅλως πνεῦμα
K708 περιεχόμενον ἐν αὐταῖς φαίνεται. καὶ γὰρ / εἰ τῇ λεπτοτάτῃ
βελόνῃ διατρήσαις ἀρτηρίαν, εὐθὺς ἐξακοντίζεται [ἂν] τὸ αἷμα.
A4 ἐχρῆν δ’ οἶμαι καὶ εἰ μὴ διὰ τοῦ μεγάλου τραύματος, ἀλλὰ
διὰ γοῦν τοῦ μετρίου μὴ ταχέως μηδ’ ἀναισθήτως, ἀλλ’ ἐν
χρόνῳ πλείονι κενοῦσθαι τὸ πνεῦμα. πρὶν γὰρ ἐκεῖνο κενω-

---

6 ἐλθόντ(ος) La: ἐλθόντα V   τε om. Va
8 ἀτμωδέστερον Ka: ἀπαλωδέστερον L: ἀπαλ. Va: πλαδωδέστερον Corn: pin-
   guior i
12 πάχ(ους) L: πάχος V
15 δὴ a: δὲ LV
16 λεπτομερῶς LV: corr. a
19 ἐκτὸς L: ἐκ Va
21 αὐτ(ῶν) L: item ambigue V: αὐτοὺς a
22 ἀθρόον a: ἀθρόαν LV
25 γε a: τε LV

For according to Erasistratus it comes into being inside the body from the air around us, having entered first into the arteries in the lungs,[7] then into the heart and the other arteries. Now, to the extent that it is associated with moist bodies, we may assume it becomes that much more coarse-grained and more vaporous.[8] It does indeed become warmer, but, ascending as / vapor, it will be neither imperceptible when emerging, nor so K707 swift. Praxagoras,[9] indeed, says it is both somewhat coarse-grained and fairly vaporous; Erasistratus, however, does not say precisely how it stands as to coarseness, though from what he says about it, one would infer that fineness is by no means one of its characters. For he says that the arteries are expanded when filled with it, as also the cavities of the muscles,[10] though neither of these could possibly occur, if it were precisely fine-grained; for it is of course appropriate that a thing of that character should not rather be retained in bodies, but escape from them. Why ever, then, is it not perceived being blown out, in just the same way as in the case of wounds on the outside of the chest or the cavity of the belly or the throat?

3. But perhaps we commit an absurdity proving this from other considerations, when it is easy to refer to the arteries themselves, from which it [pneuma] is clearly perceived being blown out whenever the blood is ejected in a mass. For as the blood of the arteries is hotter, so it is more vaporous.[11] Yet in isolation by itself, neither vapor, not air, nor aether, nor any pneuma whatever is seen to be contained in them. For / if you K708 pierce an artery with the finest needle, the blood spurts out at once. / It ought to be the case, however, I believe, that even if A4 not from a large wound, yet at any rate from a moderate one, the pneuma should be evacuated not rapidly, nor imperceptibly,

---

26 post περιεχ. lacuna in L   αὐτ(αῖς) L: αὐτῶ Va
26-27 λεπτοτ(ά)τ(η) β. διατρήσαις L: λ. β. διατρήσαιο a: λεπτότητι βελώνη
    διατρίψαιο V
27 ἄν eiecit k
A4
  2 διὰ om. Va
3-4 κενωθ(ῆ)ν(αι) L: κενωθῆ Va

θῆναι πᾶν, πῶς ἂν ἐκπίπτοι διὰ τοῦ τραύματος τὸ αἷμα, λέγοντός
5 γε αὐτοῦ τοῦ Ἐρασιστράτου τὰς πορρωτάτω κειμένας ἀρτηρίας
πρώτας ἀπολαύειν τῆς μεταχύσεως; εἰ δὲ καὶ μὴ πρὸς ἐκείνου
γεγραμμένον ἦν, ἐξ ἀνάγκης ἠκολούθησε ταῖς ὑποθέσεσιν. εἰ
γὰρ συνεχὲς αὐτῷ πάντως ἐστὶ τὸ κατὰ τὰς ἀρτηρίας πνεῦμα
καὶ οὕτως εὐκίνητόν τε καὶ λεπτὸν ὡς ἐν ἀκαρεῖ χρόνῳ
10 κενοῦσθαι ῥᾳδίως, οὐ τὸ μὲν ἐν ταῖς διαιρουμέναις ἀρτηρίαις
κενωθήσεται μόνον, τὸ δ' ἐν ταῖς ἄλλαις ἁπάσαις μενεῖ. πρόδηλον
γὰρ ὡς <τῷ> τε προτέρῳ τῷ κατὰ τὴν τετμημένην τὸ λοιπὸν
ἅπαν ἑτοίμως ἀκολουθήσει καὶ πρώτῃ ταῖς ὑστάταις ἐπίδηλος
ἡ κένωσις γενήσεται μηκέτ' ἐχούσαις ἑτέρας ὅθεν μεταληφθήσε-
15 ται. ἐν αὐταῖς οὖν πρώταις κίνδυνος τοῦ κενὸν γενέσθαι τόπον,
K709 εἰ μή τις οὐσία πληρώσειε τὴν χώραν τοῦ / μεταλαμβανομένου
πνεύματος. καὶ διὰ τοῦτ' ἐξ ἀνάγκης ἕπεται τὸ διὰ τῶν συναναστομώσεων ὡς αὐτός φησιν αἷμα τῇ πρὸς τὸ κενούμενον
ἀκολουθίᾳ καὶ τοῦτο ὥσπερ προσδεδεμένον τῷ κατὰ τὰ πέρατα
20 τῶν ὑστάτων ἀρτηριῶν πνεύματι πρῶτον μὲν ἅπαντος τοῦ
ἄλλου αἵματος, ὕστερον δὲ παντὸς τοῦ κατὰ τὰς ἀρτηρίας
πνεύματος κενωθήσεται. δύο οὖν ἄτοπα μέγιστα συμβήσεται
κατὰ τὸν λόγον, πρότερον μὲν τὸ διὰ τοῦ κατὰ τὴν βελόνην
τρήματος ἅπαν ἐκκενοῦσθαι τὸ κατὰ τὰς ἀρτηρίας πνεῦμα
25 ταχέως οὕτως ὥστε λαθεῖν, δεύτερον δὲ τὸ ζῆν ἔτι τὸ ζῷον
ἅπαντος τοῦ ζωτικοῦ πνεύματος ἐκκενουμένου. ἀλλὰ τοιαῦτα
καὶ μετ' ὀλίγον ἐξέσται διελθεῖν.

A5 3. Ἐπὶ δὲ τὸ λοιπὸν τῶν προτεθέντων μεταβάντες
ἐπιδείξομεν ὡς οὐδ' εἰ παρὰ τῆς καρδίας θλιβούσης ἐπιπέμ-
ποιτο τὸ πνεῦμα ταῖς ἀρτηρίαις, πιθανὸν οὐδ' [αὐτὸ] οὕτως ἐστὶ
τὸ τῆς παρεμπτώσεως δόγμα. τί γὰρ καὶ βούλεται; π[ρ]ότερον

---

4 πᾶν, πῶς Ka: πάντ(ως) L: πάντως οὐκ Corn: item interpretes
8 αὐτ(ῷ) LVa: corr. Alb: sibi interpr.
9 λεπτὸν La: λευκὸν V
10 οὐ τὸ a: οὔτ(ω) LV
12 <τῷ> Alb: duae vel tres litterae evanidae in L: om. Va
13 ἅπαν L quoque, sed ἅ expunxit
14 ἐχούσης LVa: corr. Corn
15 αὐτ(αῖς) L: αὐτῇ Va: in his i πρώτ(αις) L: πρώτως Va: πρῶτος Corn
16 τῆς οὐσίας LVa: corr. Corn et interpretes
19 προδεδεμένον Va
21 ὕστερον Alb: ὕστατον LVa

but over a considerable time. For before that has all been emptied out, how could blood escape from the wound, since Erasistratus himself says it is the arteries lying furthest away that first profit by the transfusion [of blood from the veins]? Indeed, even if it had not been written by him, it followed necessarily from his hypotheses. For if the pneuma in the arteries is a single continuous mass, and so easily mobile and subtle that it can easily be emptied out in a single moment, it is not the case that only the pneuma in the pierced artery will be emptied out, while that in the others will remain. For it is obvious that what is first—that is, what was in the wounded artery—will immediately be followed by the whole of the rest;[12] and the evacuation will first be apparent in the furthest arteries, since they have no others behind them whence further pneuma might be drawn. So it is there that the danger of an empty space arising will first occur, unless some substance fills the place of / the pneuma that is taken over. Hence, necessarily, as he himself K709 says, the blood will follow through the anastomoses,[13] because of the tendency to refill the void; and this blood, as though attached to the pneuma at the extremities of the furthest arteries, will be emptied out before all the rest of the blood, but after all the pneuma in the arteries. Thus two very absurd consequences will follow, according to this argument: first, that through the hole made by the needle the whole of the pneuma in the arteries will be emptied out with such speed that it is imperceptible; second, that the animal will still live when the whole of the vital pneuma is emptied out of it.[14] But it will be possible to discuss considerations of this kind in a little while. /

Chapter 3

Passing on to the rest of their assumptions, we shall prove A5 that even if it is assumed that the pneuma is transmitted to the arteries by pressure from the heart, the doctrine of transfusion [of blood] is not even then credible. For what does he mean? Is

A5

1 προτεθ(έν)τ(ων) L: προτεθεμένων Va

3 αὐτὸ La: αὐτὸ τὸ V: del. Alb

4 πρότ(ε)ρ(ον) LVa: emend. Corn

K710

5 εἰς ἔσχατον πεφυκέναι συστέλλεσθαι τὰς ἀρτηρίας ὥσπερ καὶ
τὰς φλέβας ἢ ὅπερ ἀληθές ἐστι / μέχρι τινός; ἔστω πρότερον
τὸ εἰς ἔσχατον, ἵνα μηδὲν παραλείπηται. ἀλλ' εἰ τοῦτο, μοχθηρὸς
ὁ λόγος ἔσται καὶ ἀπέραντος παρὰ τὸ τῆς διαιρέσεως ἐλλιπές.
οὐκέτι γὰρ ἔξεστι λέγειν "κενουμένου τοῦ πνεύματος ἤτοι κενὸς
10 ἔσται τόπος ἀθρόος ἢ τὸ συνεχὲς ἀκολουθήσει," ἀλλ' ὑπομνή-
σωμεν αὐτὸν ὡς καὶ τρίτον ἔστι παραλειπόμενον ἐν τῇ διαιρέσει·
"τὸ κενούμενον ἀγγεῖον συσταλήσεται," καὶ διὰ τοῦτ' ἀπέραντος
ὁ λόγος γενήσεται. προ<ς>ληφθέντος γὰρ ἑνὸς λήμματος ἀληθοῦς
τοῦ "ἀλλὰ μὴν οὐ γίγνεται κενὸς ἀθρόος τόπος" οὐκέτ' ἔξεστι
15 λέγειν "τὸ ἄρα συνεχὲς ἀκολουθήσει," ἀλλὰ τί ποτ' ἔσται τὸ
συμπέρασμα; "ἤτοι ἄρα τὸ συνεχὲς ἀκολουθήσει ἢ τὸ ἀγγεῖον
συσταλήσεται." οὕτως μὲν οὖν μοχθηρὸς ὁ τῆς παρεμπτώσεως
ἐπιδειχθήσεται λόγος, εἰ τελέως ἡ ἀρτηρία συστέλλοιτο.

2. εἰ δὲ
μέχρι ποσοῦ τινος, ἐκεῖνος αὖθις ὁ λόγος ἀποδειχθήσεται μοχθη-
20 ρός, ἐὰν τὸ κατὰ τοὺς ἁπαλοὺς καλάμους ἀναμνησθῶμεν φαινόμενον, οἷς ἐμφυσῶντες ἐπὶ τοσοῦτον αὐτοὺς διαστέλλομεν ἐφ'

K711

ὅσον πεφύκασιν, εἶτ' αὖθις ἐκκενοῦται κατὰ τὸ πέρας / ὁ ἀὴρ
τοσοῦτον εἰς ὅσον ὁ κάλαμος πέφυκε συστέλλεσθαι. πλέον γὰρ
οὐκ ἂν ὁ κάλαμος οὔτ' ἐκτείνοιτο φυσώντων οὔτ' αὖ συστέλλοιτο.
25 ὅσον γὰρ ἐνεφυσήσαμεν, τοσοῦτον ἀναγκαῖον κενοῦσθαι μόνον·
ὅσον δ' ἔφθανεν ἀέρος περιέχεσθαι καὶ πρὶν ἡμᾶς ἐμφυσῆσαι,
τοῦθ' ὑπομένειν ἀναγκαῖον. οὕτως οὖν ἔχει καὶ κατὰ τὰς
ἀρτηρίας. περιέχεται μὲν γάρ τι πνεῦμα καὶ συνεσταλμένων
αὐτῶν, ἐπιπέμπεται δ' ἕτερον ὑπὸ τῆς καρδίας πληρούσης, καὶ

A6

τοῦτ' ἐπιπληροῖ μὲν αὐτῶν τὰς κοιλίας, παρ' ὃν χρόνον εἰσέρχεται
καὶ τὴν διαστολὴν ἐργάζεται, κενούμενον δὲ συστέλλεσθαι πάλιν,
εἰς ὅσον ἐξ ἀρχῆς, ἐπιτρέψει. οὔκουν οὐκέτ' οὐδὲ κατὰ τοῦτον
τὸν λόγον οὐδεμία τῆς τοῦ αἵματος παρεμπτώσεως ἀνάγκη. τά
5 τε γὰρ ἄλλα καὶ πολὺ σφοδρότερον διὰ τοῦ στόματος ἐμφυσῶμεν

---

8 ἐλλειπές LVa: corr. Alb
11 αὐτ(ὸν) La: αὐτὸ V: eos i   tertium quiddam i: quid t. r: volebant fort. τρίτον
ἔστι τι
11–12 fort. διαιρέσει· <τὸ "ἢ"> τὸ
13 προσληφθέντος Alb: προληφθέντ(ος) L: παραληφθέντος Va
16 ἢ τὸ a: ἤτοι LV
21 οἷς Alb: οὓς LVa
24 ἂν om. Va   αὖ k: ἂν codd. a

it that the arteries are so made as to collapse utterly, like the veins; or, what is true, / that they collapse up to a certain K710 point? Let it be the former, that they collapse utterly, so that nothing may be passed over. But if so, the argument will be unsound and inconclusive by defect of disjunction.[15] For then it is no longer possible to say, "When the pneuma is emptied out, either (i) there will be a massed empty space,[16] or (ii) that which is continuous with it will follow it," but we shall remind him that a third has been passed over in the disjunction: "(iii) the vessel will collapse as it is emptied."[17] Hence the argument will become inconclusive. For although one true proposition forms the minor premise,[18] namely, "but no massed empty space occurs," it is not legitimate any longer to assert: "therefore what is continuous with it will follow it." But what then will be the conclusion? It will be: "Either, therefore, what is continuous will follow it, or the vessel will collapse." Thus the argument for transfusion will be proved defective, if the artery collapses totally.

2. If however the arteries are said to collapse up to a certain point, the argument can again be shown to be worthless, if we call to mind the phenomenon occurring with soft reeds. When we blow into them, we cause them to expand as far as they are naturally able; afterwards the air is emptied out from the end, / just so much as the reed is naturally able to contract. For the K711 reed will neither expand more, when we blow into it, nor again contract more. For it must be the case that only so much air is evacuated as we blew into it, and that just as much air as was held in it before we blew remains in it. Now the same is true of the arteries: some pneuma is held in them, even when they are contracted, but more is supplied from the heart when it fills them, / and this fills their cavities during the time it passes into A6 them and causes the swelling; then, being emptied, it will allow them to contract again to their original size. But now, according to this argument also, there will never be the least necessity for any transfusion of the blood. Apart from anything else, we blow

---

A6

1 ἐξέρχεται LVa

2 κενούμ(ε)ν(ον) L: κενουμένων Va

ἡμεῖς τοῖς καλάμοις ἢ ταῖς ἀρτηρίαις ἡ καρδία. χρὴ δὲ δήπου
τὸ σφοδρότερον ἐμφυσώμενον μᾶλλόν τε καὶ θᾶττον κενοῦσθαι.
ἀλλ' ὅμως οὐδ' εἰ τὸν κάλαμον αὐτὸν ἐπιστήσειέ τις κατὰ τῶν
ἀνέμων ἁπάντων, οὐδ' οὕτως ἔσται τις ἐν τοῖς καλάμοις τόπος
K712 / 10 κενός, ἀλλ' ἀεὶ μὲν ὁδὸν ἕξει / τὴν εὐρυχωρίαν τοῦ καλάμου τὸ
διαρρέον πνεῦμα, κενωθήσεται δ' οὐδέποθ' οὕτως ὡς δεηθῆναί
τινος ἑτέρου σώματος ἀναπληροῦντος τὴν χώραν τοῦ κενωθέντος.

4. Ἐπεὶ τοίνυν τὸ προκείμενον ἱκανῶς ἀποδέδεικται,
τί κωλύει προσθεῖναί τινα καὶ τῶν ἄλλων ἀτόπων; ἅπαντα μὲν
15 γὰρ διελθεῖν ἀδύνατον, οὕτω πολὺ πλῆθος αὐτῶν ἔστιν. ἐν μὲν
δὴ καὶ πρῶτον ἄτοπον τὸ δεῖν πάντως ἐπὶ πάσῃ τρώσει, κἂν
τὸ δέρμα μόνον ᾖ τετρωμένον ὑπὸ τῆς λεπτοτάτης βελόνης,
ἁπάσας μὲν τὰς ἀρτηρίας αἵματος πληροῦσθαι, πυρετὸν δ' ἐξ
ἀνάγκης ἕπεσθαι. φανερὸν δ' ἔσται τὸ λεγόμενον ἁρμοζομένης
20 ἡμῶν τῆς ἀποδείξεως ἐπ' αὐτῶν τῶν κατὰ τὰς ἀρτηρίας τρώσεων.
2. καὶ δὴ <διῃρη>μέν<ην> μοι νόει βελόνῃ λεπτῇ <τὴν> διὰ
τῆς μασχάλης εἰς ὅλην τὴν χεῖρα νενεμημένην ἀρτηρίαν. τί τοίνυν
συμβήσεται κατὰ τὸν Ἐρασίστρατον; ἐκκενοῦσθαι μὲν δηλονότι
τὸ κατ' αὐτὴν πνεῦμα, συγκενοῦσθαι δ' αὐτῷ καὶ τὸ τῶν πλησίον
25 ἀρτηριῶν· πλησίον δ' εἰσὶ τῆς εἰρημένης αἵ τ' ἀπ' αὐτῆς εἰς τὴν
K713 χεῖρα νεμόμεναι καὶ ἡ μεγάλη ἡ ἀπὸ τῆς / καρδίας, ἀφ' ἧς
A7 αὐτὴ πέφυκεν. ἀλλ' εἴπερ αὕτη κενωθήσεται, πᾶσα δήπουθεν
ἀνάγκη πλησίον οὖσαν αὐτῆς τὴν ἀριστερὰν κοιλίαν τῆς καρδίας
συνεκκενοῦσθαι <καὶ> τήν τ' ἐπὶ τὴν κεφαλὴν ἀνιοῦσαν καὶ
τὴν ἐπὶ τὴν ῥάχιν καταφερομένην. εἰ γὰρ ἅπαντι τῷ κενουμένῳ
5 μέρει τῆς ἀρτηρίας τὰ πλησιάζοντα συνεκκενοῦται — πλησιάζει
δ' ἀεὶ τὰ ἀπ' αὐτῆς πεφυκότα καὶ ἀφ' ὧν αὐτὴ πέφυκεν —

---

8 ἐπιστήσειέ τ(ις) μετὰ LV: ἐπ. τ. κατὰ a
11 κενωθή L
14 προσθ(εῖ)ν(αι) L: προσθῆναι Va
16 πάντ(ως) L: πάντα Va
17 λεπτοτ(ά)τ(ης) L: λεπτοτέρας Va
21 καὶ δὴ διῃρημένην μοι νόει βελόνῃ λεπτῇ τὴν διὰ Alb (nunc vers. Arab.
confirmatus): καὶ δὴ μέν μοι νόει βελόνην λεπτὴν διὰ LVa: καὶ δὴ ἐνίεσθαί
μοι νόει βελόνην λεπτὴν εἰς τὴν διὰ Corn: acum tenuem — pungere w
22 ἐνεμημένην LVa: corr. Corn
24 αὐτ(ὴν) L: αὐτῆς Va αὐτ(ῷ) L: αὐτῆς V: αὐτῇ a: cum eo w πλησίων Va
26 post καρδ. add. συνεκκενοῦσθαι V

through our mouths into the reeds much more violently than the heart into the arteries. Clearly what is more violently blown in should be emptied out more forcibly and more quickly. But nevertheless if one were to present the reed itself to all the winds, even so there would never be a vacuum in the reeds, but the pneuma flowing through them will always have a free passage / through the reed, and it will never become empty so K712 that there is need of some other body to fill up again the place of what has been emptied out.

Chapter 4

Since what we set out to prove has been sufficiently demonstrated, why should we not add some of the other absurdities [that follow from their theory]? We cannot rehearse them all; they are too numerous by far. One, however, the prime absurdity, is that always upon any wound occurring, even if only the skin is pierced by the finest needle, all the arteries should be filled with blood, and fever should supervene. What we are going to say will be obvious, since our demonstration is adapted to actual wounds in the arteries.

2. Well now, imagine, pray, the artery that passes through the armpit and is then distributed over the whole arm pierced by a fine needle.[19] What now will happen, according to Erasistratus? Clearly the pneuma in it will be emptied out, and with it the pneuma from the next arteries. Now, next to the said artery are those spreading out from it to the arm,[20] and also the great artery from the / heart, from which / it arises. But if it [the great K713 / A7 artery] is going to be emptied, of course we must necessarily suppose that the left ventricle of the heart, being next to it, will be emptied with it, and the one that goes up to the head, and the one that descends along the vertebral column. For if with every part of the artery that is emptied the next parts are emptied too, and next to it are always those arising from it and that

---

A7

1 αὐτὴ k: αὔτη LVa: cf. 1.6   κενῶ L   θ´
3 καὶ add. Alb
4 ῥάχην V   ιν
6 αὐτὴ k: αὔτη LVa

155

εὔδηλον, ὡς ἤ τ᾽ ἀριστερὰ κοιλία τῆς καρδίας καὶ τῶν εἰρημένων
ἑκατέρα συνεκκενωθήσεται τῇ κατὰ τὴν μασχάλην. ἐπεὶ τοίνυν
ἀπὸ μὲν τῆς ἑτέρας αὐτῶν αἱ κατὰ τὸν τράχηλόν τε καὶ τὴν
10 κεφαλὴν ἅπασαι πεφύκασιν, ἀπὸ δὲ τῆς ἑτέρας αἱ καθ᾽ ὅλον
τὸ λοιπὸν σῶμα, δῆλον ὡς καὶ ταύτας ἀνάγκη συνεκκενοῦσθαι
μέχρι τῶν περάτων· ἀλλ᾽ ὅταν πρῶτον ἐπὶ τὰ πέρατα τῶν
ἀρτηριῶν ἡ κένωσις τοῦ πνεύματος ἐξίκηται, μεταχεῖσθαι συμβήσεται κατὰ τὰς ἀναστομώσεις ἐκ τῶν φλεβῶν εἰς αὐτὰς τὰς
15 ἀρτηρίας αἷμα καὶ τοῦτο <ἑπό>μενον τῷ κενουμένῳ πνεύματι
τὸ μὲν ἀπὸ τῶν κάτω μερῶν τοῦ σώματος ἐπὶ τὴν κατὰ ῥάχιν
K714   ἀρτηρίαν καὶ τὴν καρδίαν ἀφικνεῖσθαι, κἄπειθ᾽ / οὕτως ἐπὶ
τὴν κατὰ μασχάλην, τὸ δ᾽ ἀπὸ τῶν κατὰ τὴν κεφαλὴν ἐπὶ
μὲν τὴν ἄνω φερομένην [τὴν] προτέραν, ἑξῆς δ᾽ ἐπὶ <τὴν
20 κατὰ> τὸν τράχηλον <καὶ> τὴν τετρωμένην. οὕτω δὲ καὶ τὸ διὰ
τῶν κατὰ τὴν χεῖρα πασῶν ἀρτηριῶν μεταληφθὲν αἷμα τῷ
πνεύματι συνακολουθοῦν ἐπὶ τὴν διῃρημένην ἀρτηρίαν ἐνεχθή-
σεται καὶ πᾶν οὕτω τὸ καθ᾽ ὅλον τὸν ὄγκον αἷμα ῥυήσεται
πρὸς τὴν διαίρεσιν.

            3. ἀλλὰ τοῦτο μὲν καὶ πάνυ ἀληθές· φαίνεται
25 γὰρ διὰ μιᾶς ἀρτηρίας ἡστινοσοῦν τῶν ἀξιολόγων, εἰ μὴ
κωλύσεις αὐτῶν τὴν ῥύσιν, ἅπαν ἐκκενούμενον τὸ καθ᾽ ὅλον
A8   τὸν ὄγκον αἷμα. μάχεται δ᾽ ὡς ἐδείξαμεν οὐ τοῖς καὶ τὰς
ἀρτηρίας αἷμα περιέχειν φάσκουσιν, ἀλλ᾽ Ἐρασιστράτῳ τε καὶ
τοῖς οἰομένοις ὄργανα τοῦ ζωτικοῦ πνεύματος ὑπάρχειν αὐτάς.
ἀναγκαῖον γὰρ ἔσται βελόνῃ τρωθείσης τῆς εἰρημένης ἀρτηρίας
5 πρῶτον μὲν ἐκκενοῦσθαι τὸ ζωτικὸν πνεῦμα πᾶν, ἔπειτα δὲ
εἰς ἁπάσας τὰς ἀρτηρίας αἷμα μεταχεῖσθαι· τὸ δὲ πάντων
δεινότατον, ὅτι καὶ εἰς αὐτὴν τὴν ἀριστερὰν κοιλίαν τῆς καρδίας.

---

11 ταύτ(ας) L: ταύτην Va: hasce i
13 πν(εύματο)ς L: πνεύμονος V ἐξίκηται Alb: ἐξεικητ(αι) L: ἐξεικῆται V:
    ἐξικνῆται a
15 ἑπόμενον Ka: μένον LV: μόνον a
16 κάτ(ω) La: κατὰ V
18 κατὰ om. Va ἀπὸ τ(ῶν) L: ἀπὸ τοῦ Va
19 τὴν ante προτ. deleri iubet Ka: in codicis L margine corruptelae signum ad-
    scriptum est
19-20 τὴν κατὰ add. Alb
20 καὶ add. c οὕτω Corn: οὔπ(ω) LVa

from which it itself arises, it is perfectly clear that both the left
ventricle of the heart and each of those mentioned will be emptied along with the one that passes through the armpit. Since
from one of them all those through the neck and in the head
arise, and from the other those to the rest of the body, it is clear
that they will necessarily be emptied at the same time, right up
to their extremities. But as soon as the emptying of the pneuma
has reached the ends of the arteries, it will happen that blood is
transfused through the anastomoses out of the veins into the
arteries themselves; and, following upon the evacuated pneuma,
the blood from the lower members of the body will reach the
artery along the spine and the heart, and so / finally the axilla; K714
while that which comes from the vessels in the head will first
reach the artery which leads upward, and then that in the neck
and the pierced artery. Thus also the blood distributed throughout all the arteries of the arm, following the pneuma, will flow to
the pierced artery; and in this way the blood throughout the
whole mass[21] will flow toward the puncture.

3. But this, indeed, is entirely true; for the blood of the
whole body is seen to be emptied out through any one artery
whatever among those of any size, unless you / prevent the A8
flow in them. This, however, is an objection, as we have shown,
not against those who believe blood to be contained in the
arteries as well [as in the veins], but against Erasistratus and
those who think they [the arteries] are organs of the vital
pneuma. For it must necessarily be the case [if what Erasistratus
says is true] that if the aforesaid artery is pierced with a needle,
first the whole of the vital pneuma will be emptied out, second
that blood will be transfused into all the arteries; the most
alarming of all being that it will flow even into the left ventricle

---

23 καθόλ(ον) L: *distinxit* a: καθόλου V
25 γὰρ *Corn*: δὲ LVa: *enim* wr: *quippe* t
A8
1 καὶ *Alb*: κατὰ LVa
1–2 contineri w: *voluit igitur* κατὰ τὰς ἀρτηρίας ... περιέχεσθαι
3 οἰομένοις L: οἰκείοις Va
6 μετοχεῖσθαι LVa: *corr.* b

157

εἶτα πῶς οὐκ ἐπνίγη τὸ ζῷον αἵματος ἐμπλησθείσης τῆς κοιλίας /
K715   ταύτης ἢ οὐκ ἀπέθανεν ἔμπροσθεν, ἡνίκ' ἐ[κ]κενοῦτο τὸ πνεῦμα
10 τὸ ζωτικόν, ἢ τὰς τῶν μυῶν κινήσεις οὐκ ἀπώλεσεν ἢ τὰς
αὐτῶν τῶν ἀρτηριῶν οὐκ ἐβλάβη ἢ πυρετὸς οὐκ ἠκολούθησεν
αὐτῷ; πάντα γὰρ ταῦτα ἀναγκαῖον ἦν συμπίπτειν κατὰ τὸν
Ἐρασίστρατον οὕτως, ὅτε μήτε τὰς κινήσεις τῶν ἀρτηριῶν
ὑπελάμβανε τεταγμένας διαμεῖναι δύνασθαι μήτε τὴν τοῦ
15 πνεύματος χορηγίαν ἐν ἅπασι τοῖς μορίοις ἀκώλυτον, ὅταν μὴ
κεναὶ παντελῶς αἵματος ὑπάρχωσιν, ἕπεσθαί τε πυρετὸν ἐξ
ἀνάγκης, ὅταν εἰς τὰς ἐντὸς τῶν βουβώνων καὶ μασχαλῶν
ἀρτηρίας αἵματος παρέμπτωσις γένηται. καὶ μὴν οὐδὲν τούτων
φαίνεται συμπῖπτον τῷ ζῴῳ.

    4. πειραθῆναι δ' ἔστι παντὶ τῷ
20 βουλομένῳ, καθότι καὶ ἡμεῖς ἐπειράθημεν πολλάκις τρώσαντες
τὴν προειρημένην ἀρτηρίαν. οὐ χαλεπῶς δὲ ἐξευρήσεις αὐτὴν
καὶ πρὶν γυμνῶσαι τὸ δέρμα τῷ σφυγμῷ τεκμαιρόμενος· δια-
σημαίνει γὰρ ἡ κίνησις ἐν μὲν τοῖς ἰσχνοῖς ζῴοις ἐπὶ πλέον,
ἐν δὲ τοῖς πίοσιν <ἐπ' ἔλαττον> πλησίον τοῦ κατ' ὀλέκρανον
25 ἄρθρου. ταύτην τοίνυν εἴπερ ἂν διασημαίνῃ, τίτρωσκε ἢ
K716 / A9 γραφεῖον ὀρθὸν καθεὶς / ἢ βελόνην ἤ τι τῶν ἰατρικῶν μαχαι-
ρίων τῶν ἰσχνῶν ἤ τι τῶν παραπλησίων ὀργάνων ὅσα βραχεῖαν
δύναται ποιῆσαι τὴν διαίρεσιν, ἵνα τά τ' ἄλλα πάνθ' ὅσα πρόσθεν
εἴρηται κατὰ τὸν τόπον ἀποδείξῃς αὐτὸν καὶ ὡς οὐδὲν οὔθ'
5 αἱ τῶν ἀρτηριῶν κινήσεις οὔθ' αἱ τῶν μυῶν παραβλάπτονται.

    5. μὴ τοίνυν ὅτι μεγάλης ἀρτηρίας τιτρωσκομένης ἀνάγκη ταῦτα
συμβαίνειν, ἀλλὰ καὶ μικρᾶς τῆς τυχούσης καὶ τοῦ δέρματος
μόνον· καὶ γὰρ τοῦτο βούλεται πλέγμα τῶν τριῶν ἀγγείων

---

8 ἐπνίγ(η) L: ἐπενέγκη V: ἐπεπνίγη a
9 ἐκκενοῦτ(ο) LVa: ἐξεκ. c: corr.
10 ἀπώλεσεν Alb: ἀ^{πλ'} L: ἀπέλειπεν Vc: ἀπέλοιπεν a
14 μήτε Alb: μὴ δὲ LVa
15 ὅταν ... ὑπάρχωσιν Ka: ὅτι ... ὑπάρχουσιν LVa
16 κε^{Ν '} L: κενωτικὰ Va: κενὰ vel κενούμενα Corn (post κενὰ littera erasa, fort. a Cornario ipso)
17 τ(ὰς) L: τὸ Va
18 τούτ(ων) La: τούτου V
22 τῶν σφυγμῶν Va
24 ἐπ' ἔλαττον add. Alb

of the heart. Then how is it that the animal was not stifled, when blood had filled this / ventricle? Or why did it not die K715 before, when the vital pneuma was being emptied out? Or why did it not lose the movements of its muscles? Or why did it not suffer damage to the movements of the arteries themselves? Or fever follow upon it? For all these things should have happened thus, according to Erasistratus, since he assumed that neither could the movements of the arteries remain regular, nor the supplying of the pneuma in the members remain unhindered, when they are not totally free of blood; and fever must necessarily supervene whenever an infusion of blood into the arteries within the groin and armpits occurs.[22] But nothing of all this is seen to occur to the animal.

4. Anyone who wishes can test this for himself, as we have often done, piercing the aforementioned artery. You will have no difficulty in finding it, even before the removal of the skin, taking the pulse as an indication: the movement reveals it more plainly in thin animals, less so in fat ones, near the joint at the top of the forearm. Puncture this artery, then, if it does show itself, / by lowering point downwards either / a scriber or a A9 / K716 needle or one of the fine knives of the physicians, or any similar instrument, of such a size as to be able to make the wound small, so that you may be able to demonstrate on the spot all the other things that have been mentioned, and particularly that neither the movements of the arteries nor those of the muscles suffer incidentally in any way.

5. Now, let alone the necessity of these things happening when a great artery is pierced, it is so also when any little one whatever or even only the skin is pierced. For he [Erasistratus] wants to say that the skin is a network of the three types of

<hr/>

25 ταύτ(ην) L: ταύτῃ Va Δ.ὄ/(=διασημαίνῃ) L (cf. l. 22–23 Δ.ὄ/=διασημαίνει L): δεήσῃ Va τίτρωσκ(ε) L: τίτρωσις V: τιτρώσεις a
A9
1 γραφίον Va: L sine accentu: corr. c ὀρθὸν καθεὶς conj. Alb: ὀρθ̓καθεις L: ὀρθώσας ᾧ καθιεὶς V: ὀρθώσας καὶ καθιεὶς a: nihil auxilii in vers. Arab.
3 τὲ τὰ ἄλλα LV: τὰ τἄλλα a: corr. c
4 αὐτὸν Furley: αὐτ(ῶν) LVa
8 καὶ L: οὐ Va

ὑπάρχειν, ὥστ' εἰ καθ' ὁτιοῦν αὐτοῦ μέρος νύξειας βελόνῃ
10 λεπτῇ, πάντως [ὡς] τὰ τρία γένη τῶν ἀγγείων τετρώσεται.
νυττέσθω τοίνυν τὸ κατὰ τὸν βραχίονα δέρμα τὸ ἐπικείμενον τῇ κατὰ
τὰς μασχάλας ἀρτηρίᾳ, εἶτ' ἐκκενούσθω τὸ διὰ τῆς ἀδήλου [μὲν]
πρὸς τὴν ὄψιν <ἀρτηρίας πνεῦμα>, ὅπερ Ἐρασίστρατος βούλεται
γίγνεσθαι τετρωμένης ἀρτηρίας [πνεῦμα], συνεκκενούσθω δ' αὐτῷ
15 καὶ τὸ συνεχὲς τὸ κατὰ τὴν ὑποκειμένην ἀρτηρίαν τὴν μεγάλην
τὴν διὰ τῆς μασχάλης. πάντῃ γάρ που τό γ' ἐπικείμενον τοῖς
μορίοις τοῦ σώματος δέρμα πρὸς τῶν ὑποκειμένων ἀρτηριῶν
ἀποφύσεις τινὰς λαμβάνει· ἀλλ' εἰ καὶ παρ' ἄλλων τινῶν, οὐδὲν
K717 ἐμοὶ / γοῦν διαφέρει. συνεκκενωθήσονται γὰρ αἵτινες ἂν ὦσι
20 ταῖς κατὰ τὸ δέρμα τιτρωσκομέναις συνεχεῖς, ἐκείναις δ' αἱ
λοιπαὶ πᾶσαι· ταῦτα γὰρ ἐδείχθη μικρῷ πρόσθεν. εἶτα πῶς
οὐκ ἄτοπον κἂν εἰ τῇ λεπτοτάτῃ βελόνῃ τρωθείη τὸ δέρμα,
εὐθὺς οὕτω πάσας μὲν ἐμπίμπλασθαι τὰς ἀρτηρίας αἵματος,
πυρετὸν δ' ἐξ ἀνάγκης ἕπεσθαι;

A10 5. Πρὸς ταῦτ' ἐγὼ μὲν ᾠόμην αὐτοὺς μήτ' ἀντι-
λέξειν μηδὲν μαθήσεσθαί τε τὰ κακῶς ἐγνωσμένα. οὐ μὴν
ἐθέλουσί γε, ἀλλ' ὥσπερ οἱ παντελῶς ἰδιῶται παλαισμάτων οὐ
γνωρίζοντες κείμενον ἐπὶ γῆς ἐνίοτε τὸν νῶτον αὐτῶν ἔχονται
5 τραχήλου τῶν καταβαλόντων οὐδ' ἐπιτρέποντες ἀναστῆναι, τὸν
αὐτὸν τρόπον καὶ οὗτοι ἀμαθεῖς ὄντες τῶν ἐν τοῖς λόγοις
πτωμάτων οὐκ ἐπιτρέπουσιν ἀπαλλάττεσθαι καινάς τινας ἀεὶ
στροφὰς στρεφόμενοι καὶ παντοίως λυγιζόμενοι μέχρι τοῦ
μισήσαντά τινα τήν τ' ἀναισχυντίαν ἅμα καὶ τὴν ἀμαθίαν αὐτῶν
10 ἀποδυσπετήσαντα χωρισθῆναι.

2. οἵ γε καὶ νῦν οὐκ αἰδοῦνται

---

9 ὑπάρχ(ειν) La: ὑπάρχει V   αὐτοῦ Furley: αὐτῶν codd.
10 παντ(ως) LVa: omnia i   ὡς delevit a   τιτρώσεται a
12-13 μὲν secl. et ἀρτηρίας πνεῦμα ins. Furley, vers. Arab. secutus: crucem posuit
  L (in marg.), Alb: v. comm.
14 πνεῦμα secl. Furley   αὐτ(ῷ) La: αὐτὸ V
19 αἵ τινες La: ὥς τινες V
20 τιτρωσκομέναις συνεχεῖς Ka: τιτρωσκομ(έ)ν(αις) συνεχέσιν L: τιτρωσκό-
  μενον συνεχέσιν Va   ἐκείνης LV: corr. a
24 πυρετ̊ (fort. = -τὸν) L: πυρετὸς V
A10
1 οἰόμην LVa: mutavit c   αὐτ(οὺς) L: αὐτὸ V: αὐτὸς a
2 μηδὲν Ka: μηδένα LVa

vessels,[23] so that in whatever part you prick it with a fine needle, the three kinds of vessels will be injured all together. Now, let the skin of the arm overlying the artery of the armpit be pricked, then let the pneuma of the invisible artery be emptied out, as Erasistratus will have it when an artery is injured;[24] and with it let the connected pneuma of the under-lying great artery of the armpit be emptied out. For everywhere the skin overlying the parts of the body receives branches from the underlying arteries; or if from some others [not immediately underlying that part of the skin], then / it makes no difference K717 to me; for whichever may be continuous with those vessels wounded in the skin will be emptied, and with them all the rest. This was proved in a passage not far back.[25] Then how can it fail to appear ridiculous that, if the skin is injured with the very finest needle, all the arteries should be filled with blood at once, and that fever should necessarily supervene? /

Chapter 5

Against these arguments I had supposed that they would raise A10 no objection, and would learn what they had misapprehended. However, they are not willing, but just as in wrestling complete amateurs sometimes do not understand that they have been floored, and hold the necks of those who have thrown them, not allowing them to rise;[26] in the same way these people, not hav-ing acquainted themselves with the falls of argument, will not let their opponents go, wriggling uselessly about and twisting and turning, until one detests both their shamelessness and their ignorance, becomes impatient, and takes himself off.

2. These people, even now, are not ashamed to say / that the K718

---

3 οἰδιῶτ(αι) L

4 κειμένον a: κειμένων LV   ἔχοντες LVa: corr. Corn

7 καινάς Cobetus Mnem. N.S. IX, 447: κενάς LVa: novos ... modos wt: novas ... circuitiones r

8 λυγιζόμενοι Cobetus l.c.: λογιζόμενοι LVa

9 μισήσαντ(ά) τινα τήν τ' L: μισήαντός τινά τήν τ' V: -ντός τινος τὴν a
   ἁμα L: ἀμάθιαν V

10 ἀποδυσπετήσαντ(α) L: -σαντες V Corn: -σαντας a: quousque aliquis ... cum illis loqui fastidiens t

K718 λέγοντες ὡς ἐκ / τῶν πλησίον μόνων συναναστομώσεων ἡ μετά-
ληψις ταῖς ἀρτηρίαις τοῦ αἵματος γίγνεται, μὴ μεμνημένοι μήθ'
ὅτι τὰς ἐσχάτας αὐτὸς Ἐρασίστρατος εἴρηκε κενοῦσθαι πρώτας
μήθ' ὅτι φαίνεται τοῦτ' ἐναργῶς ἐφ' ὧν αὐτὸς ἐκεῖνος ἔγραψεν
15 ἀνατομῶν. ἐν γὰρ τῷ διαιρεῖσθαι τὸ ἐπιγάστριον ἅμα τῷ
περιτοναίῳ κατὰ τὸ μεσεντέριον ἀρτηρίας ἰδεῖν ἔστι σαφῶς ἐπὶ
μὲν τῶν νεοθηλῶν ἐρίφων γάλακτος πλήρεις, ἐπὶ δὲ τῶν τελείων
ζῴων ἀλλοίας, οὐ μὴν πνεῦμά γε μόνον ὤφθησαν ἔχουσαι
πώποτε καθάπερ οὐδ' ἄλλη τις ἀρτηρία γυμνωθεῖσα. νομίζω
20 δ' αὐτοὺς εἰς τοσοῦτον ἀμαθεῖς εἶναι τῶν κατὰ τὰς ἀνατομὰς
φαινομένων, ὡς μηδ' αὐτὸ τοῦτο γιγνώσκειν, ὅτι καλῶς εἴρηκεν
ὁ Ἐρασίστρατος ἐσχατιὰς τὰς κατὰ τὸ μεσεντέριον ἀρτηρίας
παραβάλλων αὐτὰς δηλονότι ταῖς κατ' ἐπιγάστριον. οἴονται γὰρ
ἴσως, ὅτι τῇ θέσει πλησίον εἰσίν, οὕτω καὶ τῇ συνεχείᾳ πλησίον
25 ὑπάρχειν αὐτάς, οὐκ εἰδότες ὡς ἀπὸ τῆς ἐπὶ τῇ ῥάχει μεγάλης
K719 ἀρτηρίας ἑκάτεραι πεφύκασιν αἱ μὲν κατὰ / τὸ μεσεντέριον
A11 ἅπασαι, τῶν δὲ κατ' ἐπιγάστριον αἱ πλεῖσται. καίτοι καὶ αἱ ἀπὸ
βουβώνων ἀνιοῦσαι καὶ αἱ ἀπὸ τοῦ στέρνου κατιοῦσαι συνεχεῖς
εἰσι ταῖς κατὰ τὸ μεσεντέριον ἀρτηρίαις διὰ τῆς μεγάλης τῆς
κατὰ τὴν ῥάχιν. οὔκουν ἐνδέχεται διαδοθῆναι τὸ πάθος ἀπὸ
5 τῶν ἑτέρων ἐπὶ τὰς ἑτέρας, οὔτ' οὖν κένωσιν οὔτ' ἄλλ' οὐδέν,
μὴ διὰ τῆς ἐπὶ τῇ ῥάχει πρότερον ὁδοιπορῆσαν.

3. ᾧ γὰρ δὴ
ἔοικε μάλιστα, καὶ δὴ πειράσομαι φράσαι. νόησόν μοι τὴν μὲν
ἀρτηρίαν τὴν ἐπὶ τῇ ῥάχει καθάπερ τι δένδρου πρέμνον, τὰς
δ' ἀπ' αὐτῆς φυομένας οἷον κλάδους, ὅσαι δ' αὖθις σχιζόμεναι
10 τελευτῶσιν οἷον βλαστήματά τινα καὶ φύλλα. ὡς οὖν τὰ φύλλα
πολλάκις ἀπὸ διαφερόντων ὄντα κλάδων πλησίον μέν ἐστι τῇ
θέσει, πορρωτάτω δὲ τῇ πρὸς ἄλληλα συνεχείᾳ — διὰ μέσου γὰρ
ἑνοῦται τοῦ πρέμνου — τὸν αὐτὸν τρόπον καὶ αἱ κατ' ἐπιγάστριον ἀρτηρίαι ταῖς κατὰ μεσεντέριον ἐγγυτάτω κείμεναι διὰ

---

14 αὐτὸς om. V
18 γε Corn: τε LVa
20 ἅμα L: ἀμαθίας V: corr: a
21 αὐτ(ὸ) L: αὐτοὺς Va
26 μεσου V

162

transference of blood to the arteries occurs only from the near-by anastomoses;[27] remembering neither that Erasistratus himself said that the furthest parts of the arteries are emptied first, nor that this appears clearly from what he himself wrote on anatomy. For upon dividing the abdominal wall together with the peritoneum, it is possible to see plainly arteries running through the mesentery which, in the young kid, are seen to be full of milk;[28] while in the full-grown animals they are of various kinds, but never seen to contain merely pneuma, any more than any other exposed artery. Indeed I judge them to be so ignorant of the observed facts of anatomy that they do not know even this: that Erasistratus correctly called the arteries of the mesentery remote, comparing them, obviously, with the arteries of the abdominal wall. They appear to think that, because they are near to one another in position, therefore they are near to one another by being connected, not realizing that both arise from the great artery on the spine; those of / the mesentery / all arising from it, and most of those of the abdominal wall arising from it. Moreover, both those traveling upward from the groin and those traveling downward from the chest are in connection with the mesenteric arteries through the great artery along the spine. So it is not possible that the effect, whether it be emptying or anything else, should be transmitted from the ones to the others, unless it makes its way first through the one on the spine.

K719

A11

3. What this most resembles, I shall now attempt to state. I ask you to think of the artery on the spine as a tree trunk, and of those arteries that arise from it as branches, and those that spread out again at the ends as twigs and leaves.[29] Now, just as the leaves of different branches are often very close together in position, while they are very distantly connected (for they are united through the central trunk), so the arteries of the abdominal wall and those of the mesentery, lying very close together,

---

A11

1 καίτ(οι) L: καί τινες Va αἱ om. Va

9 ὅσαι δὲ αὖθις Corn: ἴσαι δ' αὗται LVa

11 ὄντ(α) L: ὄντων V: om. a

15 μακροτάτου συνάπτονται. εἰς οὖν τὰς ἐσχάτας ἀρτηρίας — τοῦτο
K720   γὰρ ἐξ ἀρχῆς ἐλέγετο — μεταχεῖται πρό/τερον <ἢ> εἰς τὰς ἄλλας
ἁπάσας τὸ αἷμα, καὶ διὰ τοῦτ’ ἀναγκαῖον, ἵν’ ἐπὶ τὰς τετρωμένας
ἀφίκηται, ἅπαν ἐκκενωθῆναι τὸ ζωτικὸν πνεῦμα. τοῦτο δ’ ὡς ἄτοπόν
ἐστιν, ἔμπροσθεν ἐδείχθη.

4. τάχ’ <ἂν> οὖν ἤδη τις θαυμάζοι
20 τε καὶ ζητοίη, πόθεν ἐπῆλθε συνετοῖς οὕτως ἀνδράσιν ἄτοπον
ἐσχάτως προελέσθαι δόγμα. οὐ γὰρ δὴ ἀπ’ ὄνου γε κατα-
πεσόντες, ἀλλὰ πάντως ὑπό τινων πιθανῶν ἀναπεισθέντες ἐπὶ
τοῦθ’ ἧκον. ὑφ’ ὧν μὲν οὖν ἐπείσθησαν, αὐτοὶ διὰ τῶν ἰδίων
δηλώσουσι γραμμάτων. ὅτι δὲ πιθανοῖς μέν, οὐ μὴν καὶ
25 ἀληθέσιν ἠκολούθησαν λογισμοῖς, ἐγὼ πειράσομαι δεῖξαι, πρότε-
ρόν γε τὸ καθόλου περὶ πάντας τοὺς λογισμοὺς σφάλμα διὰ
βραχέων ὑπομνήσας.

5. ἁπάντων γὰρ τῶν εἰς γνῶσιν ἀνθρωπίνην
ἠκόντων τὰ μὲν αἰσθήσει, τὰ δὲ λόγῳ φωρᾶται. καὶ τοίνυν
ὥσπερ τὰς αἰσθήσεις πολλὰ τῶν αἰσθητῶν διαφεύγει κατὰ πολλὰς
A12   αἰτίας, οὕτω καὶ τὸν λόγον. ὁ μὲν δὴ φιλαλήθης ἀνὴρ οὔτε
τῶν ἐναργῶς γιγνωσκομένων ἀφίσταται διὰ τὴν τῶν ἀδήλων
K721   ἀγνωσίαν οὔτε τοῖς ἀγνώστοις / συγκατατίθεται διὰ τὴν τῶν
ἐναργῶν γνῶσιν, ὁ δὲ μὴ τοιοῦτος ἢ τοῖς ἀδήλοις συνηπόρησε
5 τὰ γιγνωσκόμενα ἢ διὰ ταῦτα καὶ τὸ ἄδηλον προσήκατο.
πεπόνθασι δὲ τὸ μὲν πρότερον οἱ Σκεπτικοί, τὸ δὲ δεύτερον
οἱ πλεῖστοι τῶν Δογματικῶν. πῶς μὲν οὖν ἄν τις μηδὲν τοιοῦτον σφάλλοιτο, δι’ ἑτέρων δεδήλωται.

6. Νυνὶ δὲ τοῖς περὶ τὸν Ἐρασίστρατον ἐνδείξα-
10 σθαι τὸ σφάλμα πειράσομαι. οὐ γὰρ ἐξ οἰκείων ἀποδείξεων
αἵματος κενὰς τὰς ἀρτηρίας ἀπεφήναντο, ἀλλ’ ἐξ ὧν ἠπόρησαν
ἐν ἑτέροις ἀπιστήσαντες τῷ ἐναργεῖ, παραπλήσιόν [ὂν] τι πα-
θόντες <τοῖς> τὴν κίνησιν ἀνελοῦσιν, ὅτι τὸν κατ’ αὐτῆς λόγον

---

15 εἰ Va
16 μαχεῖται V   ἢ add. b: quam w
18 πνεῦμα b in marg.: αἷμα LVa
19 ἂν add. Alb
21 ἀπ’ ὄνου Alb: ἀπὸ νοῦ LVa
22 πάντες Va
23 ὑφ’ Alb: ἀφ’ LVa
24 καὶ om. Va
26 πάντ(ας) L: πάντων Va

are united at a very considerable distance. So it is into the furthermost arteries (as was said at first) that the blood is transfused before / it flows into any of the others; hence it must be K720 that for it to arrive at the injured ones the vital pneuma must be totally emptied out. But that this is absurd has been proved above.

4. Probably someone will be amazed and will desire to find out how it has occurred to such sensible men to favor such an extremely absurd opinion.[30] For indeed they have not "fallen from a donkey,"[31] but have all come to this opinion misled by plausible notions. By what they were persuaded, they shall themselves display in their own writings. But that they have followed reasonings which, though plausible, are not correct, I shall attempt to prove, first calling to mind in a few words the general mistake to which all arguments are liable.

5. Of all those things that come to human knowledge, some are discovered by sense and others by reason. Now, just as many sensible things escape the senses from many / causes, so A12 it is with reason. But he who loves the truth neither rejects those things that are clearly known because of his ignorance of what is unknown, nor gives his assent to / what is unknown K721 because of his knowledge of what is clear. He who is not of this character either has doubts about what is known along with what is not clear, or because of what is known believes what is not clear. The first happens to the Sceptics, the second to most of the Dogmatics. How one may avoid both these pitfalls I have shown in another place.[32]

Chapter 6

Now I will attempt to show those who follow Erasistratus their error. They have not demonstrated that the arteries are empty of blood from proper proofs, but have come to doubt the obvious from their perplexity in other matters—suffering much

---

29 καταφεύγει Va   κατά τὰς π. Va

A12

  5 ταῦτα Alb: τοῦτο LVa

  6 πεπόνθ(α)σ(ι) La: πεπόνθεσαν V

12 ἐναργ(εῖ) L: ἐναργῶς Va   ὄν τ(ι) LV: corr. a

13 τοῖς suppl. k   αὐτ(ῆς) L: αὐτὸν V: αὐτῶν a   κίνησιν L: κένωσιν Va

ἠπόρησαν διαλύσασθαι. βέλτιον δ' οἶμαι τὴν μὲν κίνησιν ὡς
15 ἐναργὲς πρᾶγμα τιθέναι, τὸν δὲ κατ' αὐτῆς λόγον ἐπὶ σχολῆς
πειρᾶσθαι διαλύεσθαι, ὡσαύτως δὲ καὶ τὰς ἀρτηρίας ὅτι μὲν
αἷμα περιέχουσιν ἐκ τοῦ κἂν <εἰ τῇ> λεπτοτάτῃ τρωθεῖεν βελόνῃ
K722 παραχρῆμα φαίνεσθαι προ/χεόμενον αὐτὸ συγχωρεῖν, διὰ τί δὲ
μηδὲν ἡ φύσις εἰκῇ ποιοῦσα διττὸν ἀγγείων γένος ἐδημιούρ-
20 γησεν μιᾶς ὕλης περιεκτικὸν ἰδίᾳ ζητεῖν· οὕτω δὴ καὶ τὸ πῶς
εἰς ἅπαν τὸ σῶμα κομισθήσεται τὸ διὰ τῆς εἰσπνοῆς ἑλκόμενον
πνεῦμα τῶν ἀρτηριῶν αἷμα περιεχουσῶν ἢ μὴ κομιζομένου
πῶς αἱ κατὰ προαίρεσιν κινήσεις ἔσονται ἢ πῶς ἡ κατ' αὐτὰς
τὰς ἀρτηρίας κίνησις ἀπαραπόδιστος μενεῖ μὴ δυναμένου
25 συνοικεῖν ἀμάχως πνεύματος ὑγρῷ. τὰ γὰρ τοιαῦτα προβλή-
A13 ματα μέν ἐστιν ἰδίᾳ τε καὶ καθ' ἑαυτὰ προβάλλεσθαί τε καὶ
ζητεῖσθαι δίκαια καὶ τάχ' ἂν τῷ καὶ ἄπορα νομισθέντα, οὐ
μὴν ἱκανά γε τὸ ἐναργὲς ἀνατρέπειν.

2. αὐτίκα γέ τοι τὸ πρῶτον
<ὑπ'> αὐτῶν εἰρημένον ὁμοιότατόν ἐστιν ὡς εἰ καί τις ἐν τοῖς
5 μηρυκάζουσι ζῴοις θεασάμενος πλέονας κοιλίας τὴν μὲν τῆς
τροφῆς ὑποδεκτικὴν εἶναι λέγοι, τὴν δὲ τοῦ πόματος, τὴν δὲ
τοῦ πνεύματος· οὐ γὰρ τὴν μηδὲν εἰκῇ ποιοῦσαν φύσιν ὑπο-
δοχῆς ἕνεκα μιᾶς ὕλης πολλὰς ἐργάσασθαι τὰς γαστέρας. ὡς
K723 γὰρ κἀνταῦθα χρεία τίς ἐστιν / ἑτέρα δι' ἣν αἱ πολλαὶ γεγόνασιν
10 καίτοι τὴν αὐτὴν ὕλην ὑποδεχόμεναι, οὕτως ἔχει καὶ περὶ τῶν
ἀρτηριῶν καὶ τῶν φλεβῶν. αἷμα γὰρ ἀμφότεραι περιέχουσιν
ὡς ὁ πρόσθεν λόγος ἀπέδειξεν, διάφοροι δὲ τῇ κατασκευῇ
γεγόνασι χρείας τινὸς ἕνεκεν, ἣν ἐν ἑτέροις ὑπομνήμασι διέξιμεν.
K724.5 /
A14.2 3. ἀλλὰ πῶς, φασίν, εἰς ὅλον τὸ σῶμα κομισθήσεται τὸ
διὰ τῆς ἀναπνοῆς ἑλκόμενον πνεῦμα τῶν ἀρτηριῶν αἷμα

---

15 αὐτῆς Alb: αὐτοὺς L, in marg. crux: αὐτὸν V: αὐτῶν a
                      θ'
17 εἰ τῇ supp. Alb   τρωθεῖεν a: τρω L: τρωθῆναι V   βελώνης V
19 διττῶν ἀγγ. μέρος L: διὰ τῶν ἀγγ. μέρος V: διττὸν τῶν ἀγγ. γένος a: corr.
   Alb
22 κομιζόμ(ε)ν(ον) L: κομιζομένων Va
24 μενεῖ Furley: μένει edd.   δυναμ(έ)ν(ον) L: δυναμένης Va
25 πν(εύματ)ος LV: πνεύματι a
A13
  1 ἴδια LVa: corr. Alb: privatim w
  2 τῷ καὶ ἄπορα νομισθέντ(α) L: τῷ καὶ ἄπειρα νομισθέντι Va
  3 μὴν γε ἱκανά γε L

the same fate as those who did away with motion because they were perplexed as to how to refute the argument against motion.[33] A better course, I believe, was to accept motion as an obvious fact, and try at leisure to refute the argument against it. Similarly, it is better, in the case of the arteries, to agree that they contain blood, from the fact that blood is seen / to pour K722 from them at once even if they are pierced with the finest needle, and then enquire separately why Nature, who does nothing in vain,[34] has contrived a double class of vessels to contain one single matter—and then this also, how the pneuma drawn in through respiration will be conveyed to the whole body, if the arteries contain blood; or, if it is not so conveyed, how the voluntary motions will take place; or how its motion in the arteries themselves will remain unimpeded, if pneuma cannot coexist amicably with a liquid. For such / problems as these A13 are worthy to be raised and investigated separately and by themselves; and it may be that they are thought perplexing by some, but nevertheless they are not sufficient to upset the obvious.[35]

2. Well now, the very first thing they have said is exactly as if someone considering the many stomachs of ruminants were to say that the first is to receive food, the second drink, and the third pneuma, since Nature, who does nothing in vain, did not make the many stomachs for the reception of one single matter.[36] For as in this case there is another / use for which the K723 many stomachs have come into being, although they receive the same matter, so also in the case of the arteries and the veins. Both contain blood, as the previous argument demonstrated, but they have come to be differently constituted, for a use which I have explained in another book.[37] /

3. But how, they ask,[38] will the pneuma drawn in through breathing be conveyed to the whole body, if the arteries contain A14.2 / K724.5

---

4 < > Furley τις ἐν τοῖς Alb: τοῖς ἐν τοῖς L: τοῖς Va: quis interpr.

6 πόματος a: σωμάτος LV

7 μηδενὶ L

10 καίτοι γε Va

13 διέξιμεν k (nunc vers. Arab. conf.): διέξειμ(ι) L: διέξειμεν Va

A14.2 ἀλλὰ πῶς — 16 ὅπως [αἱ κατὰ προαίρεσιν] huc transposuit Furley, ex post 14.2 αἵματος μεστάς, vers. Arab. secutus: v. comm.

περιεχουσῶν; τίς δ' ἀνάγκη τοῦτο γίγνεσθαι; δύναται γὰρ
5 ἅπαν ἀντεκπνεῖσθαι καθάπερ τοῖς πλείστοις τε καὶ ἀκριβεστά-
τοις ἔδοξεν ἰατροῖς τε ἅμα καὶ φιλοσόφοις, οἳ μὴ τῆς οὐσίας
ἀλλὰ τῆς ποιότητος αὐτοῦ δεῖσθαί φασι τὴν καρδίαν ἐμψύχεσθαι
ποθοῦσαν καὶ ταύτην εἶναι χρείαν τῆς ἀναπνοῆς. λαμβάνουσιν
οὖν οἱ περὶ τὸν Ἐρασίστρατον κἀνταῦθα τὸ ζητούμενον· αὐτὸ
10 πρὶν ἀποδεῖξαι, δέον αὐτὸ τοῦτο πάλιν ἰδίᾳ ζητεῖν ὥσπερ ἡμεῖς
πεποιήκαμεν καὶ πάντες ὅσοι τάξει περὶ τῶν πραγμάτων
σκοποῦνται μὴ πάντα ὁμοῦ ζητοῦντές τε καὶ ταράττοντες.

K725   ἀποδέδεικται δ' / ἡμῖν ἐν τῷ Περὶ χρείας ἀναπνοῆς, ὡς ἤτοι
παντελῶς ὀλίγον ἢ οὐδὲν ὅλως τῆς τοῦ πνεύματος οὐσίας εἰς
15 τὴν καρδίαν μεταλαμβάνεται.

4. τὰ δ' αὐτὰ διαμαρτάνουσι κἂν
τῷ   προβάλλειν   ὅπως   [αἱ   κατὰ   προαίρεσιν]
K723.6 /   αἱ κατὰ προαίρεσιν ἔσονται κινήσεις ἢ πῶς αἱ τῶν
A13.14   ἀρτηριῶν τεταγμέναι φυλαχθήσονται καὶ πῶς ἀμαχὶ δύναται
συνεῖναι τὸ αἷμα τῷ πνεύματι. ὥσπερ γὰρ ὁμολογούμενον
λαμβάνοντες τὸ δεῖν ἀπὸ τῆς καρδίας αὐταῖς ἐπιπέμπεσθαι τὸ
πνεῦμα τὰ λοιπὰ συμπεραίνουσιν οὐκ εἰδότες ὡς καὶ τοῦτ'
αὐτὸ μοχθηρόν ἐστι καὶ ῥᾳδίως ὅπῃ παρακρούεται φωραθῆναι
20 δύναται.

5. γυμνοῦντες οὖν ἡμεῖς ἑκάστοτε μεγάλας ἀρτηρίας ἃς
ἐνδέχεται — μάλιστα δ' ἐνδέχεται τὰς κατὰ κῶλα — τοὺς
Ἐρασιστρατείους ἐρωτῶμεν, εἰ κἂν νῦν γοῦν, ὁπότε γεγύμνων-
ται, δοκοῦσιν αὐτοῖς ἔχειν αἷμα. οἱ δ' ἐξ ἀνάγκης ὁμολογοῦσιν
K724   ἅμα μὲν ὅτι καὶ / αὐτὸς Ἐρασίστρατος ἐν αὐτῷ τῷ διαιρεῖσθαι
A13.25   τὸ   δέρμα   παρέμπτωσιν   αἵματος   εἰς   τὰς
ἀρτηρίας γίγνεσθαί φησιν, ἅμα δ' ὅτι καὶ τὸ φαινόμενον οὕτως
ἔχει. βρόχῳ γὰρ ἡμεῖς ἑκατέρωθεν τὰς γεγυμνωμένας ἀρτηρίας
A14.1   διαλαμβάνοντες,   εἶτ'   ἐκτέμνοντες   τοὖν   μέσῳ
δείκνυμεν   αἵματος   μεστάς.   <ὁμολογησάντων

---

6 οἵ La: οἷον V
12 σκοποῦνται μὴ πάντα Furley, vers. Arab. secutus (v. adn. 38): σκοπούμενοι
καὶ πάντες codd.   ταράττοντες sugg. DeLacy, vers. Arab secutus: πράττοντες
codd.
16 ὅπως: ὥπως a   αἱ κατὰ προαίρεσιν secl. Furley: v. comm.
A13.14 αἱ κατὰ προαίρεσιν κτλ post 13.13 διέξιμεν habent codd: lacunam stat.
edd.

blood? But what is the necessity that this should occur? For it [the pneuma] can all be breathed out again, as indeed has been the opinion of the majority of both physicians and philosophers and the most accurate of them, who say that the heart requires not the substance but the quality of the pneuma, since it needs to be cooled, and that this is the use of breathing.[39] So here too the Erasistrateans assume the very thing that is to be discovered, before proving it, though what they ought to do is look into this question itself again separately, as we have done and as all those have done who investigate things in due order without mixing up all their enquiries together in confusion.[40] We have shown / in *The Use of Breathing*[41] that either very little or none at all of the substance of the pneuma is transmitted to the heart. K725

4. They make the same mistake also in raising the problem of / how the voluntary motions will exist, or how the movements of the arteries will be preserved in good order and how blood can associate with pneuma without conflict.[42] For they take it for granted that the pneuma must be transmitted to the arteries from the heart, and then infer the rest, not realizing that this itself is wrong, and can easily be detected as leading into error. A13.14 / K723.6

5. On each occasion, then, we expose large arteries that are able to be exposed—especially those in the limbs—and we ask the Erasistrateans if they agree that they contain blood at least at this time, when they are exposed.[43] They agree of necessity, first because / Erasistratus himself says that there is a flow of blood into the arteries at the very moment of cutting the skin, and second because the observed fact is so—for we tie the exposed arteries in two places, / and then cut out the middle and show that it is full of blood. So when they have agreed that K724 A14

---

22 ἐρασιστρατ(είους) La: ἐρασιστράτους V ἢ κἂν LVa: *corr.* c: εἰ καὶ *Fuchs* (*Philol. 1893, p. 375*)

24 ἅμα a: αἷμα LV ἐν αὐτῷ *Furley:* αὐτὰς ἐν LVa

25 ἐκ τὰς LV: ἐκ τῆς a: εἰς τὰς *Corn:* in arteriam r: in arterias it

A14.2 μεστάς Va: μεστόν L ὁμολογησάντων οὖν αὐτῶν ὅτι *ins. Furley, vers. Arab. secutus: v. comm.*

K725.5 /
A14.18

οὖν   αὐτῶν   ὅτι>   γεγυμνωμέναι   περιέχουσιν αἷμα, δείκνυμεν ἐφεξῆς κινουμένας αὐτὰς ἀπαρα-
20 ποδίστως οὐ πρὸς τὴν ἀφὴν μόνον, ἀλλὰ καὶ πρὸς τὴν ὄψιν,
εἶτα ἐπερωτῶμεν λόγον οὗ τὰ λήμματα καὶ πρὸς αὐτῶν ἐκείνων
ὡμολόγηται.

6. φασὶ γὰρ ἀληθὲς ὑπάρχειν τουτὶ τὸ συνημμένον·
"εἰ [δὲ] καὶ αἷμα περιέχουσιν αἱ ἀρτηρίαι καὶ παρὰ καρδίας
πληροῦνται πνεύματος, διαφθαρήσεται τῶν ἐν αὐταῖς κινήσεων
25 ἡ τάξις." αὐτὸ μὲν γὰρ καθ' ἑαυτὸ τὸ τοιοῦτον συνημμένον
"εἰ αἷμα περιέχουσιν αἱ ἀρτηρίαι, διαφθαρήσεται τῶν ἐν αὐταῖς
κινήσεων ἡ τάξις" οὔτ' ἐκεῖνοι τολμῶσιν ἀληθὲς εἶναι λέγειν
οὔτ' ἄλλος τις νοῦν ἔχων, δυναμένων γε δὴ τῶν ἀρτηριῶν οὐ
A15 διὰ τὸ πληροῦσθαι παρὰ τῆς καρδίας διαστέλλεσθαι, ἀλλ' ὅτι /
K726 διαστέλλονται, διὰ τοῦτο πληροῦσθαι. χρὴ τοίνυν προωμολο-
γῆσθαι τὸ παρὰ τῆς καρδίας αὐτὰς πληροῦσθαι πνεύματος, εἰ
μέλλει τὸ συνημμένον ἀληθὲς ἔσεσθαι. ἀμφοτέρων γὰρ τεθέντων
5 τοῦ τε περιέχειν αἷμα καὶ τοῦ παρὰ τῆς καρδίας πληρουμένας
διαστέλλεσθαι, τὸ διαφθείρεσθαι τῶν κατὰ φύσιν ἐν αὐταῖς
κινήσεων τὴν τάξιν ἐξ ἀνάγκης ἕπεται, θατέρῳ μόνῳ κατ'
οὐδεμίαν ἀνάγκην ἑπόμενον.

7. ἐρωτάσθω τοίνυν ὁ λόγος ἐπὶ
τῶν γεγυμνωμένων ἀρτηριῶν ὧδέ πως· "εἰ αἱ ἀρτηρίαι καὶ
10 αἷμα περιέχουσι καὶ παρὰ καρδίας πληρούμεναι διαστέλλονται,
διαφθαρήσεται τῶν ἐν αὐταῖς κινήσεων ἡ τάξις· ἀλλὰ μὴν οὐ
διαφθείρεται· φαίνεται γὰρ καὶ τοῦτο· οὐκ ἄρα καὶ αἷμα περιέχουσι καὶ παρὰ καρδίας πληρούμεναι διαστέλλονται." οἱ δέ γε
περὶ τὸν Ἐρασίστρατον καὶ τὰ δύο λήμματα καὶ τὸ συνημμένον
15 καὶ τὸ ἀντικείμενον τοῦ λήγοντος ἐν αὐτῷ προ<σ>ιέμενοι οὐκ
οἶδ' ὅπως οὐκέτι προσίενται τὸ συμπέρασμα, τυχὸν ἴσως
ἀγνοοῦντες ἅπερ οὐδὲ τοὺς ἐπιτυχόντας λέληθεν, ὡς ἐκ συνημ-
μένου καὶ τοῦ ἀντικειμένου τῷ εἰς ὃ λήγει τὸ ἀντικείμενον τοῦ
K727 ἡγουμένου / περαίνεται. ἡγουμένου δὴ κατὰ τὸν λόγον ὄντος

A14.18 γεγυμνωμέναι κτλ *post* 14.17 αἱ κατὰ προαίρεσιν *habent codd: lacunam
stat. edd.: v. comm.*
19 δείκνυμ(εν) L: δείκνυμι Va
23 δὲ *om.* Alb   παρὰ καρδ(ίας) La: περὶ καρδίαν V
A15
2–3 προωμολογεῖσθαι LV: προομολογεῖσθαι a: *corr.* Alb
5 τοῦ τὸ ᵉ *ut vid.* L

/ the exposed arteries contain blood,[44] we show in order, first, that they are moved without interruption not only to touch but also to sight, and then we raise an argument of which the premises are accepted by them also.

6. For they say the following conditional is true: "If the arteries contain blood, and they are filled with pneuma from the heart, then the order of their motions will be destroyed." For a conditional of the following kind, taken by itself, "if the arteries contain blood, then the order of their motions will be destroyed," neither they nor anyone else in his senses dares to call true, since it is always possible that the arteries are not expanded / through being filled from the heart, but on the contrary are filled / through being expanded. So it has to be conceded first that they are filled with pneuma from the heart, if the conditional is to be true. For if both premises are posited, that they contain blood and that they are expanded through being filled from the heart, the conclusion follows of necessity that the order of their natural motions is destroyed, though there is no necessity whatever that the conclusion should follow from one of these alone.

7. So the argument concerning the exposed arteries is to be propounded as follows: "If the arteries contain blood, and they are expanded through being filled from the heart, then the order of their movements will be destroyed. But it is not destroyed (this is evident). Hence it is not the case that they both contain blood and are expanded through being filled from the heart." The Erasistrateans, accepting the two premises[45] and the conditional and the contradictory of the consequent in it, incomprehensibly fail to accept the conclusion, perhaps through ignorance of what even the man in the street knows, namely, that from the conditional and the contradictory of its consequent, the contradictory of the antecedent / follows.[46] Well, the antecedent of the

---

6 τὸ Corn et interpretes: τῷ LVa

7 θάτερον μόνῳ ... ἐπόμ(ε)ν(ον) L: θατέρω μόνω ... ἐπομένην Va: corr. Corn: sim. interpretes

15 λήγοντος Ka (annal. philol. 1897 suppl. p. 687): λήμματος LVa: consequentis interpretes προιέμενοι LVa: corr. Corn

16 οὐδέ τι V

17 ὅπερ coniecit Ka l.c.: quod interpr. τῷ Ka l.c.: οὕτως LVa

20 οὐ μόνον τοῦ περιέχειν αἷμα τὰς ἀρτηρίας, ἀλλ' ὡς ἐδείχθη
μικρῷ πρόσθεν καὶ τοῦ παρὰ καρδίας πληρουμένας διαστέλλεσθαι, τὸ συμπέρασμα γενήσεται τῆς τούτων συμπλοκῆς ἀπο-
φα[ν]τικόν. ὅταν γὰρ ἐν συνημμένῳ τῷ ὅλῳ ἀξιώματι τὸ μὲν
ἡγούμενον ᾖ τι συμπεπλεγμένον, τὸ δὲ λῆγον ἀπλοῦν, εἶτα
25 προσληφθέντος <τοῦ ἀντικειμένου> τοῦ λήγοντος τὸ ἀντικείμενον
ἐξ ἀνάγκης περαίνεται τοῦ συμπεπλεγμένου.

A16   7. Πρὸς ταῦτ' οὖν οὐδὲν ἔχοντες λέγειν ὥσπερ
ἐπί τινα βωμὸν ἐλέου καταφεύγουσι τὴν Πυρρωνείαν ἀγροικίαν,
οὐκ ὀρθῶς ἔχειν φάσκοντες ὑποβαλέσθαι διαλεκτικαῖς περιεργίαις
ἰατρικὴν θεωρίαν. εἶθ' ἡμῶν ἐρωτώντων αὖθις αὐτούς, εἰ τοῖς
5 ὡμολογημένοις λήμμασιν ἐπιφέρειν ὁτιοῦν ἔξεστιν ἢ μέθοδός
τίς ἐστι καὶ τέχνη ἡ διδάσκουσα, τίνων ὁμολογηθέντων τί περαίνεται, πρὸς μὲν ταῦτ' οὐδὲν ἀποκρίνονται, μάχης δ' ἀπέρχονται.
K728   τί γὰρ / δὴ καὶ ἔχουσιν ἀποκρίνασθαι νοῦν ἔχον; ἀρά γ' ὡς
οὐκ ἔστιν οὐδεμία μέθοδος, ἀλλ' ἔξεστιν ἁπλῶς ἐπιφέρειν ὁτιοῦν
10 τοῖς δοθεῖσι λήμμασιν ἢ ὡς ἔστι μέν, οὐ χρηστέον δ' αὐτῇ πρὸς
τὰς ἀποδείξεις; ἀλλ' ἀμφότερα δεινῶς ἄτοπα. τὸ μὲν γὰρ
πρότερον εἰ φαῖεν, ὥσπερ οὖν ἤδη τις ἀναισχυντήσας ἀπετόλ-
μησεν εἰπεῖν, ἑξῆς γε ἀκούσονται παρ' ἡμῶν τοιούτους λόγους
οἵουσπερ κἀκεῖνος ἤκουσεν· "αἱ ἀρτηρίαι διχίτωνές εἰσιν, ἀλλὰ
15 καὶ τὸ αἷμα ξανθόν ἐστιν, οὐκ ἄρα πνεῦμα μόνον, ἀλλὰ καὶ
αἷμα περιέχουσιν αἱ ἀρτηρίαι." καὶ γελασάντων γε αὐτῶν
συνείροντες ἡμεῖς ἕτερον ἐπηνέγκαμεν λόγον τοιοῦτον· "οἱ κόρακες
μέλανές εἰσιν, ἀλλὰ καὶ οἱ κύκνοι λευκοί· οὐκ ἄρα πνεῦμα μόνον
ἐν ταῖς ἀρτηρίαις περιέχεται," καὶ πάλιν γελώντων τρίτον γε
20 τοιοῦτον· "τὸ πῦρ θερμόν ἐστιν, ἀλλὰ καὶ ἡ χιὼν ψυχρὰ καὶ
σὺ μωρός· οὐκ ἄρ' ἐνδέχεται πνεῦμα μόνον ἐν ταῖς ἀρτηρίαις

---

21 μικρῷ πρόσθεν] supra l. 2
22 τοῦτ(ων) L: τούτου Va
22-23 ἀποφαντικόν LVa: corr. Ka l.c.: negatio i: negans r
23 ὅταν L: ὅπερ Va
24 τὸ συμπεπληγμένον L: τὸ συμπεπλεγμένον Va: corr. Alb   λῆγον τό ἀπλοῦν
a
25 τοῦ ἀντικειμένου add. Corn: opposito (consequentis) assumpto interpretes
A16
  2 ἐλαίου LV: ἐλέους a: corr. Cobetus Mnemos. NS IX 447   πυρων(είαν) L:
πυρωνίαν Va: ρ add. c
  3 ὑπολαβέσθαι LV: ὑποβάλλεσθαι c   περιεργ(ίαις) L: περιέργοις Va
  4 εἰ a: ἐν LV

argument is not just that the arteries contain blood, but also (as was shown a little earlier) that they are expanded through being filled from the heart; so the conclusion will be the negation of this conjunctive proposition. For when in the whole conditional proposition the antecedent is a conjunctive proposition and the consequent is a simple proposition, when the contradictory of the consequent is posited also, the contradictory of the conjunctive proposition follows of necessity. /

Chapter 7

Having nothing to say to this, they escape as it were to an A16 altar of mercy in the form of Pyrrhonian boorishness,[47] saying that it is not right to submit medical theory to dialectical subtleties. When we then ask them again whether anything whatever can be inferred from the agreed premises, or is there a method and an art that teaches what conclusion may be drawn from what premises, they make no answer to this, but withdraw from the battle. For what / sensible answer can they give? That there is K728 no method, but anything whatever may be inferred from the given premises, or that there is a method but it must not be used in demonstrations? But both are monstrously absurd. For if they say the former, which indeed one person has already had the effrontery to say, they will in their turn hear such arguments from us as he heard: "The arteries are double-coated, but the blood is yellow, therefore the arteries contain not only pneuma but also blood." And when they had had their laugh, we went on and produced another argument: "Ravens are black, but swans are white, therefore there is not only pneuma in the arteries." Another laugh, and a third argument: "Fire is hot, but snow is cold, and you are a fool, therefore pneuma alone cannot be

---

5 ὁμολογουμένοις Va

6 τίνων] τι τῶν V

7 ἀπέρχονται Alb: ὑπάρχοντ(αι) L: ὑπάρχοντες V: ὑπαρχούσης a: eodem modo peccaverunt interpretes

8 νοῦν ἔχ(ον) ἐναργῶς L: νοῦν ἔχειν ἐναργῶς Va: οὐχὶ ἀρ' ὡς Corn: corr: Alb

10 ἢ om. Va αὐτ(ῇ) L: αὐτῷ Va

13 γε a: τε LV

18 πνεύματος V

19 γελῶ͞ν L: γελῶντες Va: corr. Alb

173

περιέχεσθαι." ἂν γὰρ ὅλως ἐξῇ τοῖς δοθεῖσι λήμμασιν ὁτιοῦν ἐπιφέρειν καὶ μηδεμία μέθοδος ᾖ τῆς τοῦ συμπεράσματος εὑρέσεως, τί κωλύει τοιούτους ἐρωτᾶσθαι λόγους;

2. ἐὰν δ' ᾖ τις

K729 / 25 τέχνη καὶ μέθοδος αἷσπερ / [ὁτιοῦν] διαγιγνώσκεται, τίνων ὁμολογηθέντων τί περαίνεται, πότερον ὁ μὴ γιγνώσκων αὐτὴν ἢ ὁ γιγνώσκων μέν, μὴ χρώμενος δὲ δοκεῖ σοι σωφρονεῖν

A17 μᾶλλον ἢ ὅστις γιγνώσκει καὶ κέχρηται; θαυμάζω δ' ὑμῶν, ὦ Ἐρασιστράτειοι, πῶς ὑμνοῦντες ἑκάστοτε τὸν Ἐρασίστρατον τὰ <τ'> ἄλλα καὶ ὡς Θεοφράστῳ συνεγένετο, φεύγειν τολμᾶτε τὰς λογικὰς μεθόδους, ὧν χωρὶς οὔτε Θεόφραστος οὔτ' Ἀρι-
5 στοτέλης ἐνεχείρουν τι γράφειν.

3. ταὐτά τινες αὐτῶν μόγις αἰδε-
σθέντες καὶ ὥσπερ ἐξ ὕπνου βαθέος ἐγερθέντες οὐκ ἔτ' ἀγροίκως τε καὶ ἀγρίως, ἀλλ' ἤδη λογικῶς τε καὶ ἀνθρωπίνως ἐπι-
στραφέντες ἐπεχείρουν διαλέγεσθαι· καὶ τί, φασί, πλέον ἂν περαίνοιτο πρὸς τοῦ λόγου τοῦ "οὐχὶ καὶ αἷμα ἔχουσιν αἱ
10 ἀρτηρίαι καὶ παρὰ καρδίας πληροῦνται πνεύματος;" καὶ ἡμεῖς ἤδη μὲν ἔφαμεν αὐτὸ τοῦτο κακῶς ὑμᾶς ἐπιφέρειν· "οὐκ ἄρα αἱ ἀρτηρίαι αἷμα περιέχουσι" μὴ γὰρ τοῦτ' εἶναι τὸ περαινόμενον,

K730 ἀλλὰ τὸ μὴ δύνασθαι συνδραμεῖν εἰς ταὐτὸν αἷμά / τε περιέχειν καὶ ταύτας καὶ παρὰ καρδίας πληροῦσθαι πνεύματος. ἐφεξῆς
15 δέ τοι πάλιν ἐκ τούτου [πο]τε καὶ τοῦ περιέχειν αὐτὰς αἷμα συνάγομεν· ἔσται γὰρ ὁ λόγος τοιοῦτος· "εἰ αἷμα περιέχουσιν αἱ ἀρτηρίαι, οὐ[κ ἄρα] παρὰ καρδίας πληροῦνται πνεύματος· ἀλλὰ μὴν αἷμα περιέχουσιν αἱ ἀρτηρίαι· οὐκ ἄρα παρὰ καρδίας πληροῦνται πνεύματος." ἐφ' ᾧ πάλιν εἰ βουληθείημεν, τῶν
20 ἔμπροσθεν ἀναμνήσαντες αὖθις ἐρωτήσαμεν <ἂν> ὧδε· "εἰ αἱ ἀρτηρίαι πλήρεις αἵματος ὑπάρχουσαι καὶ αὐταὶ σφύζουσι τεταγμένως καὶ τὰς ἀπ' αὐτῶν πεφυκυίας οὐ κωλύουσιν

---

22 ὅλ(ως) L: ὅλον Va

25 αἷσπερ a: ὥσπερ LV ὁτιοῦν om. Alb

A17

3 τὰ ἄλλα LV: τἄλλα a: corr. k

6 καὶ om. Va

8 ordinem verborum ἐπεχ. διαλ. et οὐκ ἔτ' — ἐπιστρ. in V turbatum restituit qui α β γ supascripsit

13 περιέχεσθ(αι) LVa: continere w: corr. Alb

14 ἐφεξῆς — 19 πνεύματος om. vers. Arab.

contained in the arteries." For if it is possible to infer anything whatever from the given premises, and there is no method for discovering the conclusion, what prevents the propounding of such arguments as these?

2. But if there is some art and method by which / it is deter- K729 mined what is the conclusion from what given premises, who seems to you most sensible—he who does not know it, or he who knows it but does not use it, / or he who knows it and A17 uses it? I am amazed at you, Erasistrateans, who always praise Erasistratus and particularly for his association with Theophrastus,[48] and dare to run away from logical methods, without which neither Theophrastus nor Aristotle undertook to write anything!

3. Some of them, feeling belated shame at this, as if woken from a deep sleep, put aside their boorish and fierce manner for a rational and humane one, and attempted to enter upon a dialogue. "What more could be concluded from your argument," they ask, "than[49] that it is not the case, both that the arteries contain blood, and that they are filled with pneuma from the heart?" We did indeed, say this very thing, that you [Erasistrateans] concluded wrongly, "Therefore the arteries do not contain blood," since that was not the conclusion, but that the two propositions could not stand together, namely, that / these vessels too contain blood, and that they are filled with K730 pneuma from the heart. However, we go straight on again with our inferences, from this and from the proposition that the arteries do contain blood. The argument will be as follows: "If the arteries contain blood, then they are not filled with pneuma from the heart. But they do contain blood. Therefore they are not filled with pneuma from the heart." Further to this, if we wish, we shall recall former points, and propose this argument: "If the arteries, being full of blood, both pulsate regularly and do not prevent those others which grow from them from pulsat-

---

15 ποτε LVa: corr. Ka   καὶ τὸ LVa: emendavit Corn
17 οὐκ ἄρα LV: corr. a
18 μὴ a
19 πληροῦντ(αι) La: πληροῦντες V
20 ἐρωτήσοιμεν L: -σομεν V: -σωμεν a: corr. Alb (cf. l. 25)   ἂν add. Alb
21 ὑπάρχουσαι Ka: ὑπάρχουσι LVa   αὗται LVa: corr. Alb
22 ταῖς LVa: corr. Corn   πεφυκυίας V: -κύας L: -κυίαις a

ὡσαύτως κινεῖσθαι, οὐ διὰ τὸ πληροῦσθαι παρὰ τῆς καρδίας
πνεύματος σφύζουσιν ἀλλὰ δι' ἄλλην αἰτίαν· ἀλλὰ μὴν τὸ
25 πρῶτον· τὸ ἄρα δεύτερον." ἐφεξῆς δ' ἂν αὖθις ἐρωτήσαιμεν
A18 ὡδί· "ἢ διὰ τὸ πληροῦσθαι τοῦ παρὰ καρδίας πνεύματος αἱ
ἀρτηρίαι διαστέλλονται ἢ ὅτι διαστέλλονται πληροῦνται· ἀλλὰ
μὴν οὐ τὸ πρῶτον· τὸ ἄρα δεύτερον" τῷ γὰρ εἶναί τινα δύναμιν
ἐν τοῖς χιτῶσιν αὐτῶν, ὑφ' ἧς διαστέλλονται, πᾶν ἕλκεται τὸ
5 συνεχὲς ἐκ παντὸς μέρους [αὐτῶν] ὅθεν ἂν ἐγχωρῇ.

4. νοήσαις /

K731 δ' ἂν ἔτι μᾶλλον ἐπὶ παραδειγμάτων τὴν διαφορὰν τοῦ πληρού-
μενον διαστέλλεσθαι καὶ διαστελλόμενον πληροῦσθαι. οἱ μὲν
γὰρ ἀσκοὶ καὶ οἱ θύλακοι πληρούμενοι διαστέλλονται, αἱ φῦσαι
δὲ τῶν χαλκέων διαστελλόμεναι πληροῦνται. τὰς τοίνυν ἀρτηρίας
10 ὅτι μὲν ἢ κατὰ τὸν πρότερον ἢ κατὰ τὸν δεύτερον τρόπον
ἀναγκαῖον πληροῦσθαι, παντὶ δῆλον. ὅπως δ' ἔχει τἀληθές,
ἐπιδέδεικται μὲν ἡμῖν καὶ δι' ἄλλων ὑπομνημάτων αὐτάρκως,
ἀτὰρ οὐχ ἥκιστα καὶ νῦν πέφανται τὸ διαστελλομένας αὐτὰς
ἕλκειν ἐκ παντὸς τοῦ πλησιάζοντος διὰ τῶν περάτων τε καὶ
15 τρημάτων ὅτι περ ἂν ἑτοιμότατα δύνηται πληρῶσαι τὴν διαστολὴν αὐτῶν. ἢ γὰρ τοῦτο πάντως ἢ θάτερον· ἐδείχθη δὲ
ψεῦδος ἐκεῖνο· δῆλον <οὖν> ὡς τοῦτ' ἀληθές.

8. Ὥσθ' ὅταν ἀπορῶσι, πῶς εἰς ὅλον τὸ σῶμα
παρὰ τῆς καρδίας κομισθήσεται τὸ πνεῦμα πεπληρωμένων
20 αἵματος τῶν ἀρτηριῶν, οὐ χαλεπὸν ἐπιλύσασθαι τὴν ἀπορίαν
αὐτῶν, μὴ πέμπεσθαι φάντας, ἀλλ' ἕλκεσθαι μήτ' ἐκ καρδίας
K732 μόνης, ἀλλὰ πανταχόθεν, ὡς Ἡροφίλῳ τε καὶ / πρὸ τούτου
Πραξαγόρᾳ καὶ Φιλοτίμῳ καὶ Διοκλεῖ καὶ Πλειστονίκῳ καὶ
Ἱπποκράτει καὶ μυρίοις ἑτέροις ἀρέσκει.

---

23 οὐ — 24 ἀλλὰ Furley, vers. Arab. secutus: ἢ — ἢ cett.: v. comm.
24 post μὴν add. οὐ Alb: μὴ vel οὐ Corn: atqui non primum w: negativum non
habet vers. Arab.
25 τὸ ἄρα LV: ἄρα τὸ a: eodem modo p. 18.3 ἐρωτήσωμεν LVa: corr. Alb
A18
1 ἢ Corn: εἰ LVa παρὰ καρδ(ίας) La: περικαρδίον V
3 τὸ γὰρ L: τὸ V: τῷ a: corr. Corn
4 perversus verborum χιτῶσιν — παραδειγμάτων (l. 6) ordo restituitur litteris α β
γ suprascriptis in V
5 aut αὐτῶν deleri aut <πλησιάζοντος> αὐτῶν (cf. l. 14) scribi iubet Ka
νοῆσαι LV: corr. a

ing likewise, then they pulsate not through being filled with pneuma from the heart but from some other cause. But the first. Therefore the second."[50] Continuing again we shall argue / thus: "Either the arteries are expanded through being filled with pneuma from the heart, or they are filled because they are expanded. But not the first. Therefore the second." For because there is a certain power in their coats through which they are expanded, all that is continuous is drawn in from every part, wherever it is possible.[51]   A18

4. You might grasp / the difference between being expanded through being filled and being filled through being expanded still better with the help of examples. Wineskins and bags are expanded through being filled; bronzesmiths' bellows are filled through being expanded. Now it is obvious to everyone that the arteries must be filled either in the first or in the second of these two ways. How the truth stands has been demonstrated by us independently elsewhere;[52] but the present argument is not the most insignificant proof that through being expanded they draw from their whole neighborhood, through their extremities and their pores, whatever can most readily fill their expanded size.[53] For either this is entirely true, or the other; but the other has been shown to be false; so clearly this is true.   K731

Chapter 8

Hence, when they are perplexed as to how the pneuma will be conveyed to the whole body from the heart if the arteries are full of blood, it is not hard to settle their perplexity by telling them that it is not driven but drawn, and not from the heart alone but from everywhere—as is the opinion of Herophilus and / before him Praxagoras, Philotimus, Diocles, Pleistonicus, Hippocrates, and innumerable others.[54]   K732

---

6 τοῦ om. Va

6–7 πληρώμ(ε)ν(ον) L ut vid.: πληρωμένου Va

7 διαστελλόμ(ε)ν(ον) L: διαστελλομένου Va

12 μέν om. Va

17 οὖν add. Alb

23 φιλοτίμῳ LVa: Φυλοτίμῳ Alb: cf. Kaibel, Athenaei dipnosoph. praef. XLI

24 ἱπποκράτ(ει) La: ἱπποκράτη V τε om. Va

2. ὅτι μέντοι τῆς δια-
25 στελλούσης τὰς ἀρτηρίας δυνάμεως οἷον πηγή τίς ἐστιν ἡ καρδία,
καὶ τοῦθ᾽ ἑτέρωθί τε πρὸς ἡμῶν ἐπιδέδεικται καὶ τοῖς προ-
A19 ειρημένοις ἅπασιν ἀνδράσιν ὡμολόγηται, καὶ πολλῷ φυσικώτερόν
ἐστιν οὕτω δοξάζειν ἢ ὡς διά τινων ἀψύχων σωμάτων ἡγεῖσθαι
φέρεσθαι δι᾽ αὐτῶν τὸ πνεῦμα· δυνάμεως γὰρ μεταλήψει τὸ
ζῷον τοῦ μὴ ζῶντος, οὐκ οὐσίας περιοχῇ διαφέρει.

3. ἀλλ᾽ οὐ
5 νῦν περί γε τούτων πρόκειται λέγειν οὐδ᾽ <ἵν᾽> ἐπεξέλθοιμι
τελέως τὸν λόγον ὑπηρξάμην αὐτοῦ — δέδεικται γὰρ ἐν ἑτέροις
ἱκανῶς περὶ τούτων καὶ μάλιστ᾽ ἐν τοῖς Περὶ τῶν Ἱπποκράτους
καὶ Πλάτωνος δογμάτων ὑπομνήμασιν —, ἀλλ᾽ ὑπὲρ τοῦ δεῖξαι,
τίσιν ἀπατηθέντες οἱ περὶ τὸν Ἐρασίστρατον οὕτως ἄτοπον
10 δόξαν προσήκαντο, καὶ τούτων τῶν δογμάτων ἠναγκάσθην
μνημονεῦσαι. καὶ νῦν ἔτι προσθεὶς αὐτοῖς ἕν τι τῶν ἐξ ἀνα-
K733 τομῆς φαινομένων ἐνταῦθά που καταπαύσω τὸν / λόγον.

4. ἔστι
δὲ τὸ φαινόμενον τόδε. τῶν προφανῶν τε ἅμα καὶ μεγάλων
ἀρτηριῶν εἰ ἐθελήσεις <ἥντιν>οῦν γυμνῶσαι πρῶτον μὲν τοῦ
15 δέρματος, ἔπειτα δὲ καὶ τῶν ὑποκειμένων τε καὶ παρακειμένων
σωμάτων, ὡς περ<ι>βάλλειν αὐτῇ δύνασθαι βρόχον καὶ μετὰ
ταῦτα κατὰ μῆκος χαλάσας κοῖλον ἐνθεῖναι κάλαμον ἤ τινα
χαλκοῦν αὐλίσκον εἴσω τῆς ἀρτηρίας διὰ τοῦ χαλάσματος ὡς
ἐπιφράττεσθαι πρὸς αὐτοῦ τὸ τραῦμα καὶ κωλύεσθαι τὴν αἱμορ-
20 ραγίαν, ἄχρι μὲν ἂν οὕτως ἔχουσαν ἐπισκέπτῃ, θεάσῃ σφύζουσαν
ὅλην, ἐπειδὰν δὲ βρόχον περιβαλὼν σφίγξῃς τὸν χιτῶνα τῆς
ἀρτηρίας πρὸς τὸν κάλαμον, οὐκ ἔτ᾽ ὄψει τὰ μετὰ τὸν βρόχον
ἐπισφύζοντα, καίτοι <γ᾽> ἡ τοῦ αἵματός τε καὶ τοῦ πνεύματος
φορὰ διὰ τῆς τοῦ καλάμου κοιλότητος ἐπὶ τὰ πέρατα τῆς
25 ἀρτηρίας ὡσαύτως ἐπιγίγνεται. καὶ εἴπερ οὕτως εἶχον αἱ
ἀρτηρίαι τὸ σφύζειν, ἔσφυζον ἂν καὶ νυνὶ τὰ πρὸς τοῖς πέρασιν
αὐτοῖς μόρια τὰ μετὰ τὸν βρόχον. οὐ μὴν γιγνόμενον <τούτου>, δή-

---

A19

1 ἢ om. V

5 τούτ(ων) L: τούτου Va: de his *interpretes, cf. l.* 7 ἵν᾽ add. a

11 ἕν τι a: ἕν τε LV

14 ἐθελήσει Va   ἥντιναοῦν a: οὖν LV   πρῶτον a: πρῶ L: πρώτην V

2. That the heart, however, is a source, as it were, of the faculty[55] that expands the arteries, has been shown elsewhere by us,[56] and has been / agreed by all the men mentioned above. Moreover it is a much more natural view than that the pneuma is taken through the arteries as through inanimate bodies;[57] for the living differs from the nonliving by its participation in faculties, not by its superiority in substance. A19

3. But this is not the time to speak of these things, nor did I raise the subject in order to carry the argument through to a conclusion (this has been dealt with sufficiently elsewhere, especially in *The Doctrines of Hippocrates and Plato*),[58] but for the sake of showing what has misled the Erasistrateans into such an absurd view; so I was compelled to mention these doctrines. I will now add to them a fact that appears in anatomy, and then end the / argument. K733

4. It is this. If you will expose any one of the large and obvious arteries, freeing it first from the skin and then from the matter that lies over it and around it, so as to be able to put a ligature round it; then open it along its length and insert a hollow reed or small bronze tube into the artery through the opening, so as to mend the wound with it and prevent hemorrhage; then so long as you study it in this condition, you will see the whole artery pulsating. But when you put a ligature round and press the coat of the artery against the reed, you will no longer see the part beyond the ligature pulsating, although the passage of the blood and the pneuma through the hollow of the reed proceeds as before to the end of the artery. If the arteries got their pulsation in this way, then even now pulsation would be continuing in the parts beyond the ligature near their ends. Since this does not happen, it is clear that the faculty that

---

16 ὥσπερ βάλλειν LV: corr. a

20 ἐπισκέπτ(η) L: ἐπισκέπτης Va

23 γ' inseruit Mueller scr. min. II praef. LXVI

26 πρὸ Va

27 αὐτῶν pro. Alb: αὐτοῖς LV

27–28 οὐ μὴν γιγνόμενα δῆλον ὡς ἡ μὲν δύναμις ἀτρεμείη οὐ κινεῖσθαι παρὰ τ. κ. codd.: ex vers. Arab. corr. Furley: v. adn. 57

K734 λον ὡς ἡ [μὲν] δύναμις ἡ τὰς ἀρτηρίας κινοῦσα παρὰ / τῆς καρδίας
A20 αὐταῖς διὰ [δὲ] τῶν χιτώνων ἐπιπέμπεται.

5. τὰ δ' ὑπ' Ἐρασι-
στράτου περὶ κινήσεως τῶν ἀρτηριῶν εἰρημένα ψευδῆ παντελῶς
ἐστιν. πρὸς γὰρ τῷ παύσασθαι τῆς γεγυμνωμένης ἀρτηρίας
τὴν κίνησιν ἐν τοῖς μετὰ τὸν βρόχον μέρεσιν, ὅπερ οὐκ ἐχρῆν
5 γίγνεσθαι, καὶ πρὸ τοῦ βρόχον αὐτῇ περιβαλεῖν ἔνεστι θεάσα-
σθαι πᾶσαν ἑνὶ χρόνῳ κινουμένην, οὐ τὸ μὲν αὐτῆς πρότερον
μόριον, τὸ δ' ὕστερον, ὅπερ Ἐρασίστρατος βούλεται. καίτοι καὶ
ταῦτ' αὐτῷ δεινῶς ἄτοπα. πρὶν μὲν γὰρ αἷμα περιέχειν αὐτὴν
ἴσως ἄν τις οὕτως ὠκεῖαν εἶναι τὴν τοῦ πνεύματος φορὰν
10 συνεχώρησεν ὡς λανθάνειν τὴν αἴσθησιν, ποιά ποτ' ἐστὶ μόρια
τῆς ἀρτηρίας τὰ διαστελλόμενα πρότερα· πεπληρωμένης <δ'>
αἵματος οὐκ ἐγχωρεῖ τὸ πνεῦμα ταχέως οὕτως ὡς πρόσθεν
ἀπὸ τῆς καρδίας ἐπὶ τὰ πέρατα τῆς ἀρτηρίας διεξέρχεσθαι.
ἀλλ' εἰ καὶ τοῦτο οὕτως <ὡς> ἔφην ἴσως οὐ συγχωρήσειεν, ἤ
15 γε μετὰ τὸ καθεῖναι τὸν κοῖλον κάλαμον εἰς τὴν ἀρτηρίαν τῶν
κάτω μερῶν αὐτῆς κίνησις πρὶν περιβληθῆναι τὸν βρόχον,
ἀκινησία δὲ περιβληθέντος ἐναργῶς ἐνδείκνυται δύναμιν ἀπὸ /
K735 καρδίας ἐπιπέμπεσθαι τοῖς χιτῶσι τῶν ἀρτηριῶν τὴν δια-
στέλλουσαν αὐτούς, οὐχ ὕλην διὰ τῆς κοιλότητος. ὡς γὰρ καὶ
20 τὸν τοῦ ποδὸς δάκτυλον κινῆσαι προελόμενοι παραχρῆμα
κινοῦμεν αὐτὸν οὐ τὸν λογισμὸν ἔχοντες ἐν αὐτῷ τῷ μορίῳ,
διαδοθείσης δέ τινος ἐπ' αὐτὸν ἐν ἀκαρεῖ χρόνῳ δυνάμεως,
οὕτω κἀπὶ τῆς καρδίας καὶ τῶν ἀρτηριῶν γίγνεται. ταῖς μὲν
γὰρ δυνάμεσι τὸ τάχος τῆς κινήσεως ὁμολογεῖ, ταῖς δ' ὕλαις
25 ἀντιμαρτυρεῖ. ταῦτ' εἴ τις <μὴ> φυλάττοι[το] θέσιν, ὡς Ἀρι-
στοτέλης εἴωθε λέγειν, οἶδ' ὅτι βεβαίως ἀποδεικνύναι τὸ προκεί-
A21 μενον αὐτῷ δόξει, [μὴ] φυλάττοντι δὲ φιλονείκως ἅπερ ἔθετο μήθ' ὑπὸ
τούτων πείθεσθαι μήθ' ὑφ' ἑτέρας ἀποδείξεως ἀναγκαῖόν ἐστιν, ἀλλὰ

A20

1 αὐταῖς Furley: αὐ^{τ̂} L: αὐτοῦ V: αὐτάς a   post αὐτ. adiecit ἀλλὰ διά τινος
δυνάμεως Corn: sed ob virtutem i δὲ secl. Furley   ante ἐπιπέμπ. addidit
αὐτὴν a   ἐπιπέμπεται Furley: -εσθαι LVa   ὑπ' L: ὑπὲρ Va
3 πρὸς τὰρ τὸ LV: πρὸ γὰρ τοῦ a: corr. Alb
5 καὶ om. a
6 αὐτ(ῆς) L: αὐτῶν Va: eius t
11 δὲ a: om. LV   ταχ(έως) L: τάχα Va
14 ὡς supplevit Corn   ἥ] ἢ V

causes the movement of the arteries / is transmitted to them K734
from the heart through their coats.[59]   A20

5. But what Erasistratus says about the motion of the arteries
is wholly false. For apart from the fact that the motion of the
exposed artery ceases in the parts beyond the ligature, which
ought not to happen, even before putting the ligature round it it
is possible to observe the whole of it in motion at a single time,
not one part after another, as Erasistratus wants. This idea of
his, too, is wildly absurd. For before it contains blood one might
concede that the motion of the pneuma is so rapid that which
parts of the artery are the first to be expanded escapes perception. But when it is full of blood, the pneuma cannot proceed
from the heart to the end of the artery as rapidly as before. But
even if, perhaps, he refuses to concede that it is as I have said,
the motion of the lower parts of the artery after the insertion of
the hollow reed into it before the ligature was passed round it,
and its motionlessness after being ligatured, clearly show that a
faculty is transmitted from / the heart by the coats of the arter- K735
ies, and that this is what expands them, not matter in the hollow. For just as people choose to move their toe and do so at
once, not because they have rationality in the part itself but
because a faculty is transmitted to it in a moment of time, so it
happens in the case of the heart and the arteries. For the speed
of the motion is consistent with [the assumption of] faculties,
but it contradicts that of material substances.

If one is not taking this position as a debating champion, as
Aristotle used to say,[60] I know that these considerations will be
thought / to demonstrate our case; on the other hand, if he   A21
defends his position from contentious love of victory, then
necessarily he is persuaded neither by these arguments nor by

---

15 καθ(εἰ)ν(αι) L: καθεσθῆναι V: καθεστῆναι a
17 περιβληθ(έν)τ(ος) L: περιβληθέντων Va
19 αὐτούς L: αὐτάς Va
25 μὴ ins. Ka (nunc vers. Arab. conf.: v. adn. 58)   φυλάττοιτ(ο) corr. Alb
A21
1 αὐτ(ῷ) L: αὐτοῦ Va
2 τούτ(ων) L: τούτου Va

181

πρὸς <ταῖς ἄλλαις μωρίαις οὐκ ἐτόλμησεν Ἐρασίστρατος> τῶν
φαινομένων ἐξ ἀνατομῆς καταψεύδεσθαι. γεγράφασι μὲν γὰρ πολλοὶ
5 τρόπους τινὰς ἀνατομῶν οἷς δείξειν ἐπαγγέλλονται κενὰς αἵματος
εἶναι τὰς ἀρτηρίας. εἶτ᾽ οὐδὲν ἐξ αὐτῶν ἀληθές ἐστιν. εἴροιτ᾽ <ἂν>
K736   δήπου καὶ πρὸς Ἐρασιστράτου / πολὺ μείζονα τούτων τῶν ἀναι-
σχύντως ψευδομένων ἐν ταῖς ἀνατομαῖς ἐξουσίαν πεπορισμένου.
ἀλλ᾽ οὐκ ἦν εἰς τοσοῦτον Ἐρασίστρατος ἀναίσχυντος, ὡς γράφειν
10 ἐπιχειρεῖν, ὃ δὴ ἰδεῖν ἦν ἀδύνατον <ὄν>.

---

3 πρὸς τοῖς φαινομένοις LVa ταῖς — Ἐρασίστρατος ins. Furley, vers. Arab.
secutus   τῶν φαινομένων sugg. DeLacy
4 ἀνατομ(ῆς) L: ἀνατομῶν Va   γεγράφασι LV: καὶ γράφουσι a   γὰρ om. Va
6 οὐδὲν — ἀληθές Furley, vers. Arab. secutus: οὐδεὶς — ἀληθής LVa (ἀληθές
L)   εἴροιτ᾽ ἂν Furley, vers. Arab. secutus: εἴρηται γὰρ LVa
7 τῶν Furley: τοίνυν LVa

any other demonstration. But Erasistratus, with all his other follies, did not dare to tell lies about anatomy.[61] Many have written Anatomies of one kind or another, in which they claim that they will show the arteries to be empty of blood.[62] But nothing in them is true.[63] For it would surely have been stated by Erasistratus also, / who was possessed of much greater ability than they who shamelessly tell lies in their Anatomies.[64] But Erasistratus was not so shameless as to undertake to write what he could observe to be impossible.[65]

K736

---

8 ψευδο^{μν}' L: ψευδόμενος Va   ἐξουσίαν πεπορισμένου Furley, vers. Arab. secutus: ἐξ.ν πεπορισ^{μν} L: ἐξ ὧν πεπορισμένος Va

9 γράφων Va

10 ὅ — <ὅν> sugg. Delacy: ἅ — LVa

in fine: γαληνοῦ εἰ κατὰ φύσιν ἐν ἀρτηρίαις αἷμα περιέχεται L: τέλος γαληνοῦ εἰ περιέχεται κατὰ φύσιν ἐν ἀρτηρίαις αἷμα V

DE USU PULSUUM

INTRODUCTION

Title and Text

Galen refers to this work several times under the title Περὶ χρείας σφυγμῶν (e.g. *De plac. Hipp. et Plato.* VI 3 (K V 572); and VIII 8 (K V 709); *De usu partium* IV 12 (K III 300).

There are two extant Greek manuscripts that preserve the whole of this work: Scorial. Φ III 11, of the fourteenth to fifteenth centuries, f.16ʳ-20ᵛ, of which I have collated a photocopy (S); and Cantabrigensis, Caius Coll. 355, of the fifteenth to sixteenth centuries, f.16-42, which I have collated in the original (C). Bound with C is a copy of the same manuscript, in an elegant fine hand, from the beginning to 164.11. I have also collated this, but it is of no value for establishing the text. It is not mentioned in Diels's list of the Greek medical manuscripts.

There are thirty-nine places[1] where S first hand left a space, a few words long, which was filled in later in a different ink (but by the same hand, I think). All the spaces are roughly commensurate with

[1]The gaps are as follows: 150.11 ὠφέλουν ἕκαστον, 151.15 διαφέρειν ἡμῖν φαινομένης, 152.10 τοῖς καυσώδεσι πυρετοῖς, 153.1 ὅσον γὰρ ἐνδεέστερον, 153.15 τῶν λόγων ὁ ἕτερος παραλογίζεται, 155.1 ἐπεὶ δὲ μέχρι μὲν πολλοῦ, 155.10 ὡς εἰ νοήσεις ἀλλήλοις ἐπικείμενα, 156.15 παραπλησίως δ' αὐτῷ, 157.8 τῶν δ' ἄλλων οὐδὲν στερῆσαι, 158.1 ἰατρικαῖς σικύαις ἡ μὲν φλόξ, 158.9 τὸ σκέπασμα αὐτῆς διελών 159.2 ὑπάρχει κατὰ φύσιν ἔχουσι, 159.15 περὶ δὲ τοῦ μὴ δι' ἀρτηριῶν, 160.12 εἰ δὲ καὶ χωρὶς τραύματος ἐθελήσαις, 161.3 ὥσθ' ὅπερ ἐκ τῆς ἀναπνοῆς, 162.5 τεκμαίρομαι μάλιστα, 162.12 οὔθ' ὑγιαίνοντος οὔτε νοσοῦντος, 163.5 εἰ δὲ πρὸς τῷ μηδὲν ὠφελεῖσθαι, ἔτι καὶ, 163.13 καὶ κατὰ τοῦτον ἀναλογίαν εἶναι, 164.6 ἡ γὰρ ἐν τῷ σώματι τῆς καρδίας δύναμις ὑφ' ἧς, 164.12 συστελλόμενα δ' ἐκθλίβουσι, 165.13 τούτου πολλάκις ἡμεῖς τοῦ φαινομένου, 166.12 ἀλλ' ἐκεῖνος μὲν ἔοικεν, 167.9 τὴν καρδ. παντάχοσε, 167.16 καὶ καθαίρεσθαι 168.4 περιέχεσθαι, 168.14 τοῦτο μὲν δὴ πολλάκις τε καὶ, 169.18 χαλεπώτερον δή τι τὸ τῆς εὑρέσεως, 170.13 παντοίως οὖν ἀπόρου τοῦ ζητουμένου, 171.6 οὐδέτερον δ' οὕτως ἔχει καὶ πρόσεστιν, 172.1 ἐν αὐτῇ καθὰ ἐν ταῖς ἐκπνοαῖς, 173.7 εὐλογώτερον οὖν μακρῷ, 173.13 κἂν ταῖς ἀρτηρίαις, 174.13 καὶ κάλλισθ' ὅταν, 175.12 δεύτερον δὲ τὸν ἐκ τῆς κινήσεως ὅρον, 176.14 ἐκείνων κινηθέντων, 177.13 ὅσῳ δ' ἂν ἕκαστον, 178.7 φαίνεται γὰρ 179.5 εἴρηταί μοι τὸ πᾶν ἤδη περὶ χρείας σφυγμῶν.

the words omitted. C left spaces at exactly these points, but measured the gap less efficiently, almost always underestimating it. The gaps are filled in, in C, in such a way that the difference from the main manuscript is always detectable, because of a different ink, different hand, or different size of writing; but the insertions are not themselves homogeneous. The insertions in C differ a little from the insertions in S: 158.1 συκῆαις S, σικείαις C; 164.12 φαινομένου S, φαινομένην C; 167.16 καθαίρεσθαι S, -εται C; 172.1 καθὰ ἐν S, καθ' ἐν C; 175.12 δεύτερον δὲ τὸν ἐκ S, δευτέρως δ' ἐκ C.

C was evidently copied from S. S is rather badly written, and frequently abbreviates the ends of words. C is in a much better hand: abbreviations are avoided, but where the abbreviation in S is difficult to decipher, C often interprets it wrongly and on occasion simply transcribes the symbol, more or less accurately. The relation between S and C is revealed at once in the sixth line of the text (K 149.6), where the correct word στερηθέντες is written in such a way in S that it can easily be mistaken for περιτίθεντες, the meaningless reading of C. The fact noted in the last paragraph, that S left spaces of the right size to fit the insertions whereas C generally underestimated also suggests that C copied S without direct access to the archetype.

Since C is a copy of S, its readings have been entered in the *apparatus* only when they are particularly revealing.

The Aldine edition of 1525 has a better text than S, and is not simply a corrected copy of S. Its manuscript source is now lost.

The present edition, the first since Kühn's (1822), incorporates the results of a study of an Arabic translation contained in the Aya Sofya manuscript no. 3690. According to the colophon, this translation was made by Iṣṭefan (Iṣṭefan ibn Bāsīl) from an original version (from Greek into Syriac) by Ḥunain ibn Isḥāq. J.S.W. has collated this manuscript. The existence of only a single manuscript in this case, as opposed to the two Arabic manuscripts of *An in arteriis*, makes it more difficult to be sure of the Arabic text. Although the results are less dramatic than in *An in arteriis*, there is no doubt that the Arabic translation preserves a better tradition than the Greek vulgate, and the text is much improved by this discovery: see notes 8, 13, 19, 20, 25, 26, 31, 36, 43.

There is a Latin translation by Mark of Toledo, printed in the Juntine edition of 1528 and elsewhere, and another by Thomas Linacre (London: R. Pynson, 1522; and many other printed editions, including Kühn's).

We acknowledge with gratitude many helpful comments by Dr. Maurice Pope, who expects soon to publish some work of his own, in collaboration with Dr. Hymie Gordon, on this treatise.

Pages and lines are numbered according to Kühn's edition.

Summary

Chapter 1

Examination of the common view, that the use of the pulse is the same as that of breathing.

If so, why is deprivation of the pulse relatively harmless to the parts concerned, while deprivation of breathing is fatal? Experiments with ligatures of arteries show that this is the case.

Whence comes the diagnostic value of the pulse? Can it be only as sign, not cause, of harm?

The reason for believing both pulse and breathing to have the same use is that both change in similar conditions. Examples of this.

Chapter 2

The brain has been shown to profit from breathing both because of the preservation of the innate heat, and because of the nourishing of the psychic pneuma. Ligaturing the carotid arteries therefore makes little difference. Experiment shows this.

The retiform plexus works up the stuff in the arteries, and keeps up the supply of pneuma to the brain.

Similarly in the case of other parts, if arteries are ligatured: sufficient warmth is conveyed to the parts through their coats or through the veins. Contrast the heart itself, which needs greater heat than other parts, and has only breathing to maintain it.

Chapter 3

Proof that heat flows into the parts by routes other than the arteries, from experience with ligatures.

So there is nothing after all against the thesis that the use of the pulse and of breathing is the same — preservation of heat, and restoration of the psychic pneuma.

Expansion of arteries, like breathing in, draws in airy stuff; contraction, like breathing out, discharges smoky residue.

Chapter 4

Criticism of the view of Archigenes' school, that arteries are filled on contractions and emptied in expansions. Their analogy with the contraction of the mouth and nostrils in breathing is turned against them.

Motion of the arteries is governed by the heart, whose power flows through the coats.

Chapter 5

Arteries draw in from all sides on expanding, and expel on all sides on contracting, through vents in their coats, through "pores" connecting them with each other and the heart, through junctions with the veins. Proof of these junctions, from the fact that all the blood in both veins and arteries flows out of a wounded artery.

Through all these, the arteries draw in air or blood and eliminate wastes; except that they do not give much to the heart, since the valves hinder it. They do, however, give something to the heart, because the valves do not completely prevent it; Erasistratus was wrong about this.

Erasistratus was also wrong in thinking that the filling of the arteries is what expands them; on the contrary, their expansion fills them.

Chapter 6

Are both expansion and contraction activities or is one a passive return to normal after the activity? The analogy with breathing may not help here, because breathing is caused by the psychic power, and pulse by the vital power.

Why do arteries not collapse, at death, like veins?

190

Arguments to show that expansion is an activity: (a) the volume of expansion varies with pulsative power; (b) fullest pulse occurs when one is about to recover from a disease.

Chapter 7

There are two kinds of breathing out: passive relaxation of the expanded thorax, and active blowing out of the breath. Are there likewise two kinds of contraction of the artery? That there are two kinds is suggested by the fact that all organs have contrary powers, by the analogy with breathing, and by the fact that Nature needs this way of getting rid of wastes.

This is confirmed by examples: in sleeping after eating; in childhood and old age, and so on.

A contrary view: deeper contractions of the artery are explained by the greater softness of the coats.

But although this may be true in the case of old age, it will not explain more rapid changes in the contractions. The truth is that softer coats respond more readily to the power acting on them, but they are slower to return to their natural state.

Chapter 8

Summary.

Sigla

S = codex Scorial III 11.
C = codex Cantabrigensis, Caius Coll. 355
D = codex Cantabrigensis, Caius Coll. 355 (appendix)

a = editio aldina (1525)
K = editio Kühniana (1822)
Lin. = Tho. Linacri interpretatio

In commentario citatur versio Arabica:
Istanbul: A.S. 3590^8, 51^a–65^b

ΓΑΛΗΝΟΥ ΠΕΡΙ ΧΡΕΙΑΣ
ΣΦΥΓΜΩΝ ΒΙΒΛΙΟΝ

K149 1. Τίς ἡ χρεία τῶν σφυγμῶν; ἆρά γε ἤπερ
καὶ τῆς ἀναπνοῆς, ὡς σχεδὸν ἅπασιν ἰατροῖς τε καὶ φιλοσόφοις ἔδοξεν, ἤ τις ἑτέρα παρὰ ταύτην;
2. οὐ γὰρ δὴ ἀβα-
σανίστως πειστέον αὐτοῖς, ἐναντιοῦσθαι δοκούντων ἄλλων
5 τέ τινων οὐκ ὀλίγων φαινομένων, καὶ τοῦ νῦν εἰρῆσθαι
μέλλοντος οὐχ ἥκιστα. στερηθέντες μὲν γὰρ τῆς ἀναπνοῆς
εὐθέως ἀποθνήσκομεν, ἄσφυκτα δ' ἀπεργάσῃ πολλὰ τῶν
μορίων ἄνευ μεγάλης βλάβης. εἰ γοῦν ἐθελήσῃς ἢ τὰς διὰ
K150 τῶν βουβώνων ἐπὶ τὰ σκέλη καθηκούσας ἀρτηρίας, ἢ τὰς
διὰ τῶν μασχαλῶν εἰς τὰς χεῖράς βρόχῳ διαλαβεῖν, ἀσφύκτους μὲν εὐθέως ἐργάσῃ τὰς ἐν τοῖς κώλοις ἁπάσας, οὐ
μὴν παραλύσεις ταῦτα τῆς καθ' ὁρμὴν κινήσεως, ὥσπερ
5 οὐδὲ τῆς αἰσθήσεως. εἰ δ' ἐν τῷ χρόνῳ ναρκώδη τε καὶ
ψυχρὰ καὶ ὠχρὰ καὶ ἄτροφα γίνεται, τάχ' ἂν τοῦτο κατὰ
συμπάθειαν μᾶλλον ἢ τὴν τῶν σφυγμῶν ἀπώλειαν συμβαίνοι. εἰ δὲ τὰ νεῦρα βρόχοις διαλάβοις, ἀκίνητά τε παντελῶς καὶ ἀναίσθητα παραχρῆμα ποιήσεις τὰ μόρια. ἐχρῆν
10 οὖν καὶ τὰς ἀρτηρίας ὁμοίως τοῖς νεύροις κακωθείσας, εἰς
ἅπερ ἔμπροσθεν ὠφέλουν ἕκαστον τῶν μορίων, εἰς ταῦτα
καὶ βλάπτειν εὐθέως. τὸ δὲ δὴ πάντων ἀτοπώτατον, εἰ
τὰς κατὰ τὸν τράχηλον ἀρτηρίας βρόχοις διαλάβοις, οὐδὲν
σαφὲς βλάψεις τὸ ζῷον, καίτοι συνάπτουσιν αὗται καρδίαν
15 ἐγκεφάλῳ, τὸ κυριώτατον τῶν ζωτικῶν ὄργανον τῷ κυριω-
τάτῳ τῶν ψυχικῶν. εἴπερ οὖν τῶν οὕτως ἐπικαίρων
ἀρτηριῶν ἡ βλάβη μηδὲν σαφὲς ἀδικεῖ τὸ ζῷον, σχολῇ γ'
ἂν τῶν ἄλλων τις ἀδικήσειεν. εἰ δ' οὐδὲν βλάπτουσιν
K151 παθοῦσαι, παντί που δῆλον, ὡς οὐδ' ὠφελοῦσιν, οὐδ' ἂν
ἐρρωμέναι τύχωσιν.
3. πῶς οὖν ἐκ σφυγμῶν τὸ μέγιστον προ-

K149
6 στερηθέντες Sa: περιτίθεντες C

ON THE USE OF THE PULSE

Chapter 1[1]

What is the use of the pulse? Is it the same as that of breathing, as nearly all physicians and philosophers have supposed, or something else apart from this?[2]

2. We must not believe them uncritically, seeing that many of the appearances are against them, and not least the following: that we die at once if deprived of breathing, but it is possible to cause many of the limbs to become pulseless without doing great harm. For if you ligature either / the arteries descending K150 through the groin to the legs, or those through the armpits into the hands, you will at once make pulseless all the arteries in the limbs; but you will not deprive the limbs of voluntary motion,[3] nor even of feeling. And if in the course of time they become numb and cold and pale and deprived of nourishment, it may be that this is rather from some connected affection[4] than from loss of pulse. But should you ligature the nerves, you will immediately make the parts both completely motionless and without feeling; so it should have been the case[5] that the arteries, no less than the nerves, when damaged, at once do harm to each of the parts they formerly did good to. But, what is most striking, if you ligature the arteries in the neck you will do the animal no harm that can be detected, although these arteries join the heart to the brain—the principal vital organ to the principal psychic organ.[6] If then the damage done to these most important arteries does no clear hurt to the animal, scarcely would any damage done to the others hurt it. But if they do no / harm when injured, then everyone must see that they do no K151 good either, even when they are well and whole.

3. How is it then that we most often make our prognosis

K150
  8 συμβαίνοι K: -ει Sa
  12 εἰ a: εἰς S
  14 βλάψεις K, -οις Sa
K151
  2 τύχωσιν a: τυγχάνουσι S

195

γινώσκομεν; οὐχ ὡς ἐξ αἰτίων πολὺ δυναμένων, φήσει τις, ἀλλ' ὡς σημείων ἐπικαίρων, ὡς εἰ καὶ γρυπουμένοις τοῖς
5 ὄνυξι καὶ μελαινομένοις τεκμαίροιτό τις περὶ θανάτου. ὅταν γὰρ τοῖς χρησίμοις εἰς τὴν ζωὴν ἕπηταί τινα κατ' ἀνάγκην, ὁ μὲν κίνδυνος ἐπὶ τῇ τοῦ χρησίμου βλάβῃ, τὸ δ' ἐξ ἀνάγκης ἑπόμενον σημεῖον γίνεται τοῦ κινδύνου. κύριον μὲν οὖν σπλάγχνον ἡ καρδία, ἐκπεφύκασι δ' ἀπ' αὐτῆς αἱ
10 ἀρτηρίαι, καὶ κινοῦνται δὲ τὸν αὐτὸν ἐκείνῃ τρόπον· ὥστε καὶ βλάπτονται τὸν αὐτόν, καὶ ταύτῃ μέγα δηλοῦν πεφύκασιν. ἐδείχθη δὲ οὐ ταὐτὸν ὂν τὸ δηλοῦν μεγάλα τῷ δύνασθαι μεγάλα.

4. πόθεν οὖν ἐπῆλθεν ἅπασιν ἰατροῖς τε καὶ φιλοσόφοις εἰς τὴν αὐτὴν χρείαν ἀνάγειν τήν τε ἀναπνοὴν καὶ
15 τοὺς σφυγμούς, τῆς μὲν οὕτως εἰς μέγα διαφέρειν ἡμῖν φαινομένης, τῶν δ', ὡς ἔοικεν, ἢ παντάπασιν εἰς οὐδέν, ἢ παντελῶς μικρόν;

5. ἐμοὶ μὲν οὖν δοκοῦσιν, ὥσπερ οὖν καὶ
K152 γράφουσιν οἱ πλείους αὐτῶν, ἐκ τοῦ τρέπεσθαι παραπλησίους τροπὰς ἐπὶ τοῖς αὐτοῖς αἰτίοις ἀμφότερα κοινὴν εἶναι καὶ τὴν χρείαν αὐτῶν ὑπονοῆσαι· τῶν τε γὰρ γυμναζομένων καὶ λουομένων, καὶ τῶν ὁπωσοῦν ἄλλως θερμαι-
5 νομένων, οὐ τὴν ἀναπνοὴν μόνον ὠκυτέραν τε καὶ πυκνοτέραν καὶ μείζονα γινομένην ἔστιν ἰδεῖν, ἀλλὰ καὶ τοὺς σφυγμοὺς ὡσαύτως τρεπομένους, τῶν τ' ἀργούντων, καὶ τῶν ὁπωσοῦν ἄλλως ψυχομένων, οὐ τὴν ἀναπνοὴν μόνην ἀραιοτέραν τε καὶ βραδυτέραν καὶ μικροτέραν, ἀλλὰ καὶ τοὺς
10 σφυγμούς. καὶ ἐν τοῖς καυσώδεσι πυρετοῖς πλεῖστον μὲν καὶ τάχιστον καὶ πυκνότατον ἀναπνέουσι, μεγίστους δ' ἔχουσι καὶ ταχίστους καὶ πυκνοτάτους τοὺς σφυγμούς. εἰ δ' ἐπὶ ταῖς ἀσυμμέτροις τροφαῖς οἱ μὲν σφυγμοὶ μείζονες, αἱ δ' ἀναπνοαὶ γίνονται μικρότεραι, οὐδὲ τοῦτο ἀπόρημα
15 τῷ λόγῳ· μικρότερον μὲν γὰρ ἀναπνέουσιν ἢ σφύζουσι στενοχωρίᾳ τῶν φρενῶν, ἀλλ' ὅσῳ μικρότερον, τοσούτῳ πυκνότερον, ἰώμενοι τὴν μικρότητα τῆς ἀναπνοῆς τῷ συνε-

---

6 ὅταν a: οὔτε S
10 δὲ S: *om.* aK
14 αὐτὴν a: τοιαύτην S   ἀνάγειν K: ἀγαγεῖν a

from the pulse? Not, it will be said, as from causes that have great power, but as from relevant signs; as, for example, one might make a forecast of death from the fact that the nails are curved and blackened. For whenever the things that are useful for life are necessarily accompanied by other things, then any danger is dependent on damage to what is useful, but the necessary accompaniment is a sign of the danger. The heart, now, is the principal viscus; and the arteries spring from it, and they move just as it moves, so that they suffer the same hurts, and thus they are naturally able to reveal something important. But it has been shown that to reveal something important is not the same as to have the power to produce it.

4. Whence, then, has it occurred to all physicians and philosophers to assign to one common use both breathing and the pulse, since the former is apparently of such great importance to us, and the latter, or so it seems, good either for nothing or for very little?

5. They seem to me / to believe both to have the same use, K152 as indeed most of them write, because both are subject to changes of the same kinds from the same causes. For when people take exercise or a bath or otherwise become heated, it is clear to all that not only does the breathing become quicker and more frequent and deeper, but the pulse also changes in the same manner;[7] whereas when they are at rest or are cooling off in any other way, not only does the breathing become less frequent and slower and more shallow, but the pulse also. And in burning fevers people breathe very deeply and rapidly and frequently, and they also have a pulse that is very full, rapid, and frequent. If it happens that after immoderate eating the pulse is greater while the breathing is shallower, even this presents no problem to the argument: for they breathe more shallowly than they pulsate because of the constraint of the midriff; but they breathe as much more frequently as more shallowly, making up by the continuity of the activity what the

---

K152

7 ἀργούντων a: ἀλγούντων ἤ S: algent Lin.
10 καὶ a: om. S

K153 χεῖ τῆς ἐνεργείας. ὅσον γὰρ ἐνδεέστερον ἀπέλαυσεν ἡ φύσις
ἀέρος, οὐ δυνηθέντος ἐπὶ πλεῖστον διαστῆναι τοῦ θώρακος,
τοῦτο ἐπανορθοῦται τῇ πυκνότητι. καὶ διὰ τοῦτο ἴσον
δύναται τὸ μικρότερόν τε ἅμα καὶ πυκνότερον πνεῦμα τῷ
5 μείζονί τε ἅμα καὶ ἀραιοτέρῳ. λέγομεν δὲ νῦν ἀραιότερον
σφυγμὸν τὸν ἐπὶ τροφαῖς, οὐ πρὸς τὸν πρὸ τῆς τροφῆς, ἐκείνου
μὲν γὰρ πυκνότερός ἐστιν, ἀλλὰ τῇ τῆς ἀναπνοῆς ἰδέᾳ πα-
ραβάλλοντες.

6. εἰ τοίνυν τρέπεται μὲν ὡσαύτως ἐπὶ τοῖς αὐτοῖς αἰτίοις ἡ ἀναπνοὴ τοῖς σφυγμοῖς, βλάπτεται δ' οὐχ
10 ὡσαύτως ἀπολλυμένη, καὶ γὰρ τοῦτ' ἔμπροσθεν ἐδείχθη,
περαίνοιτ' ἂν οὐδὲν ἧττον ὁμοίως ἀλλήλοις τὰ ἀντικείμενα,
τό τε τῆς αὐτῆς ἕνεκα χρείας ἄμφω γεγονέναι καὶ τὸ μὴ
τῆς αὐτῆς. ἀλλ' οὐκ ἐνδέχεται· χρὴ γὰρ θάτερον αὐτῶν
ἀληθὲς ὑπάρχειν, οὐκ ἄμφω.

15 **2.** Ζητητέον οὖν, ὅπῃ τῶν λόγων ὁ ἕτερος παραλογίζεται, κάνονα τῆς κρίσεως ποιησαμένοις ἡμῖν
τὴν χρείαν τῆς ἀναπνοῆς, ἣν ἐδείξαμεν ἐν τοῖς περὶ
αὐτῆς λόγοις διττὴν οὖσαν, ὡς ἐδόκει καὶ Ἱπποκράτει·
K154 τὴν μὲν γὰρ ἑτέραν, τὴν μείζω, φυλακὴν τῆς ἐμφύτου θερμασίας, τὴν δὲ ἑτέραν, τὴν ἐλάττονα, θρέψιν τοῦ ψυχικοῦ πνεύματος. ἀλλ' εἰς ἄμφω ταῦτα παρὰ τῆς διὰ τῶν
ῥινῶν εἰσπνοῆς ὠφελεῖσθαι τὸν ἐγκέφαλον ἐλέγομεν. ὥστ'
5 οὐδὲν θαυμαστόν, ὀλίγης αὐτῷ παρὰ καρδίας χορηγουμένης
τῆς ἐπικουρίας, ὀλίγην εἶναι καὶ τὴν βλάβην, τῶν καρωτίδων λεγομένων ἀρτηριῶν βρόχοις διαληφθεισῶν. ἀλλ'
ἴσως τις φήσει, μηδ' ἐλαχίστην φαίνεσθαι· δι' ὅλης γὰρ
ἡμέρας τὸ ζῷον, ὡς ἐπειράθημεν πολλάκις, ἀβλαβὲς δια-
10 μένει. καὶ ὀρθῶς γε φήσει. καὶ δὴ τοῦθ' ἡμεῖς ἀποροῦν-
τες ἐπενοήσαμεν τοιούτου τινὸς ἀποπειραθῆναι φαινομένου.
πρότερον δ' ἐρῶ τὸν λογισμόν, ὅθεν εἰς τοῦθ' ἥκομεν.
2. ἐπεὶ γὰρ ἐν ἑτέροις ἡμῖν ἀποδέδεικται, τὰς κατὰ τὸν ἐγκέφαλον κοιλίας πνεύματος εἶναι ψυχικοῦ μεστάς, τροφῆς

K153
1 ἀπέλαυσεν a: ἀπόλλυσιν S
6 πρός a: om. SK: v. comm.   πρὸ τῆς a: προὸν S
9 αἰτίοις ἡ a: αἰτίαν C: om. S
13 αὐτῶν a: αὐτοῖς ut videtur S

198

breathing lacks in depth. / By so much as Nature goes short of   K153
air because the chest is not able to expand very much, by so
much she puts things right by the frequency. And in this way
shallower breathing that is at the same time more frequent is
equivalent to that which is deeper but at the same time less
frequent. We say now that the pulse is less frequent after food,
not in comparison with its rate before food, for it is more frequent than that, but in comparison with the breathing.[8]

6. If, then, the breathing changes as the pulse changes, and
from the same causes, but does not do harm of the same order
when it is brought to a stop[9] (and certainly that has been proved
already), then with equal validity and by similar arguments
contradictory conclusions would be reached—namely, that both
came into being for the same purpose, and that they did not.
But this is impossible; one or the other must be true, not both.

Chapter 2

We must find, then, in what way one of the two arguments
is fallacious, using as our criterion the use of breathing, which
we have shown in our book on the subject to be twofold, as
Hippocrates also believed:[10] / one, the more important use, the   K154
conservation of the innate heat; the other, the less important,
the nourishing of the psychic pneuma. We said that the brain
profits by the inbreathing through the nostrils in respect to both
of these.[11] It is not surprising, then, that since little profit is
supplied to it [the brain] from the heart, it suffers but little
harm if the arteries called "carotids" are ligatured. But someone
may say, "but not even the very least harm is observed; certainly the animal remains a whole day unhurt, as we have made
trial of it many times." And he will be right. Indeed, being
puzzled by this, we devised a way of putting such an observation to the proof. First, however, I will tell the reasoning by
which we came upon it.

2. Since it has been proved by us elsewhere[12] that the hollows in the brain are full of psychic pneuma that requires con-

---

18 Ἱπποκράτει K: -ης Sa
K154
4 ἐλέγομεν a: λέγομεν S

15 χρῄζοντος συνεχοῦς, ἀποδέδεικται δὲ καὶ ὡς δαπανᾶται
τοῦτο ἐν ταῖς καθ᾽ ὁρμὴν κινήσεσιν, ἄμεινον ἐδόκει
τρέχειν ἀναγκάζειν τὸ ζῷον, ᾧ τὰς ἀρτηρίας βρόχοις
K155 διελάβομεν. ἐπεὶ δὲ μέχρι μὲν πολλοῦ καλῶς ἔτρεχε, μέχρι
παντὸς δ᾽ οὐκ ἠδύνατο, ζητεῖν ἐδόκει τὴν αἰτίαν δι᾽ ἥνπερ μέχρι
πολλοῦ ἔτρεχε, χρῆναι γὰρ οὐδὲ μέχρι πολλοῦ
διαρκεῖν, ἀλλ᾽ εὐθέως ἐκλύεσθαι, δαπανωμένου τοῦ
5 ψυχικοῦ πνεύματος.

3. ἀλλὰ καὶ αὐτοῦ τού-
του τὸ δικτυοειδὲς πλέγμα πρὸς τῶν ἀμφὶ τὸν Ἡρόφιλον
κληθὲν ἐδόκει τὴν αἰτίαν ἔχειν. ἐκεῖ γὰρ αἱ ἐπὶ τὸν ἐγκέφαλον ἀνιοῦσαι καρωτίδες ἀρτηρίαι, πρὶν διελθεῖν τὴν σκλη-
ρὰν μήνιγγα, σχίζονται πολυειδῶς ὑπ᾽ αὐτῆς, περιπλεκόμε-
10 ναι κατὰ πολλοὺς στίχους, ὡς εἰ νοήσαις ἀλλήλοις ἐπικείμενα δίκτυα πλείω, καὶ χώραν παμπόλλην, ἣν καλοῦσιν
ἐγκεφάλου βάσιν, καταλαμβάνουσιν, ἐνὸν αὐταῖς εὐθὺς μὲν
διεκπεσεῖν τὰς μήνιγγας, ἐμφῦναι δὲ εἰς τὸν ἐγκέφαλον, οὗ-
περ ἐξ ἀρχῆς ἴενται. τοῦτ᾽ οὖν τὸ θαυμαστὸν πλέγμα πρὸς
15 τῆς μηδὲν εἰκῆ ποιούσης φύσεως ἐν οὕτως ἀσφαλεῖ χώρᾳ
ταχθῆναι, μεγάλης τινὸς ἐδόκει χρείας ἐνδεικτικὸν ὑπάρχειν.
ἀλλ᾽ ἐπειδὴ τὴν τῶν ἐντέρων ἕλικα καὶ τὴν τῶν εἰς τοὺς
K156 ὄρχεις ἐμφυομένων ἀγγείων ἀκριβοῦς τε πέψεως ἕνεκα τῶν
περιεχομένων ὑλῶν καὶ προσέτι δαψιλοῦς παρασκευῆς ταῖς
ἑξῆς ἐνεργείαις ἑωρῶμεν γεγενημένην, εὔλογον ἐδόκει κἀνταῦθα τοιοῦτόν τι μεμηχανῆσθαι τὴν φύσιν, ἅμα τε κα-
5 τεργαζομένην πολλῷ χρόνῳ τὴν ἐν ταῖς ἀρτηρίαις ὕλην, αἷμα
θερμὸν καὶ λεπτὸν καὶ ἀτμῶδες ὑπάρχουσαν, ἅμα τε κα-
τασκευάζουσαν τροφὴν δαψιλῆ τῷ κατὰ τὸν ἐγκέφαλον ψυχικῷ πνεύματι. καὶ διὰ τοῦτο, κἂν στερηθῇ τῆς πρὸς τὴν
καρδίαν συνεχείας ὁ ἐγκέφαλος, ἐξαρκεῖν αὐτῷ τὸ δικτυοει-
10 δὲς πλέγμα μέχρι πολλοῦ, καὶ μάλισθ᾽ ὅταν ἀτρεμῇ τὸ
ζῷον, ὡς ἂν μὴ δαπανωμένου τηνικαῦτα τοῦ ψυχικοῦ πνεύματος εἰς τὴν καθ᾽ ὁρμὴν ἐνέργειαν.

4. τὸ μὲν δὴ χα-
λεπώτατόν τε καὶ ἀπορώτατον δοκοῦν, τὸ κατὰ τὰς καρω

K155

1 καλῶς ἔτρεχε ... 4 διαρκεῖν sic Furley, vers. Arab. secutus: καλῶς ἔτρεχε,
μέχρι παντὸς δ᾽ οὐκ ἠδύνατο, ζητεῖν ἐδόκει χρῆναι πάλιν αὐτό, τὸ μέχρι

tinual nourishment, and it has also been proved that this is expended during voluntary movement, we decided to ligature an animal's arteries and then force it to run about. / Well, he K155 ran well for a good while, but could not keep it up for ever; so we decided to inquire why he ran for a good while, since it seemed that he ought not to hold out even for a while, but should collapse at once, as the psychic pneuma was consumed.[13]

3. But the "net-like" plexus, as it is called by the followers of Herophilus, appeared to be the cause of just this thing.[14] For there the carotid arteries, on their way to the brain, before they pass through the hard membrane, are split into many branches by it, weaving together in many layers, like a number of nets one above the other; and they occupy the ample space called the base of the brain, for they are able at once to penetrate the membranes and to root themselves into the brain, which they are making for from the first. The fact that this wonderful plexus was placed by Nature, who does nothing in vain, in such a well-protected situation, seemed to be an indication of some great use. Since we find the spiral of the guts and that of the vessels that enter / the testes made for the meticulous concoc- K156 tion[15] of the matters contained in them and for the abundant provisioning of their subsequent activities, it seemed reasonable to suppose that here also Nature has contrived something of the kind, to work up for a long time the stuff in the arteries, which is hot, thin, vaporous blood, and also to provide abundant nourishment to the psychic pneuma in the brain. And on this account, even if the brain is deprived of connection with the heart, the net-like plexus suffices it for a good while, particularly if the animal is at rest; for then it is not expending the psychic pneuma upon voluntary movements.[16]

4. So what seemed the hardest and most puzzling thing, the

πολλοῦ διαρκεῖν a: ζητεῖν ἐδόκει χρῆναι γὰρ οὐδὲ μέχρι καλῶς ἔτρεχε, μέχρι παντὸς δ᾽ οὐκ ἠδύνατο, πάλιν αὐτό τὸ μέχρι πολλοῦ διαρκεῖν S: v. comm.

14 ἰέντai Sa: ἰέναι K

17 ἐπειδὴ a: ἐπεὶ καὶ C (S illeg.) τῶν om. a

τίδας ἀρτηρίας, οὐδὲν ἔχειν ἄπορον ἔτι φαίνεται.

5. παραπλη-

15 σίως δ' αὐτῷ καὶ τὸ κατὰ τὰς ἄλλας ἁπάσας, ὧν ἑκάστης βρόχῳ διαληφθείσης οὐδὲν ἐν τῷ παραυτίκα βλάπτεται τὸ μέρος. ἐχρῆν γάρ, οἶμαι, κἀνταῦθα σκοπεῖν, ὡς οὐκ ἴσον K157 ἐστίν, ἢ τὴν ἀρχὴν αὐτὴν τῆς ἐμφύτου θερμασίας παθεῖν, ἤ τι τῶν ὑπ' αὐτῆς θερμαινομένων. τὴν μὲν γὰρ ἀεὶ χρὴ θερμὴν ἱκανῶς ὑπάρχειν· καὶ γὰρ ἑαυτὴν καὶ τἄλλα κινεῖ τε ἅμα σφυγματωδῶς καὶ θερμαίνει· τοῖς δὲ ἀπόχρη
5 βραχείας εὐπορεῖν θερμασίας εἰς τὸ διασώζεσθαι. καὶ τὴν μὲν εἰ στερήσαις τῆς ἐμφύτου θερμασίας, αὐτήν τε ψύξεις καὶ τἄλλα πάντα, ὅσα πρότερον ὑπ' αὐτῆς ἐθερμαίνετο· τῶν δ' ἄλλων οὐδὲν στερῆσαι τελέως δυνήσῃ τῆς θερμασίας, κἂν βρόχοις διαλάβῃς τὰς ἀρτηρίας· διά τε γὰρ τῶν
10 χιτώνων ἐπιρρυήσεταί τι, καὶ γὰρ σύμπνουν ἐστὶ καὶ σύρρουν ἑαυτῷ πᾶν τὸ σῶμα κατὰ τὸν Ἱπποκράτους λόγον. ὥστε, κἂν μὴ διὰ τῶν ἀρτηριῶν, ἀλλά γε διὰ τῶν ἄλλων καὶ μάλιστα διὰ φλεβῶν τῷ συνεχεῖ τῆς μεταλήψεως εἰς πᾶν μόριον ἐνεχθήσεταί τι τῆς θερμασίας.
15 6. ἅπαντα οὖν τὰ τοιαῦτα τοῖς φαινομένοις ὁμολογεῖ, καὶ θαυμαστὸν οὐκ ἔτι δόξει τὴν ἀρχὴν τῆς θερμασίας μᾶλλον τῶν ἄλλων βλάπτεσθαι στερηθείσης τῆς ἀναπνοῆς. K158 καὶ γὰρ ἐν ταῖς ἰατρικαῖς σικύαις ἡ μὲν φλὸξ ἀπόλλυται παραχρῆμα, μένει δ' ἄχρι πλέον ἡ θερμασία περί τε τὸν ἐντὸς ἀέρα καὶ κατ' αὐτὸ τὸ σῶμα, οὐ τραφεῖσα. οὕτω δὲ κἂν τοῖς οἴκοις τοῖς ὑπὸ πυρὸς θερμανθεῖσιν ἡ θερμα-
5 σία φαίνεται διαμένουσα, τοῦ πυρὸς ἐσβεσμένου πολλάκις.

7. οὐχ ὅμοιον οὖν ἐστι τὸ κατὰ φύσιν τῇ τε καρδίᾳ καὶ τοῖς ἄλλοις μορίοις· τὴν μὲν γὰρ ζεῖν ἀεὶ χρή, τοῖς δ' ἀρκεῖ τὸ μὴ παντάπασι καταψύχεσθαι.

8. μάθοις δ' ἂν ἐναργῶς

---

problem about the carotid arteries, appears puzzling no longer.

5. And it is much the same with the problem about the other arteries, that if any of them is ligatured, the part which it supplies suffers no sudden hurt. For we ought, I think, to have taken this also into consideration: that it makes no small / difference whether it is the source itself of the innate heat that K157 suffers, or one of those things that are warmed by it. For in it [the heart] there must always be warmth in plenty, for it both moves itself and the other parts at the same time with its pulse, and it also warms them. But for their part they have need of only a little warmth for their preservation. Again, if you deprive the heart of innate heat, you will make it cold itself, and with it all the other parts that were formerly warmed by it; but you cannot completely deprive these other parts of their warmth if you ligature the arteries, because some flows into them through the coats. For, as Hippocrates has it,[17] the whole body breathes and flows together. Hence some of the warmth will be conveyed into each and every part, even if not through the arteries, yet through the other parts, and particularly through the veins, because of the continuous chain of participation.

6. Now all this agrees with the observed facts, nor will it now seem at all strange that the source of innate heat suffers hurt, if breathing is stopped, to a greater degree than the other parts. / For in the cupping instruments of physicians also the flame is K158 quenched at once, but the warmth remains longer, both in the contained air and in the body itself,[18] without being nourished. In houses also that have been heated by fire the warmth is often found to endure when the fire has been put out.

7. So what is natural for the heart is not the same as what is natural for the other parts. The heart must always be on the boil, while as for the others, it suffices them not to be entirely cooled.

8. You will see clearly what has been described if you will lay

---

K158

1 σικύαις a: σικήαις S: σικείαις C

3 τραφεῖσα a: γράφεται S

4 ἡ om. K

7 ζεῖν a: ζῆν S   χρὴ a: χρῆν S

τὸ λεγόμενον, εἰ γυμνώσαις καρδίαν ζῴου, αὐτῆς διελὼν
10 τὸ σκέπασμα, ὃ καλοῦσι περικάρδιον χιτῶνα, χωρὶς τοῦ τὸν
ἄλλον θώρακα συντρῆσαι. τάχιστα γὰρ ἀποθνήσκει τὸ
ζῷον, εἰ καταψύξεις τὴν καρδίαν· εἰ μέντοι θερμὴν φυ-
λάττεις, οὐδὲν πάσχει. ψύξεις μὲν οὖν αὐτὴν ἐν ἀέρι τὴν
χειρουργίαν ψυχρῷ ποιούμενος καὶ ψυχρὸν καταρραίνων
15 ὕδωρ· φυλάξεις δὲ ὡς πλείστου θερμὴν διὰ τῶν ἐναντίων.
ἀλλ' εἰ, κατεψυγμένης ἤδη, καὶ διὰ τοῦτο τοῦ ζῴου τεθνεῶ-
τος, ἐθέλοις παραχρῆμα τρώσας ὁποτερανοῦν τῶν κοιλιῶν,
καὶ μᾶλλον τὴν ἀριστεράν, καθεῖναι δάκτυλον εἰς αὐτήν,
K159 αἰσθήσῃ πολλῆς τῆς θερμασίας, καὶ πολύ γε πλέονος, ἢ
ἐν τοῖς ἄλλοις μορίοις τοῖς κατὰ φύσιν διακειμένοις. τὸ
γὰρ ἴσον μέρος τῆς θερμασίας ἐλάχιστον μὲν τῇ καρδίᾳ,
πάμπολυ δὲ τοῖς ἄλλοις ἐστί. καὶ τοίνυν, ὅταν μὴ φυλάτ-
5 τηται τοῦτο, τὸ μὲν ἐκ τῆς καρδίας οἷον φλὸξ διαφορεῖται,
τὸ δ' ἐν τοῖς ἄλλοις ἄχρι πολλοῦ παραμένει. φυλακὴ δὲ
ἦν ἐκείνῃ μὲν ἡ ἀναπνοὴ μόνη, τοῖς δ' ἄλλοις διττή·
σφυγμὸς μέν, οἷον πρὸ ἀναπνοῆς, τό τε ἀπὸ τῆς ἀρχῆς
ἐπιρρέον ἐξ ἐπιμέτρου. κατὰ δύο τοίνυν αἰτίας ἕκαστον τῶν
10 μορίων πλεονεκτεῖ τῆς καρδίας εἰς τὸ μὴ ταχέως βλάπτεσθαι θερμασίας ἐνδείᾳ. καὶ γάρ, ὅτι πλείστης μὲν ἐκείνη
χρῄζει, τὰ δ' ἄλλα βραχείας, καὶ ὅτι τῇ μὲν οὐδαμόθεν
ἐπιρρεῖ, τοῖς δ' ἀπ' ἐκείνης, ἡ μὲν ἑτοίμως ἐξίσταται τοῦ
κατὰ φύσιν, τὰ δὲ οὔ.

15 3.   Περὶ δὲ τοῦ μὴ δι' ἀρτηριῶν μόνον,
ἀλλὰ καὶ διὰ τῶν φλεβῶν καὶ τῶν ἄλλων ἁπάντων ἐπιρρεῖν
ἐκ τῆς καρδίας τοῖς μορίοις τὴν θερμασίαν, ἐπεὶ διὰ
K160 βραχέος εἴρηται πρόσθεν, αὖθις ἡμῖν ἀναληπτέον τε καὶ
ἀποδεικτέον, εἰποῦσι πρότερον τὰ φαινόμενα, δι' ὧν ἄν
τις αὐτὸ συλλογίσαιτο.

2.   πολλοὺς οὖν ἤδη πολλάκις μονο-
μάχους [μονάρχους] τε καὶ στρατιώτας καὶ κυνηγέτας οὕτω

---

9 αὐτῆς διελὼν τὸ σκέπασμα a: τὸ σκεπασμένον αὐτῆς διελὼν S
14 ψυχρὸν a: ψυχρῶν S
18 τὴν a: εἰς τὴν S
K159
2 ἐν a: om. S   διακειμένοις a: ἔχουσι S

bare the heart of an animal, taking off the covering that they call the "pericardium," without penetrating the rest of the thorax. For the animal dies very swiftly if you chill the heart; but if you conserve the heat it suffers no ill. You will cool the heart if you perform the operation in cold air, and if you pour on cold water; you will keep it hot as long as possible if you do the contrary. But if when it is already chilled and the animal is therefore dead you will at once cut open either one of the ventricles, but particularly the left, and put your finger into it, / you will feel that the heat is considerable, and indeed much K159 more than in the other parts in a state of nature. For that same quantity of heat which is very small for the heart is very great for the other parts. So when this heat is not conserved, that which is like a flame in the heart is dissipated, but what is in the other parts lingers a long while. For the first of these two has only the breathing to foster it, while the second has two guardians: the pulse, as it were in place of breathing,[19] and what overflows from the source, in addition. From these two causes, then, each of the other parts has an advantage over the heart in avoiding immediate damage from a sudden loss of heat. Because the heart needs a great deal while the other parts need much less, and second, because there is nowhere whence the heart receives an influx of heat, whereas they receive one from it, therefore the heart easily loses its natural state, but they do not.

Chapter 3

However, as to the fact that the heat flows from the heart to the members not only through the arteries but also through the veins and all the other parts, since / this was mentioned some- K160 what briefly above, we must take it up again and give the proof of it, telling first the observed facts from which one may infer it.

2. It has often happened, then, to those who fight in single combat[20] and to soldiers and to huntsmen to be so wounded in

---

6 πολλοῦ a: πολλὰ S

8 πρὸ ἀναπνοῆς Furley, vers. Arab. secutus: προαναπνοὴ SaK: v. comm.

12 τῇ a: om. S

K160

2 μονάρχους om. vers. Arab., recte

5 τρωθῆναι συνέβη φλέβας καὶ ἀρτηρίας, ὥστε ἀναγκασθῆ-
ναι τοὺς ἰατροὺς βρόχῳ διαλαβεῖν αὐτάς. καὶ οὗτοι πάντες οὐ μετὰ πολὺν χρόνον ψυχροτέρων αἰσθάνονται τῶν
μορίων, πρωιαίτερον μέν, εἰ τὰς φλέβας καὶ τὰς ἀρτηρίας
βρόχῳ διαλάβοις, ὀψιαίτερον δέ, εἰ τὰς ἀρτηρίας μόνον,
10 ἥκιστα δέ, εἰ μόνας τὰς φλέβας. ἐξ ὧν δῆλον, ἥκειν μέν
τινα καὶ διὰ τῶν φλεβῶν εἰς τὰ μόρια θερμασίαν, ἀλλ'
ἐλάττονα μακρῷ τῆς διὰ τῶν ἀρτηριῶν. εἰ δὲ καὶ χωρὶς τραύματος ἐθελήσαις μόριόν τι τοῦ σώματος λαβὼν ἰσχυρῶς
καταδῆσαι, παραχρῆμα πελιδνόν τε καὶ ψυχρὸν αὐτὸ γινό-
15 μενον θεάσῃ, δῆλον ὡς στερηθὲν τῆς ἄνωθεν ἐπιρρεούσης
διὰ πάντων τῶν μερῶν αὐτοῦ θερμασίας.

3. ὁπότ' οὖν καὶ
τοῦτο δέδεικται, καὶ φαίνεται μηδὲν ἐναντιούμενον τῷ μὴ
K161 μίαν εἶναι τὴν χρείαν τῆς ἀναπνοῆς καὶ τῶν σφυγμῶν, ἔτοι-
μον ἤδη συλλογίσασθαι, φυλακῆς ἕνεκα τῆς καθ' ἕκαστον
μόριον θερμασίας γεγονέναι τοὺς σφυγμούς. ὥσθ', ὅπερ ἐκ
τῆς ἀναπνοῆς τῇ καρδίᾳ μόνῃ, τοῦτ' ἐξ ἐκείνων τῷ καθ'
5 ὅλον τὸ ζῷον ὑπάρχειν θερμῷ, εἶναι δὲ καὶ τὸ τῆς πέψεως
τοῦ ψυχικοῦ πνεύματος κοινὸν μὲν ἀμφοῖν, ἀλλ' ἰδιαίτα-
τον τῶν ἀρτηριῶν, εἴ γε δὴ μεμνήμεθα τῶν ὀλίγον πρόσθεν εἰρημένων περὶ τοῦ δικτυοειδοῦς πλέγματος.

4. ἐπεὶ τοί-
νυν ἐν τῷ περὶ χρείας ἀναπνοῆς ἐδείκνυτο διὰ μὲν τῆς
10 εἰσπνοῆς ἐμψυχόμενον τὸ ἔμφυτον θερμόν, διὰ δὲ τῆς
ἀναπνοῆς οἷον καθαιρόμενον, ἐκκρινομένου τοῦ καπνώδους
περιττώματος, ἄμφω δὲ ταῦτ' εἰς τὴν φυλακὴν αὐτοῦ συν-
τελεῖν, δῆλον ὡς κἀπὶ τῶν σφυγμῶν ἐροῦμεν, ἐν μὲν ταῖς
διαστολαῖς ἕλκεσθαί τινα οὐσίαν ἀερώδη, κατὰ δὲ τὰς
15 συστολὰς ἐκκρίνεσθαι τὸ ἐκ τῆς τῶν χυμῶν συγκαύσεως καθ' ὅλον τὸ ζῷον γινόμενον οἷον καπνῶδες περίττωμα.

K162 **4.** Καίτοι γινώσκω τοὺς περὶ τὸν Ἀρχιγένην
καί τινας ἔτι πρότερον ἐν μὲν ταῖς συστολαῖς πληροῦσθαι
τὰς ἀρτηρίας οἰομένους, ἐν δὲ ταῖς διαστολαῖς κενοῦσθαι.
πρὸς γὰρ τὴν ἕλξιν ἐπιτηδειοτάτην εἶναι νομίζουσι τὴν συ-

8 εἰ a: εἰς S
9 εἰ a: εἰς S

the veins and arteries that the physicians are compelled to ligature them. All these soon feel the limbs growing colder— sooner if you ligature both arteries and veins, later if only the arteries, and least of all if only the veins. Hence it is clear that a certain heat comes even through the veins to the members, though much less than through the arteries. But even without any wound, if you take any part of the body and bind it tightly, you will see it immediately grow pale and cold, clearly because the heat flowing down through all the parts has been cut off.

3. Now, when this has been shown, and it is also apparent that there is nothing against / there being one and the same use K161 for both breathing and the pulse, it is readily concluded that the pulse occurs to conserve the heat in each part. So what breathing does for the heart alone is done by the pulse for the warmth that is all over the body; moreover, to both breathing and the pulse the concoction of the psychic pneuma is common, but this particularly belongs to the arteries, if we call to mind what was said a little before concerning the netlike plexus.[21]

4. Now since it was shown in the book *On the Use of Breathing*[22] that on the one hand the innate heat is cooled by breathing in, and on the other by breathing out it is in a way purged, the , smoky residue being voided, and that both of these actions are for its preservation, it is clear that we shall say of the pulse, too, that in the expansions some airy substance is drawn in, and that in the contractions there is voided the stuff that is, as it were, a smoky residue from the burning up of the juices throughout the whole animal.[23] /

Chapter 4

I am fully aware that the school of Archigenes,[24] and some K162 others before them, believed that the arteries are filled in their contractions and emptied in their expansions. They supposed

---

10 καὶ S: *om.* aK
17 τῷ K: τὸ Sa
K161
  2 φυλακῆς a: φυλακὴ S
  5 ὑπάρχειν S: -ει a
K162
  4 ἑλξιν a: ἴλξιν S

5 στολήν, τεκμαιρόμενοι μάλιστα τῷ τε στόματι καὶ ταῖς
ῥισὶν κατὰ μὲν τὰς εἰσπνοάς, ὡς ἐκεῖνοί φασι, συστελλο-
μένοις, κατὰ δὲ τὰς ἐκπνοὰς διαστελλομένοις· ὅπερ ἐπὶ
τῶν ἀρρώστων μὲν τὴν δύναμιν ὁρᾶται γινόμενον. οὐδ'
οὖν οὐδ' ἐπὶ τούτων κατ' ἄλλο τι μόριον ἢ ἐν τοῖς ὑστά-
10 τοις καὶ χονδρώδεσι τῶν ῥινῶν. ὁρᾶται δέ ποτε κἀπὶ τῶν
δραμόντων ὠκέως ἢ ἄλλως πως συντόνως γυμναζομένων, οὐ μὴν ἐπ' ἄλλου γε οὐδενός, οὔθ' ὑγιαίνοντος,
οὔτε νοσοῦντος. χρὴ δὲ τὴν φυσικὴν κατάστασιν, ἥτις ἂν
ᾖ, τοῖς ἀπαραποδίστως τε καὶ ἀκριβῶς ὑγιαίνουσι μᾶλλον
15 ἤπερ τοῖς ἄλλοις φαίνεσθαι. ἀλλ' ἔστω γίνεσθαι πᾶσιν
ὁμοίως, καὶ φαινέσθωσαν αἵ τε ῥῖνες καὶ τὰ χείλη συστέλλεσθαι τοῖς εἰσπνέουσι, τίς ἡ ἐκ τούτου πίστις τῷ ζητου-
μένῳ; οὐ γὰρ δὴ ἀνάλογον φήσουσιν ἔχειν ταῖς ἀρτηρίαις
K163 τὰ χείλη καὶ τὰς ῥῖνας. ἀλλὰ τούτοις μὲν ἀνάλογον τὰ
πέρατα τῶν ἀρτηριῶν, αὐταῖς δὲ ταῖς ἀρτηρίαις αἱ ἀπὸ
τούτων ἐπὶ τὴν καρδίαν οἷον ὁδοὶ τοῦ πνεύματός εἰσιν.
εἰ μὲν οὖν ἐκείνας ἔχουσι δεῖξαι συστελλομένας ἐν ταῖς
5 εἰσπνοαῖς, εἴη ἄν τι πλέον αὐτοῖς τοῦ παραδείγματος· εἰ
δὲ <μή>, πρὸς τῷ μηδὲν ὠφελεῖσθαι, ἔτι καὶ καθ' ἑαυτῶν αὐτῷ
ἐφέλκονται, ἐρούντων ἂν ἡμῶν, ὥσπερ ἡ φάρυγξ, καὶ ὁ
πνεύμων, καὶ σύμπας ὁ θώραξ ἐν ταῖς εἰσπνοαῖς διαστέλλεται, καὶ τὰς ἀρτηρίας οὕτω χρῆναι διίστασθαι, καθ' ὃν
10 ἕλκουσι καιρόν, οὐ καθ' ὃν ἐκπέμπουσι τὸ πνεῦμα. ἀλλὰ
καὶ ἡ μετὰ τὴν συστολὴν αὐτῶν ἡσυχία πολλῷ μακροτέρα
γινομένη τῆς μετὰ τὴν διαστολήν, ὥσπερ καὶ ἡ πρὸ τῆς
εἰσπνοῆς τῆς μετ' αὐτήν, ἐνδείκνυταί τινα καὶ κατὰ τοῦτο
ἀναλογίαν εἶναι τοῖς σφυγμοῖς πρὸς τὴν ἀναπνοήν. οἷον
15 γοῦν τι ἡ εἰσπνοὴ τοῖς ἀναπνευστικοῖς ὀργάνοις, τοιοῦτον
ἡ διαστολὴ ταῖς ἀρτηρίαις, καὶ οἷον γοῦν τι ἐκείνοις ἡ
ἐκπνοή, τοιοῦτον ταῖς ἀρτηρίαις ἡ συστολή.

2. ταύτης δὲ τῆς
διπλῆς καὶ συνθέτου τῶν ἀρτηριῶν κινήσεως, ἣν δὴ καὶ

---

9 κατ' ἄλλο τι μόριον ἢ Furley, vers. Arab. secutus: κἂν ... ᾖ SaK: alia ulla in
parte quam Lin.
18 ἀνάλογον a: ἀναχ^ολ S
K163
6 μὴ Furley, vers. Arab. secutus; om. SaK: sin minus Lin. αὐτῷ Furley: αὐτὸ
SaK ἡμῶν a: ἡμῖν S

that the contractions are more suited to attraction, citing in evidence particularly that both mouth and nostrils contract, or so they say, in breathing in, but expand in breathing out. This is seen in those who are enfeebled with respect to this faculty — even in their case, however, in no other part[25] than in the extreme, cartilaginous parts of the nostrils. It is seen sometimes also in those who run swiftly, or take strenuous exercise of some other kind, but in no others, either well or sick. But the natural condition, whatever it may be, must appear more clearly in those whose health is unimpaired and perfect than in others. But suppose that the same thing happens to all, and that both mouth and nostrils are observed to contract in those who breathe in: what persuasion do we draw from this in our inquiry? For they will not say that there is some analogy between the arteries / and the lips and nostrils, but only that there is an analogy between these latter and the ends of the arteries; while to the arteries themselves correspond the pathways (so to speak) for the pneuma that lead down from the mouth and nostrils toward the heart. So if they can show these to be contracted in breathing in, the comparison will be of some service to them. But if not, they are not only not helped by it, but in addition are brought by it to oppose themselves;[26] for we shall say that, just as the pharynx, the lung, and the whole thorax expand in breathing in, so it is necessary for the arteries to expand when they draw in, not when they breathe out the pneuma. Furthermore, the pause after the contraction of the arteries is much greater than that after their expansion, just as that before breathing in is greater than that after it; and this shows that in this respect, too, there is an analogy between the pulse and breathing. What inbreathing is to the organs of breathing, then, expansion is to the arteries, and what outbreathing is to the former, contraction is for the arteries.

K163

2. This double and compounded motion of the arteries which

---

12 ἡ a: *om.* S
13 τῆς K: *om.* Sa
16 γοῦν *om.* S

K164 σφυγμὸν ὀνομάζομεν, ἐξηγεῖται μὲν ἡ καρδία, καθάπερ
καὶ ἡμῖν ἐν ἑτέροις καὶ μυρίοις ἄλλοις πρὸ ἡμῶν ἀποδέδεικται, οὐ μὴν καθ' ὃν Ἐρασίστρατος ὑπελάμβανεν τρόπον, ἀλλ' ὡς Ἡρόφιλός τε καὶ Ἱπποκράτης, καὶ σχεδὸν
5 οἱ δοκιμώτατοι πάντες τῶν παλαιῶν ἰατρῶν τε καὶ φιλοσόφων. ἡ γὰρ ἐν τῷ σώματι τῆς καρδίας δύναμις, ὑφ' ἧς
διαστέλλεται καὶ συστέλλεται, διὰ τῶν χιτώνων ἐπιρρέουσα
ταῖς ἀρτηρίαις ἁπάσαις, οὕτως αὐτὰς διαστέλλει καὶ συστέλλει,
καθάπερ καὶ αὐτὴν τὴν καρδίαν. ὡς οὖν ἐκείνη διαστελλομένη
10 μὲν εἰς ἑαυτὴν ἕλκει τὰ πλησιάζοντα τοῖς στόμασιν αὐτῆς,
συστελλομένη δὲ ἐκθλίβει, οὕτω καὶ αἱ ἀρτηρίαι διαστελλόμεναι μὲν ἕλκουσι πανταχόθεν, συστελλόμεναι δ'
ἐκθλίβουσι πανταχόσε.

5. Τί δὴ τοῦτ' ἔστι πανταχόθεν καὶ πανταχόσε,
15 σαφέστερον ἔτι διαιρήσω σοι. πάμπολλοι πόροι ταῖς ἀρτηρίαις,
οἱ μὲν ἐν αὐτοῖς τοῖς χιτῶσιν οἷον ὀπαί τινες, ἄλλοι δὲ δίκην
στομάτων εἰς ἔντερα καὶ γαστέρα καὶ τοῦτο δὴ τὸ ἐκτὸς
δέρμα περαίνονται. ἀλλὰ καὶ συνεχεῖς ἀλλήλαις τε καὶ τῇ
K165 καρδίᾳ κατὰ μεγίστους εἰσὶ πόρους, [κατὰ τὰς αὐτὰς ἀρτηρίας,] μᾶλλον δὲ κατὰ τοὺς ἔνδον χιτῶνας ἅπαντας. ταῖς γε φλεψὶν
οὔπω κατὰ μεγάλους, ἀλλ' ἐκφεύγουσι μὲν τὰς αἰσθήσεις αἱ
συναναστομώσεις αὐτῶν. ὥστε, κἂν ἀπιστοίης δικαίως, ὡς οὐκ
5 οὔσαις, πιστεύσαις ἂν διὰ τὰ ἄλλα τὰ πρὸς τῶν παλαιῶν
εἰρημένα, καὶ οὐχ ἥκιστα διὰ τόδε τὸ φαινόμενον. εἰ γάρ
τις λαβὼν ζῷον ὁτιοῦν τούτων δὴ τῶν μεγάλας τε καὶ σαφεῖς τὰς φλέβας τε καὶ τὰς ἀρτηρίας ἐχόντων, οἷον βοῦν,
ἢ σῦν, ἢ ὄνον, ἢ ἵππον, ἢ πρόβατον, ἢ ἄρκτον, ἢ πί-
10 θηκον, ἢ πάρδαλιν, ἢ ἄνθρωπον αὐτόν, ἤ τι τῶν ἄλλων τῶν παραπλησίων, κατὰ μεγάλας καὶ πολλὰς ἀρτηρίας τρώσειεν, ἐκκενώσει δι' αὐτὰς ἅπαν τοῦ ζῴου τὸ αἷμα.
τούτου πολλάκις ἡμεῖς τοῦ φαινομένου πεῖραν ἐποιησάμεθα,

K164

2 πρὸ ἡμῶν K: πρὸς ἡμῖν a: πρὸ ἡμῖν S: ante nos Lin.

8 διαστέλλει ... συστέλλει a: -ειν ... -ειν S

15 διαιρήσω σοι a: διαιρήσωσι S   πόροι a: πόνοι S

K165

1 κατὰ τὰς αὐτῶν ἀρτηρίας om. Furley, vers. Arab. secutus: αὐτῶν S: αὐτὰς aK: v. comm.

we / call the pulse is governed by the heart, as we ourselves   K164
elsewhere,[27] and many others before us have demonstrated; it is
not so, however, in the manner supposed by Erasistratus, but as
both Herophilus and Hippocrates,[28] and nearly all the most
esteemed of the ancient physicians and philosophers believed.
For that power which is in the body of the heart,[29] by which it
expands and contracts, flowing out through their coats to all the
arteries expands and contracts them, just as it does the heart; so
just as it, being expanded, draws in what is near its openings,
and squeezes it out in contracting, so also do the arteries when
expanding draw in from all sides, and contracting squeeze out
on all sides.

Chapter 5

Well, now, I will explain to you more clearly what is meant by
this "from all sides" and "on all sides." There are many pores in
the arteries, some in the coats themselves—vents, as it were—
others, like mouths, open either into the guts or the stomach or
into this outer skin.[30] Moreover, the arteries are linked continu-
ously with each other and / with the heart by means of very   K165
large pores, or rather, by means of all of their inner coats.[31] To
the veins, however, they are not linked through large pores, for
these junctions cannot be perceived. Even if, therefore, you are
sceptical of their existence, as you well might be, you may yet be
convinced by what the ancients have said, and not least from the
following observed fact. If anyone will take any animal of those
that have both veins and arteries large and conspicuous (such as
an ox, a pig, an ass, a horse, a sheep, a bear, an ape, a leopard,
or even a man, or any other of the same kind), and wound it in
its many large arteries, he will empty out all the blood of the
animal through them. Of this fact we have often made trial,[32]

---

2 κατὰ τοὺς ἔνδον χίτωνας ἅπαντας Furley, vers. Arab. secutus; εὐρυχωρίας
ἁπάσας SaK: v. comm.
3 μεγάλους Furley: -ας aK. μεγ· S
4 ὥστε a: om. S
5 πρὸς a: πρὸ S
7 μεγάλας a: μεγάλως S
12 αὐτὰς a: αὐτῶν S
13 τούτου ... φαινομένου S: τοῦ φαινομένου ἡμεῖς aK

καὶ διαπαντὸς εὑρίσκοντες ἐκκενουμένας τὰς φλέβας
15 ἅμα ταῖς ἀρτηρίαις ἀληθὲς τὸ τῶν συναναστομώσεων ἐκ
τούτων ἐπείσθημεν δόγμα.

2. διὰ γοῦν τούτων τῶν ἀναστο-
μώσεων ἐκ τῶν φλεβῶν ἕλκουσι μὲν ἐν ταῖς διαστολαῖς
αἱ ἀρτηρίαι, ἐκθλίβουσι δὲ εἰς αὐτὰς ἐν ταῖς συστολαῖς, ὥσπερ
διὰ τῶν εἰς τὸ δέρμα περαινομένων στομάτων ἐκκρίνουσι
K166 μὲν ἔξω πᾶν ὅσον ἀτμῶδές τε καὶ καπνῶδες περίττωμα,
μεταλαμβάνουσι δὲ εἰς ἑαυτὰς ἐκ τοῦ περιέχοντος ἡμᾶς
ἀέρος οὐκ ὀλίγην μοῖραν. καὶ τοῦτ' ἔστι τὸ πρὸς Ἱπποκράτους λεγόμενον, ὡς ἔκπνουν καὶ εἴσπνουν ἐστὶν ὅλον τὸ
5 σῶμα. κατὰ δὲ τὸν αὐτὸν τρόπον ἔκ τε τῆς γαστρὸς καὶ
τῶν ἐντέρων ἕλκουσί τε καὶ αὖθις ἐκκρίνουσιν. οὕτω δὲ
καὶ ἐκ τῶν περιεχουσῶν αὐτὰς χωρῶν διὰ τῶν οἷον ὀπῶν
τῶν καθ' ὅλους τοὺς χιτῶνας αὐτῶν ἐν μέρει μὲν ἕλκουσιν, ἐν μέρει δ' ἐκκρίνουσι. παρὰ δὲ τῆς καρδίας λαμ-
10 βάνουσι μὲν πλεῖον, διδόασι δ' ἔλαττον. αἰτία δὲ αἱ
τῶν ὑμένων ἐπιφύσεις, ὑπὲρ ὧν αὐτάρκως Ἐρασιστράτου
διειλεγμένου, περιττὸν ἡμᾶς νῦν γράφειν. ἀλλ' ἐκεῖνος μὲν
ἔοικεν ὑπολαμβάνειν, μηδὲν ὅλως εἰς τὴν καρδίαν ἐκ τῶν
ἀρτηριῶν μεταλαμβάνεσθαι, πλήν γε διὰ τῶν ἐν πνεύμονι·
15 τὸ δὲ οὐχ οὕτως ἔχει. τάχα μὲν γὰρ καὶ [τὰ] κατ' αὐτὸν
τὸν τῆς φύσεως νόμον διοικουμένου τοῦ ζῴου μεταλαμβά-
νεταί τι μικρόν. οὐχ οὕτως γάρ μοι δοκοῦσιν ἀκριβῶς ἀπο-
φράττειν τὸ στόμα τῆς μεγάλης ἀρτηρίας οἱ ὑμένες, ὡς
K167 μηδὲν ἐξ αὐτῆς εἰς τὴν καρδίαν παλινδρομεῖν· εἰ δὲ μή,
ἀλλά τοί γε, βιαίας τινὸς περιστάσεως καταλαβούσης τὸ
ζῶον, ἀναγκαῖον οὕτως γίνεσθαι παντὸς [δὲ] μᾶλλον ἀληθὲς
εἶναί μοι δοκεῖ. τοῦτο δὲ καὶ δι' ἑτέρων ἡμῖν γραμμάτων
5 ἀποδέδεικται, καὶ οὐ μεγάλη τις αὐτοῦ χρεία πρὸς τὸν
ἐνεστῶτα λόγον. εἰ μὲν γάρ τι καὶ τῇ καρδίᾳ μεταδιδόα-
σιν αἱ ἀρτηρίαι, πανταχόθεν ἂν οὕτως ἕλκοιέν τε καὶ αὖ-

---

18 αἱ S: om. CaK
K166
 9 παρὰ a: περὶ S
10 αἱ ... ἐπιφύσεις a: ἡ ... -ις S
11 ὧν a: τῶν S
15 τὰ secl. Furley

and having always found the veins empty along with the arteries, on these grounds we have accepted as true the teaching concerning the junctions.

2. For through those junctions the arteries draw from the veins, when they [the arteries] expand, and squeeze into them on contracting; just as they eliminate through the mouths that end in the skin / all the waste matter that is vaporous and K166 smoky, and take up into themselves in exchange no small part of the air that surrounds us. And this is what Hippocrates says: that the whole body breaths in and out.[33] Moreover, in the same way they [the arteries] draw from the stomach and the guts, and again eliminate into them. And so also, through the ventlike openings everywhere in their coats, by turns they draw in from the spaces around them and eliminate into them.[34] As for the heart, they receive much from it, but give up little to it; the cause being the membranous outgrowths, about which, since Erasistratus has written sufficiently,[35] it is superfluous for us to write more. He, however, seems to be of the opinion that nothing whatever passes to the heart from the arteries, except those which are in the lung. But that is not so. It may well be that, from the very fact that the animal is made subject to Nature's law, a little passes. For the membranes do not seem to me to close the mouth of the great artery so exactly / that nothing may K167 run back from it to the heart; and if this is not so, nevertheless when some violent circumstance constrains the animal, it seems to me unquestionably true that this must happen.[36] However, this has been expounded in others of our writings;[37] and there is no great need of it in the present argument. Now, if the arteries give something to the heart also, they could then draw in from all sides and send out again on all sides; if not, then they will

---

17 μοι a: με S

K167

2 τοι a: τι S

3 γίνεσθαι παντὸς μᾶλλον Furley, vers. Arab. secutus: γίνεται πάντως δὲ μᾶλλον a: γίνεσθαι παντὸς δὲ μᾶλλον S: v. comm.

4 δὲ aC: μὲν S

6 τῇ καρδίᾳ a: τῆς καρδίας S

θις ἀντιπέμποιεν· εἰ δὲ μή, πανταχόθεν μὲν ἕλξουσιν, ἐπι-
πέμψουσιν δέ, πλὴν εἰς τὴν καρδίαν, πανταχόσε.

                    3. καὶ

10 μοι δοκεῖ πολλῷ βέλτιον εἶναι τοῦτο τὸ δόγμα τῶν Ἐρα-
σιστρατείων ὑποθέσεων· οὐδὲ γὰρ οὐδὲ σύμπνουν οὐδὲ
σύρρουν εἶναι τὸ σῶμα δυνατὸν ἑαυτῷ, τῶν ἀρτηριῶν ἑλ-
κουσῶν μὲν πανταχόθεν, μὴ ἐκπεμπουσῶν δὲ πανταχόσε.
καὶ μὲν δὴ τὸ τῆς ἐνεργείας αὐτῶν χρηστὸν ὧδ' ἂν μᾶλ-
15 λον εἰς ἅπαν ἐκταθείη τὸ ζῷον. οὕτω γὰρ ἅπαν μόριον
ἀναψύχεσθαί τε καὶ καθαίρεσθαι δυνήσεται ταῖς τῶν ἀρτηριῶν διαφόροις κινήσεσι ἐπιστατούμενον.

                    4. ὡς δ' Ἐρασί-
στρατος ὑπελάμβανεν, ὀχετῶν ἀψύχων ἔργον, οὐκ ὀργάνων
K168 ζωτικῶν, αἱ ἀρτηρίαι τοῖς ζῴοις ὑπηρετοῦσιν. ἡμεῖς δὲ καὶ
δι' ἑτέρου τινὸς ὅλου βιβλίου πολυειδῶς ἀπεδείξαμεν,
αἷμα κἂν τῷ κατὰ φύσιν ἔχειν τὸ ζῷον ἐν ταῖς ἀρτηρίαις περιέχεσθαι. εἰ δὲ τοῦτο, παντί που δῆλον, ὡς οὐχ,
5 ὅτι πληροῦνται τοῦ παρὰ τῆς καρδίας ἐπιπεμπομένου πνεύματος, ὡς Ἐρασίστρατος ἐνόμιζε, διὰ τοῦτο διαστέλλονται
μᾶλλον ἤ, ὅτι διαστέλλονται, διὰ τοῦτο πληροῦνται. κενῶν
μὲν γὰρ αἵματος οὐσῶν, ἐνδέχοιτ' ἂν ἴσως ἐν ὀλίγῳ χρόνῳ
τὸ ἀπὸ τῆς καρδίας ἐπιρρυὲν ἐξικέσθαι μέχρι τῶν περά-
10 των· αἷμα δὲ εἴπερ ἔχοιεν, οὐδαμῶς ἐγχωρεῖ τὸ τάχος τῆς
κινήσεως ὁμολογεῖν τῷ παρὰ τῆς καρδίας πληρουμένας αὐτὰς διαστέλλεσθαι.

                    5. οὐ γάρ, ὅτι πληροῦνται, διὰ τοῦτο
διαστέλλονται, ἀλλ' ὅτι διαστέλλονται, διὰ τοῦτο πληροῦνται. τοῦτο μὲν δὴ πολλάκις τε καὶ πανταχοῦ καὶ
15 ἡμῖν καὶ πολλοῖς τῶν ἔμπροσθεν ἀποδέδεικται, τὸ τὰς
ἀρτηρίας ἐνεργεῖν αὐτάς, ὡς καὶ ἡ καρδία, συστελλομένας
τε καὶ διαστελλομένας ἐν μέρει κατὰ τὴν αὐτὴν ἐκείνῃ
K169 δύναμιν, ἣν ἐκ τῆς καρδίας ὁρμωμένην διὰ τῶν χιτώνων αὐτῶν ἐλέγομεν πέμπεσθαι.

   6.   Κάλλιον δ' εἶναί μοι δοκοῦσι ποιεῖν οἱ ζη-
τοῦντες, ἆρά γε τὴν διαστολήν, ἢ τὴν συστολήν, ἢ ἀμ-

---

9 καὶ ante πλὴν habent aK   εἰς τὴν καρδίαν a: καρδ. S
10 τοῦτο a: om. S
15 μόριον S: μόνον CaK

indeed draw in from all sides, but they will send out on all sides except into the heart.

3. This doctrine seems to me better than the suppositions of the Erastrateans. For neither can the body breathe nor can it flow all together, each part with all the others, if the arteries draw in from all sides but do not send out on all sides. And certainly the benefit of their activity would in this way be better extended over the whole animal. For thus every part will be able to be cooled and purged under the direction of the complex motions of the arteries.[38]

4. But according to Erasistratus, the arteries play for animals the part of lifeless drains, / not of living organs. However, in a K168 book wholly devoted to this subject, we have shown in many ways that the arteries contain blood, even when the animal is in its natural state.[39] But if so, it is clear to everyone that it is not by being filled with pneuma dispatched from the heart, as Erasistratus thought, that they are made to expand: it is because they expand that they are filled. For if they were empty of blood, then it would of course be possible that what had flowed from the heart would reach the extremities in a very short time: if, however, they have blood in them, it could never be that the speed of the motion would agree with the expansion being due to their being filled from the heart.[40]

5. So they do not expand because they are filled; they are filled because they expand. Indeed it has been proved again and again, both by us and by many of our forerunners, that the arteries are themselves active, just as the heart is, contracting and expanding by turns by the same power as does the heart, / which power we described as originating from the heart and K169 being transmitted through their coats.

Chapter 6

Those who inquire whether the expansion or the contraction, or both, should be considered activities of the arteries seem to

K168

3 ταῖς S: αὐταῖς a: αὐταῖς ταῖς K

4 οὐχ a οὐχ ὅς S

5 παρὰ a: περὶ S τῆς a: om. S

215

5 φοτέρας ἐνεργείας χρὴ νομίζειν τῶν ἀρτηριῶν, ὥσπερ, οἶμαι, καὶ περὶ τῶν τῆς ἀναπνοῆς μερῶν εὐλόγως ἐζη- τήθη, πότερον τὴν ἐκπνοήν, ἢ τὴν εἰσπνοήν, ἢ ἀμφοτέ- ρας ἐνεργείας ὑποληπτέον ὑπάρχειν. ἀλλὰ περὶ μὲν ἐκείνων ἐν ἑτέροις εἴρηται τὰ εἰκότα, περὶ δὲ τῆς τῶν σφυγμῶν

10 κινήσεως νῦν ζητητέον.

2. εἰ μὲν οὖν, ὥσπερ εἴρηται, τῆς αὐτῆς ἐνεργείας ἕνεκα γεγόνασιν ἀναπνοή τε καὶ σφυγμὸς καὶ πρὸς τῶν αὐτῶν δημιουργουσῶν δυνάμεων, ῥᾴδιον ἂν εἴη τῇ πρὸς ἐκείνην ὁμοιότητι καὶ περὶ τῶν σφυγμῶν τι τεκμήρασθαι. ἐπεὶ δὲ τῶν μὲν σφυγμῶν ἡ ζωτικὴ δύνα-

15 μις ἡ ἀπὸ τῆς καρδίας ὁρμωμένη δημιουργός, τῆς δ' ἀνα- πνοῆς, ὡς ἐδείξαμεν, ἡ ἀπ' ἐγκεφάλου ψυχική, οὐδὲν ἂν ἡμῖν ἐκ τῶν ὑπὲρ ἐκείνης εὑρημένων εὐποροίη πρὸς τὰ πάροντα. †χαλεπώτερον δή τι τὸ τῆς εὑρέσεως, καὶ† διότι μετὰ

K170 τὸν θάνατον οὐχ ὥσπερ τὰς φλέβας ἔστιν ἰδεῖν εἰς ἑαυτὰς συμπιπτούσας, οὕτω καὶ τὰς ἀρτηρίας. αἱ μὲν γάρ, ὅταν κενωθῶσι τοῦ αἵματος, εἰς ἑαυτὰς συνιζάνουσι τελέως, ὥστε τοὺς ἄνωθεν αὐτῶν χιτῶνας ἐπιπίπτειν τοῖς κάτωθεν,

5 αἱ δ' ἀρτηρίαι μέχρι παντὸς διεστηκυῖαι ' φαίνονται, διὰ τὸν ἕτερον δηλονότι τῶν ἐν αὐταῖς χιτώνων τὸν σκληρόν. καίτοι τινὲς καὶ αὐτὸ τοῦτο μετὰ τὸν θάνατον γίνεσθαί φασι, πηγνυμένων ὑπὸ τῆς ψύξεως αὐτῶν καὶ οὐ φύσει τοιούτων οὐσῶν. ἕτεροι δὲ εἰς θερμὸν ὕδωρ ἐμβαλόντες,

10 εἶτ' ἔτι διεστώσας ὁρῶντες, οὕτω πείθονται διακεῖσθαι καὶ πρὸ τοῦ θανάτου· ἐπανελθεῖν γὰρ ἂν εἰς τὴν ἀρχαίαν φύσιν, ἀπελθούσης τῆς ψύξεως, εἰ δὴ ταύτῃ τι ἐνενεωτέ- ριστο.

3. παντοίως οὖν ἀπόρου τοῦ ζητουμένου ὄντος, οἷς τεκμαιρόμενος ἀμφοτέρας τὰς κινήσεις τῶν ἀρτηριῶν ἐνερ-

15 γείας εἶναι νομίζω, καὶ δὴ φράσω. τὴν μὲν διαστολήν, ἔτι

K169
5 ἀμφοτέρας ἐνεργείας K: -αν -αν Sa
7 πότερον a: πρότερον S τὴν εἰσπνοὴν a: εἰς τὴν πνοὴν S
9 τῆς τῶν σφυγμῶν a: τῆς σφυγμῆς S
12 δημιουργουσῶν K: ἐδημιουργούντων Ca: ἐδημιουργ... S
15 τῆς καρδίας a: καρδίας S
17 εὐποροίη Furley: ἀποροῖ τᾶν ut videtur S: εὐπορεῖν τῆς a: ad proposita con- ducat Lin.; fortasse εὐποροιτ' ἄν: v. comm.

me to do better; just as, so I believe, it was reasonable to inquire concerning the parts of breathing, whether breathing out or breathing in, or both, must be supposed active. But what is probably the case about the latter has been spoken of elsewhere;[41] here we have to inquire about the movements of the pulse.

2. If, as has been said, both breathing and the pulse exist for the same activity and through the same fashioning powers, it would be a simple matter, from the similarity with breathing, to conclude something concerning the pulse. However, since the productive principle of the pulse is the vital power that springs from the heart, while on the other hand, as we showed, that of the breathing is psychic and from the brain,[42] nothing that has been found out about the latter <would assist us at present.[43] In fact, a somewhat difficult problem arises in this connection,> / namely, why it is that we do not see the arteries after death   K170 fallen in upon themselves like the veins. For they, when emptied of blood, collapse altogether on themselves, so that their upper coats fall upon their lower, but the arteries appear uncollapsed forever; clearly because of one of their two coats, which is stiff. Some, however, say this very thing[44] occurs after death because they coagulate on cooling, not being thus [stiff] by nature. While others, having put them [the arteries of the dead animal] in hot water, and seeing them still remain expanded, are persuaded that they are in this condition before death; for when the cold is taken away they would have returned to their former state, if there had in fact been any alteration because of the cold.

3. The problem being of the most dubious, I shall now declare by what evidence I judge both motions of the arteries to be active. It is clear to all that so long as the power is in full

---

18 post πάροντα interpunx. vers. Arab. et Latin.   χαλεπώτερον δή τι τὸ S^{corr}:   ●
χαλεπωτέρος δήπου a: v. comm.
K170
11 ἂν K: om. Sa
12 τι ἐνενεωτέριστο K: τινὶ νεωτέριστο Sa
15 εἶναι S: ἦ a   ἔτι a: ὅτι S

τῆς δυνάμεως ἐρρωμένης, μεγάλην γίνεσθαι, ὥσπερ τοὐναντίον, αὐτῆς ἀσθενούσης, μικρὰν εἶναι, πᾶσι πρόδηλον.

K171 ἔχρην δέ, εἴπερ, ὥς τινες οἴονται, τὸ μὲν συστέλλεσθαι τῶν
ἀρτηριῶν ἐνέργεια, τὸ δὲ διαστέλλεσθαι εἰς τὴν κατὰ φύσιν
τῶν χιτώνων διάστασιν ἐπάνοδος αὐτόματος, πρῶτον μὲν
ἴσον ἀεὶ τὸν ὄγκον ὑπάρχειν τῶν διαστολῶν, ἔπειτα μηδὲν
5 μᾶλλον ἐρρωμένης ἢ ἀρρώστου δυνάμεως εἶναι ἔργον τὸ
μέγεθος· οὐδέτερον δ' οὕτως ἔχει.

4. καὶ πρόσεστιν ἕτερον
τεκμήριον οὐ μικρὸν εἰς ταὐτὸν συντελοῦν. μέγιστοι καὶ
ὑψηλότατοι σφυγμοὶ τοῖς κάλλιστα κριθησομένοις γίνονται.
καίτοι τότ' οὐκ ἄν τις οὐδὲ μαινόμενος εἴποι τὴν δύνα-
10 μιν ἀρρωστεῖν. εἰ γὰρ τὸ καλῶς κριθῆναι γίνεται ἐνδείᾳ
δυνάμεως, τὸ κακῶς δι' εὐρωστίαν δηλονότι γενήσεται·
εἰ δὲ τοῦτο, καὶ τὸ ἀποθανεῖν αὐτὸ ῥώμης ἔργον εἶναι
φήσομεν. τί οὖν ἂν εἴη γελοιότερον;

5. ἀλλὰ καὶ τὸ σφο-
δρὸν τῆς πληγῆς ἐν τῷ διαστέλλεσθαι τοῖς μὲν μᾶλλον,
15 τοῖς δὲ ἧττον ὑπάρχειν τῶν σφυγμῶν ἐπίτασιν καὶ ἄνε-
σιν ἐνεργείας ἐνδείκνυται. εἰ δέ τις παῦλα τῆς ἐνεργείας
ἦν ἡ διαστολή, καθάπερ ἡ ἐκπνοή, οὔτ' ἂν τὸ μᾶλλόν τε
K172 καὶ ἧττον ἦν ἐν αὐτῇ, καθὰ ἐν ταῖς ἐκπνοαῖς, οὔθ' ὅλος
ὁ τόνος τε καὶ ἡ σφοδρότης τῆς προσβολῆς.

6. ἡ μὲν
οὖν διαστολὴ διὰ ταῦτά τε καὶ ἄλλα παραπλήσια τούτοις
ἐκ τοῦ τῶν ἐνεργειῶν εἶναί μοι φαίνεται γένους, καὶ σώ-
5 ζοιτ' ἂν ἔτι καὶ κατὰ τοῦτο ἡ πρὸς τὴν ἀναπνοὴν τῶν
σφυγμῶν ὁμοιότης.

7. Ἐφεξῆς ἂν εἴη σκεπτέον, εἰ, ὥσπερ ἡ ἐκπνοὴ ἄνεσίς ἐστι καὶ οἷον ἀνάπαυσις τῆς ἐνεργείας τοῦ
θώρακος, ἡ ἐκφύσησις δὲ ἐνέργεια, καὶ διὰ τοῦτο τὸ μᾶλλόν
10 τε καὶ ἧττον ἔχει, τῆς ἐκπνοῆς οὐκ ἐχούσης, οὕτως καὶ ἡ

---

16 ὥσπερ ... 17 πρόδηλον K: om. Sa: sicuti e diverso sub imbecillis viribus
parva, manifeste cernitur Lin.
K171
  3 αὐτόματος a: -η S
  7 post ταὐτόν, ὅτι δυνάμεως ἐρρωμένης εἰσὶν οὗτοι S
  13 τὸ secundum om. a

vigor, the expansion is great; whereas on the other hand it is small when the power diminishes. / But if, as some pretend, it K171 is the contraction of the arteries that is active, whereas the expansion is an automatic rebound to the naturally expanded state of the walls, in the first place, the bulk of the expansions should be constantly the same, and second, the size should not be dependent upon the strength or weakness of the power; but neither of these is the case.

4. And there is another sign pointing firmly the same way. The strongest and fullest pulse belongs to those who are about to pass most successfully through the crisis of a disease, and no one, however mad, would say that the power was feeble then. For if a successful crisis is due to lack of power, it is clear than an unsuccessful one would be due to strength; and if that were so, we should go on to say that death itself is the product of strength. Now what could be sillier?

5. Moreover, the fact that the vehemence of the stroke in expansion is greater in some and less in others proves both the straining and the slackening to be activities of the pulse. For if the expansion were a remission of the activity, like breathing out, there would be no more or less / in it, just as in breathing K172 out,[45] nor all the spring and vigor of the impulse.

6. And so the expansion, from these and other like considerations, seems to me to belong to the class of active operations; and this again would preserve the similarity between pulse and breathing.

Chapter 7

The next question to be considered is this: breathing out is a relaxation and, as it were, a pause in the activity of the thorax, whereas blowing out the breath with force is an activity, and hence has degrees, which breathing out has not; now in the

---

16 τις παῦλα *Furley:* τὸ φαῦλον SaK: remissio Lin.
K172
  3 διὰ ταῦτα a: δι' αὐτὰ S
  7 ἂν Ca: δ' ἂν S
  8 ἐπνοὴ Ca: ἐκπνοὴ μὲν S
  9 ἡ K: *om.* Sa

συστολὴ μὲν ἐν τοῖς σφυγμοῖς ἔκλυσις τῆς ἐνεργείας ἐστὶ
τῶν ἀρτηριῶν, ἕτερον δέ τι ταύτῃ παρακείμενον ἀνάλογος
ταῖς ἐκφυσήσεσιν ἡ ἐνέργεια. καί μοι δοκεῖ καὶ τοῦτο
παντὸς μᾶλλον ἀληθὲς εἶναι. τεκμαίρομαι δὲ ἔκ τε τῶν
15 κοινῇ περὶ πασῶν ἡμῖν τῶν ζωτικῶν δυνάμεων ἑτέρωθι δε-
δειγμένων, κἀκ τῆς πρὸς αὐτὴν τὴν ἀναπνοὴν ἀναλογίας.
ἐν μέντοι γε τοῖς περὶ τῶν δυνάμεων λογισμοῖς ἕκαστον
K173 τῶν ὀργάνων ἐμφαίνει ἐναντίας ἔχειν ἐμφύτους δυνάμεις.
ἡ δ’ αὖ τῆς ἀναπνοῆς ὁμοιότης ζητεῖ τὴν ἐνέργειαν ἐν
ταῖς ἀρτηρίαις ἀνάλογον ταῖς ἐκφυσήσεσιν.

2. καὶ γὰρ ἀτο-
πώτατον ἂν εἴη, μᾶλλον δ’ ἀδύνατον, ὑπάρχειν μέν τινα
5 χρείαν τῇ φύσει τῆς συστολῆς τῶν ἀρτηριῶν, μηδεμίαν δ’
αὐταῖς δοθῆναι σύμφυτον δύναμιν, δημιουργὸν τῆς τοιαύ-
της κινήσεως. εὐλογώτερον οὖν μακρῷ, καθάπερ ἐν τοῖς
περὶ δυσπνοίας ἐδείκνυμεν, ὁπόταν μὲν ἡ ἐκ τῆς τῶν χυμῶν συγκαύσεως ἀθροιζομένη λιγνυώδης ἀναθυμίασις ἀξιό-
10 λογος ᾖ, τηνικαῦτα μὲν ἐκφυσήσεως τὸ ζῶον ἐφίεσθαι,
ὁπόταν δ’ ἤτοι διὰ τὴν εὔχυμον, ἢ τὴν τοῦ θερμοῦ με-
τριότητα μηδὲν τοιοῦτον ὑποτρέφηται περίττωμα, μόνης
τῆς ἐκπνοῆς, κἂν ταῖς ἀρτηρίαις τὴν μὲν ἀνάλογον ταῖς
ἐκφυσήσεσι συστολὴν ἐν ταῖς πλεονεξίαις τοῦ τοιούτου περιτ-
15 τώματος γίνεσθαι, τὰς δ’ ἄλλας, ὅταν ἀτμῷ μᾶλλον ἢ καπνῷ παραπλήσιον ᾖ τὸ κενούμενον ἐξ αὐτῶν.

3. ἐναργῶς δὲ μαρτύρια πάμπολλα τῶν ἐν τοῖς
σφυγμοῖς φαινομένων, οἷον εὐθέως τὰ κατὰ τοὺς ὕπνους
K174 ἐπὶ τῶν ἐδηδοκότων δαψιλῶς. ἐν τούτοις γὰρ ἐκλύεται
μὲν ἡ διαστολὴ μικροτέρα τε ἅμα καὶ βραδυτέρα γινομένη, ἐπιτείνεται δὲ κατ’ ἄμφω ἡ συστολή, καὶ γὰρ ὠκυ-
τέρα ἢ πρόσθεν καὶ ἐπὶ πλέον εἴσω κατιοῦσα φαίνεται.
5 ἔοικε γὰρ ταῦτα γίνεσθαι κατὰ τοὺς ὕπνους εὐλόγως θ’
ἅμα καὶ ἀνάλογον ταῖς ἐκπνοαῖς. εἴσω γὰρ μᾶλλον ἢ

---

15 ἑτέρωθι K: -θεν Sa
17 ἕκαστον Furley: -ῳ SaK
K173
1 ἐναντίας ut videtur S: ἐναντίως aK
3 ἐκφυσήσεσι Furley, vers Arab. secutus: ἐμ- SaK: flatui Lin.

case of the pulse, is the contraction similarly a cessation of the activity of the arteries, whereas alongside this there is something analogous to blowing out the breath, which is the activity? This seems to me to be certainly the case. I judge both by what has been shown elsewhere about all our vital powers together,[46] and also by the analogy with breathing. In our studies on the natural faculties it appears that each of the organs / has contrary K173 innate powers; again, the comparison with breathing requires that activity of the arteries which is analogous to blowing out the breath.

2. For it would be most strange, nay, impossible, for Nature to have need of the contractions of the arteries, and yet to give them no innate power to produce such a source of motion. It is much more reasonable, as we have shown in our book *On Difficulties in Breathing*,[47] that whenever the smoky vapor rising from the burning up of the humors becomes considerable, the animal desires then to blow out its breath; but when, either from the wholesomeness of the humors or the due moderation of the heat, no such waste matters are fostered, the animal desires only to breathe out; and so in the arteries the contraction that is like blowing out the breath occurs when such waste matters are in excess, but the other contractions happen when what is voided from them [the arteries] resembles mist rather than smoke.

3. There are clearly very many evidences of what the facts are in relation to the pulse; such as (an example that springs to mind) what happens in those who sleep / after eating copiously. K174 For in these the expansive beat of the pulse is faint, becoming both lower and slower;[48] the contraction, on the other hand, increases in both ways, appearing both faster than before and reaching more deeply in. That this happens in sleep seems both appropriate and analogous to what happens in breathing out. For

---

7 κινήσεως K: κοινώσεως Sa: motum Lin.
10 τὸ ζῷον K: ἡμᾶς S: ἡμῶν a: animal Lin.
14 συστολὴν a: συστολαῖς S
16 κενούμενον K: καινούμενον S: καιούμενον a
K174
5 θ' ἅμα a: τέμα S

ἔξω κινουμένης τῆς ἐμφύτου θερμασίας, καὶ διὰ τοῦτο
πολλῆς ἀθροιζομένης κατά τε τὰ σπλάγχνα καὶ τὴν γαστέρα κατεργαζομένην τούς τε χυμοὺς καὶ τὰ σιτία,
10 πλείων ἀνάγκη καὶ τὸ περίττωμα γενόμενον δεῖσθαι τῆς
φυσικῆς κενώσεως. καὶ διὰ τοῦτο ἐν μὲν ταῖς ἀναπνοαῖς
ἡ ἐκπνοὴ θάττων τε καὶ μείζων, καὶ ὡς ἐπὶ τὸ πολὺ μετ'
ἐκφυσήσεως τοῖς [κάμνουσι] κοιμωμένοις, καὶ μάλισθ' ὅταν
ἐδηδοκότες ὦσιν ἱκανά. κατὰ δὲ τοὺς σφυγμοὺς ἡ συ-
15 στολὴ τὸν αὐτὸν διατίθεται τρόπον.

4. οὕτω τοι καὶ τοῖς
παισὶν ἄμφω πλεονεκτεῖ· πλείστη γὰρ καὶ ἡ τῶν χυμῶν
ἐργασία τοῖς τοιούτοις διὰ τὴν αὔξησιν. ἔμπαλιν δὲ ἡ
K175 τῶν γερόντων ἡλικία βραδυτάτην τε καὶ μικροτάτην ἔχουσα
φαίνεται τὴν συστολήν, ὡς ἀμυδρὰν καὶ περὶ τὰς πέψεις
ἀσθενοῦσαν καὶ τοὺς χυμοὺς ἥκιστα κατεργαζομένην, ὡς
μὴ ἀναγκαίαν.

5. ἀνάλογον δὲ τούτοις καὶ τὰς ὥρας τε καὶ
5 χώρας καὶ πάσας ἁπλῶς τοῦ περιέχοντος ἡμᾶς
ἀέρος τὰς μεταβολὰς εἰς κρύος τε καὶ θάλπος ἀλλοιοῦσθαί φασι τοὺς σφυγμούς. οὕτω δὲ καὶ τῶν ψυχικῶν πα-
θῶν καὶ τῶν ἐπιτηδευμάτων τε καὶ νοσημάτων ἕκαστον
ἤτοι τὴν ἔξω κίνησιν αὐξάνει τῶν ἀρτηριῶν, ἢ τὴν εἴσω.
10 καίτοι γ' ἐχρῆν, εἰ διὰ παντὸς ἀνάπαυσίς τις ἦν ἡ διαστολή, πρῶτον μηδαμῶς μήτ' ὠκυτέραν ἑαυτῆς μήτε
βραδυτέραν ταύτην γίνεσθαι· δεύτερον δὲ καὶ τῆς κινήσεως ὅρον ἕνα διὰ παντὸς ὑπάρχειν, ὃν ἐκ τῆς φυσικῆς
κατασκευῆς αἱ ἀρτηρίαι κέκτηνται. τὸ δὲ καὶ τοῦτο
15 προσωτέρω κινεῖν αὐτὰς ἐνδεικτικόν ἐστι τῆς τότε γινο-
μένης ἐνεργείας.

6. ἀλλ' οὐκ ἐνεργοῦσα, φασίν, ἡ ἀρτηρία
θᾶττόν τε καὶ μέχρι πλέονος εἴσω προσέρχεται, ἀλλὰ διὰ
τῶν χιτώνων μαλακότητα· πεφύκασι γὰρ οἱ τοιοῦτοι τῆς
K176 διαστολῆς ἀφεθέντες ἐπὶ πλεῖόν τε καὶ θᾶττον τῶν σκλη-
ρῶν εἰς ἑαυτοὺς συνιζάνειν. ἀλλὰ τοῦτο, φήσομεν, ὦ γεν-
ναῖοι, τῇ μὲν κατὰ τὰς ἡλικίας ἐξαλλαγῇ τῶν ῥυθμῶν

---

13 κάμνουσι *secl. Furley, vers. Arab. secutus* μάλιστα a: κάλλιστα S
K175
 2 ἀμυδρὰν a: ἀναγκαίαν S

since the innate heat moves inward rather than outward, and on that account much collects around the guts and stomach, engaged as the latter is in working up the humors and the nourishment, the superfluities, having grown much larger, must be in need of natural expulsion. And hence, with respect to breathing, it is the breathing out that is more rapid and deeper, and is usually accompanied in those who are asleep[49] by blowing out the breath, and particularly when they have eaten their fill; and as for the pulse, the contraction is disposed in the same manner.

4. Both of these things are dominant in children; for the working up of the humors is particularly great in them, on account of their growth. On the other hand, / old people are K175 found to have the contraction very slow and shallow, because it is sluggish and weak in concoction and does little to work up the humors, since it is unnecessary.

5. Analogously with this, they say that seasons and places and all changes to cold or warm of the air around us affect the pulse. Moreover, the affections of the psyche, its habitual activities, and its illnesses, all increase either the outward or the inward motion of the arteries. But if the expansion were in all cases a cessation of the activity, the following ought to be the case: first, it would never become faster or slower; then the limit of the arteries' motion should always remain the same, namely, that which they have from their natural constitution. But they move beyond this limit, which is a proof that there is then an activity.

6. Yet, it is said, it is not by being active that the artery goes more quickly or further in, but because of a softness in the coats: for such coats, / on leaving off the expansion, naturally K176 fall in upon themselves both to a greater degree and more quickly than hard coats. But this, we beg to remark, Gentlemen, may perhaps be consistent with that change of rhythm

---

5 ἡμᾶς S: ἡμῶν aK
12 καὶ τῆς a: τὸν ἐκ τῆς S
13 ὃν a: ἦν C (S illeg.)
K176
2 τῶν ῥυθμῶν K: τὸν -ὸν Sa: modulorum Lin.

223

ἴσως ὁμολογεῖ· καίτοι δείξομεν ὀλίγον ὕστερον, ὅπως δια-
5 φέρεται· παμπόλλαις δ' ἄλλαις διαθέσεσιν ἐναργῶς δια-
φωνεῖ, καθ' ἃς ἐξαιφνίδιος ἡ ἀλλοίωσις γίνεται τῶν ῥυθμῶν, οὐδὲν μέγα τῶν χιτώνων ἐν οὕτως ὀλίγῳ χρόνῳ
μεταβάλλειν εἰς μαλακότητά τε καὶ σκληρότητα δυναμένων. ἐξαπατᾷ δὲ οὐχ ἥκιστα ὑμᾶς καὶ τὸ καλῶς ὑπὸ
10 τῶν παλαιῶν ἰατρῶν εἰρημένον, οὐ συνιέντας αὐτὸ προση-
κόντως. ἑτοιμότεροι γάρ εἰσι πρὸς τὰς κινήσεις οἱ μα-
λακοὶ χιτῶνες, ὅταν ἐνεργῶσί τι δι' αὐτῶν αἱ δυνάμεις·
εὐπειθέστεροι γὰρ οὕτως αὐταῖς εἰσι καί, ὡς ἂν εἴποι τις,
εὐαγωγότεροι πρὸς ὅ τι ἂν ἐθέλωσιν. ὅταν δ' ὑπ' ἐκείνων
15 κινηθέντες αὖθις ἐαθῶσιν εἰς τὴν ἑαυτῶν κατάστασιν ἐπα-
νιέναι, τόθ' οἱ σκληροὶ θᾶττον ἐπανέρχονται τῶν μαλακωτέρων, ὥσπερ καὶ τῶν φυτῶν τὰ σκληρότερα τῶν
K177 μαλακωτέρων χαλεπώτερον μὲν ὑπείκει τοῖς βιαζομένοις
καὶ μόλις ἕπεται τοῖς ἕλκουσιν, ἀφεθέντα δ' αὖθις εὐ-
κολώτερον εἰς τὴν ἔμπροσθεν ἐπανέρχεται κατάστασιν.

7. ἀλλὰ καὶ λόγον ἔχον ἐστὶ τοῦτο πρὸ τοῦ φαίνεσθαι γι-
5 νόμενον οὕτως. ἑκάστῳ γὰρ τῶν σωμάτων ἐστί τις ἴδιος
λόγος συστάσεως ἄλυπός τε καί, ὡς Ἱπποκράτης ἔλεγεν,
ἀκάματος, ἐν τῷ μέσῳ δηλονότι τῶν ἀμέτρων αὐτοῦ κινήσεων καθεστηκυίας, καὶ ταύτης οὐκ ἄνευ καμάτου τινὸς
ἐξίσταται. καὶ μείζων δὲ κάματος καὶ αὐτῷ τῷ κινου-
10 μένῳ σώματι καὶ τῇ κινούσῃ δυνάμει τότε μᾶλλόν ἐστιν,
ὅταν σκληρόν τε καὶ ξηρὸν ὑπάρχῃ. τὸ γὰρ οὕτω συνεστηκὸς ἰσχυροτέραν ἔχει τὴν ἕξιν τοῦ μαλακωτέρου τε καὶ
ὑγροτέρου· ὅσῳ δ' ἂν ἕκαστον τῶν ὁτιοῦν πάσχειν μελ-
λόντων ἰσχυρότερον ᾖ, τοσοῦτον τῷ διατιθέντι δυσκινη-
15 τότερον γίνεται. εἴπερ οὖν πάσχει μὲν τὸ κινούμενον
ὑπὸ τοῦ κινοῦντος, ἐνεργεῖ δὲ καὶ δρᾷ περὶ αὐτὸ τὸ
κινοῦν, εὔλογον ἦν, ὅσον δυσπαθέστερόν ἐστι τὸ σκλη-
ρότερον, εἰς τοσοῦτον καὶ δυσκινητότερον αὐτὸ γενέσθαι.
K178 καὶ διὰ τοῦτο, εἴτε φυτὸν ὁτιοῦν, εἴτε τῶν ὀργανικῶν
τι τοῦ ζῴου μορίων ὑπὸ δυνάμεώς τινος κινοῖτο, τὸ
μὲν σκληρόν, ὡς ἂν δυσπαθέστερόν τε καὶ δυσκινητό-

---

4 ἴσως K: ἴσον Sa: fortasse Lin.
9 ἐξαπατᾷ K: ἐξαπατᾶται ut videtur S, a ὑμᾶς K: ἡμᾶς Sa: nos Lin.
15 ἐαθῶσι K: ἐλθῶσι S: ἔλθωσιν ἐαθῶσιν a: permittuntur Lin.

which follows the aging of the subject, though we shall show a little later how it differs; but it is clearly discordant with many other conditions, in which the change of rhythm takes place rapidly, and the coats could not, in so short a time, change greatly with respect to hardness and softness. You are not a little misled by the admirable saying of the ancient physicians, which you have failed to understand in its true sense.[50] For when they are soft, the coats are readier to move when the powers are performing some action through them [as instruments]; in this soft state they are more obedient to them and, as one might say, more yielding to their every wish. When, however, having been moved by them, they are permitted to return to their original condition, then the hard return more rapidly than the softer: just as with plants; the harder / yield less K177 readily to pressures than the softer, and follow attractive forces less easily; but when released again they return more smartly to their previous state.

7. And this is what reason would lead us to expect even before it is observed to happen. For each body has a certain constitutional temper that is proper to it and unforced; and, as Hippocrates said,[51] effortless; and this, it is clear, lies in the middle between the excessive motions of the body, and from this temper it is not displaced without effort. And the effort, both on the part of the body moved and of the moving force, is greater just exactly when the body moved is hard and dry. For what is so constituted has a stronger habitus than what is soft and moist.[52] And the stronger anything is which is to suffer change, the more difficult it is for the disposing agent to move it. So, if that which is moved suffers a change through the agency of the mover, and the mover is active and at work on it, then it is after all reasonable that the harder body is as much more difficult to move as it is resistant to change. / And for this K178 reason, any plant or any of the organic parts of an animal, if it is moved by some power, is less malleable if it is hard, as being more resistant to change and harder to move, and easier if it is

K177
11 συνεστηκὸς a: συνεστὼς S

225

τερον, ἧττον ἀκολουθεῖ, ῥᾷον δὲ τὸ μαλακώτερον. τοῦ
5 μαλακωτέρου δὲ τὸ σκληρὸν θᾶττον εἰς τὴν ἑαυτοῦ
κατάστασιν ἐπανέρχεται, ὡς ἂν ἰσχυροτέρᾳ συνεχόμενον
ἕξει. φαίνεται γὰρ ἐν τοῖς φυτοῖς, ὅσα μὲν ἁπαλὰ καὶ
νέα, λυγιζόμενά τε καὶ βραδύνοντα κατὰ τὰς εἰς τὴν φύσιν ἐπανόδους, ὅσα δ᾽ ἤδη τέλεα καὶ σκληρά, μετὰ
10 πλείονος τοῦ τόνου καὶ θάττονος τῆς κινήσεως
ἐπανερχόμενα.

8. πρὸς τῷ τοίνυν, ὡς ἔφην, καταβάλλειν
αὐτῶν τὸν λόγον τὰς ἐξαίφνης γιγνομένας μεταβολὰς τῶν
ῥυθμῶν οὐδ᾽ ἄλλως ἔοικεν ὁμολογεῖν τοῖς φαινομένοις
ἡ ὑπόθεσις, δειχθέντος τοῦ μὲν μαλακωτέρου σώματος
15 καὶ ἀσθενεστέρου ῥᾷον μὲν ἑπομένου τῷ κινοῦντι, βραδύτερον δ᾽ εἰς τὴν φύσιν ἐπανερχομένου, τοῦ δὲ σκλη-
ροτέρου διὰ συντονίαν μόγις μὲν νικωμένου, καὶ διὰ
K179 τοῦτο βραδύτερον ἑπομένου, θᾶττον δέ, ὅταν ἀφεθῇ, πρὸς
τὴν οἰκείαν ἐπειγομένου φύσιν. συνελόντι δὲ φάναι, καὶ
ταῖς μαλακαῖς ἀρτηρίαις ἄμφω συμβέβηκε πάσχειν ἐν μέρει καὶ ταῖς σκληραῖς.

5 8. Εἴρηταί μοι τὸ πᾶν ἤδη περὶ χρείας
σφυγμῶν. καὶ γὰρ ὅτι φυσικῆς ἕνεκα τῆς καθ᾽ ὅλον τὸ
ζῶον θερμασίας, καὶ ὅτι κατὰ μὲν τὰς διαστολὰς δια-
ψύχεται τοῦτο, κατὰ δὲ τὰς συστολὰς καθαίρεται, καὶ
ὡς αἱ κινήσεις αἵδε ταῖς ἀναπνευστικαῖς ἐοίκασι πάν-
10 τη, καὶ ὡς καὶ τῷ ψυχικῷ πνεύματι χρήσιμοι, καὶ ὡς
καθ᾽ ἓν μόνον ἀναπνοὴ καὶ σφυγμὸς διαφέρουσι, τῷ
τὴν μὲν ὑπὸ τῆς ψυχικῆς δυνάμεως, τὸν δ᾽ ὑπὸ τῆς
ζωτικῆς γίνεσθαι, τὰ δ᾽ ἄλλα πάντα καὶ χρείας ἕνεκα
καὶ τρόπου κινήσεως ὁμοίως ἔχουσιν, εἴρηταί τε καὶ
15 δέδεικται.

2. ῥᾷστον δὴ ταῦτ᾽ ἐπιμελῶς ἀναλεξαμένῳ διακρίνειν δύνασθαι τά τε καλῶς ὑπὸ τῶν ἔμπροσθεν
K180 εἰρημένα καὶ τὰ μή. ῥᾴδιον δὲ τῷ τοιούτῳ, καὶ ὅσα
κατὰ μέρος ὑπὲρ ἀμφοτέρων ζητεῖται τῶν ἐνεργειῶν, ἐξευ-
ρίσκειν.

K178
10 θάττονος K: θᾶττον Sa

softer. But the hard returns to its natural state more rapidly than the softer, as being constituted with a stronger habitus. For it is apparent among plants, that those which are young and tender are both pliable and slow to return to their own nature; while those which are full grown and hard return with more spring and with a swifter motion.

8. Besides their theory being upset, as I was saying, by the sudden change of the rhythm, in other respects also their hypothesis does not seem to fit the observed facts; for it has been shown that it is the softer and weaker body which is more readily affected by the mover and returns more slowly to its own nature; whereas it is the harder which, because of its springiness, is overcome with difficulty, / and on that account K179 affected more slowly, but which, nevertheless, when released, speeds more swiftly back to its proper nature. Summing up, we may say that both of these things happen in due turn to soft and to hard arteries.

Chapter 8

I have now told all about the use of the pulse. That it is for the sake of the natural heat that is all over the whole animal, and that it cools this during the expansions and purges it in the contractions; that these motions are in every way like those of breathing; that they are useful to the psychic pneuma; that breathing and the pulse differ in only one way, in that the one is moved by the psychic power and the other by the vital power, though they are like in all other ways, both as to use and manner of motion: all this has been described and proved.

2. Anyone who reads this carefully will very easily be able to decide what has been said well by previous authors, / and what K180 has not. And such a reader will easily discover whatever is required in detail about the two activities.

---

11 τῷ K: τὸ Sa: praeter Lin.
K179
2 δὲ om. S

DE CAUSIS RESPIRATIONIS

INTRODUCTION

The Text

The following Greek manuscripts of this short work are known:

A = Marcian. 276; s. xii. f. 268 (only as far as K IV 486.6)
R = Rom. Reg. Suec. 175; s. xiv. f. 240^v
M = Marcian. App. Cl. V 4; s. xv. f. 433
P = Parisin. 2165; s. xvi. f. 187.
Z = Modena. Mutinens 237 (III G 18); s. xvi. f. 247^v

I have collated all of these from microfilms kindly supplied by their respective librarians. I acknowledge gratefully the help of Mr. David Blank in the work of collation.

No Arabic translations are known to us.

There are Latin translations by Niccolo da Reggio, J. Vassaeus, and J. Cornarius (references are given in Durling, "Census," p. 290). Cornarius' translation is printed in Kühn's edition, with a few changes. We have consulted all of these translations, but not found it necessary to record their versions in the apparatus.

Galen refers to a work of his with this title elsewhere, but it seems unlikely that he is referring to the little treatise that survives. In *De usu partium* VII 20 (K I 432), he says:

Next I should speak about the thorax, though here too I should first remind you of what I have demonstrated in my book *On the Causes of Respiration*.... In that treatise I have demonstrated the many wonderful devices Nature has employed in the action of the thorax. I have shown that in inspiration some of its parts are moved upward and others downward, and that in expiration those that were earlier moved downward rise back up again, and those formerly elevated return now to their original position. I have shown, too, that there are many sources for the movement of the thorax, that one kind of respiration is unforced and another forced, and that each kind has its own proper muscles. After giving the action of these muscles, I also demonstrate their usefulness. (Trans. M. T. May)

231

His view of the position of *De causis respirationis* in his own writings is explained more clearly in *De placitis Hippocratis et Platonis* II 4, in the course of a discussion of speech and its relation to forced and unforced breathing:

> Perhaps someone may wish to learn about the organ proper to each of the activities mentioned, the muscles that move it—which ones they are, how many, where located, and how large—the nerves received by these muscles—their number and size, and the part of the brain from which they especially come—and the nature of the motion in the organs moved by them. I said earlier that I do not approve of writing many times about the same things, but anyone who is really a lover of learning has other works of mine written on all these matters. First, he has my work *On the Motion of the Thorax and Lungs*, where we show that when the lungs are moved by the thorax and distended as it expands, they draw the outside air in, and this is inhalation; but when they are contracted by its contractions, they force the air they contain into the windpipe and mouth and thus expel it, and that is exhalation. Next after this he has another treatise, *On the Causes of Respiration*, in which I pointed out all the muscles, the organs moved by them, and the nerves that transmit the power of the mind from the brain to the muscles. Then after these he has still another treatise, *On Speech*, in which I wrote about the organs of speech, the muscles that move these (organs), and the nerves that come down to these (muscles) from the brain. (Trans. P. De Lacy)

Neither of the other two works referred to here, *On the Motion of the Thorax and the Lungs* and *On Speech*, survives.

The subject matter of the surviving booklet is dealt with in *Anatomical Procedures* V 3–10 (K II 491–531), where he twice refers to *De causis respirationis* by name (K II 499, 503).

All of these references give the impression that Galen has in mind a substantial work, in which the subject matter is explained and Galen's analysis defended at length. Some have called the surviving booklet a fragment of this longer work, but since it contains a brief survey of most of the topics set out in the *De usu partium* reference, quoted above, and in the same order, it is more likely to be a summary of the longer treatise. Possibly it is by someone other than Galen.

Pages and lines are numbered according to Kühn's edition.

The Muscles of Respiration (J.S.W.)

The interpretation of our text is made easier by the fact that it is closely related in content to a relatively short passage of *Anat. Proc.* (K II 492–98; pp. 128–30 in Singer's translation). Thus if we disregard those parts of our text that require no special effort for their interpretation (those dealing with the diaphragm, the abdominal muscles, and the intercostal muscles), we are left with a set of brief notes on the respiratory muscles such that the whole set can be treated as a summary of no more than seven pages of Kühn's or three of Singer's text. This greatly strengthens our confidence in the interpretation of some very obscure passages.

Let us now consider in order the various items of information given in our text about the muscles of respiration.

1. The diaphragm, the principal organ of quiet breathing, requires no special notice. It is described in *Anat. Proc.* V, v and viii.

2. The twenty-two muscles of the ribs are certainly intercostal muscles. The expression ἐν ταῖς μέσαις χώραις (467.4) seems to mean "in the interspaces"; the supposition that it might mean "attached along the middle region of the length of each rib," that is, "not attached to the extreme ends," could be accepted only if Galen were referring exclusively to the external parts of the intercostals. The fact that, in our text, the intercostal muscles are called "double" seems to show that the number twenty-two means eleven on each side of the body: the internal and external intercostals being taken as two parts of one muscle. The intercostal muscles are described in *Anat. Proc.* V, iv.

3. The two belonging to the first ribs are the *scalenus brevis anterior* on the two sides of the body. See *Anat. Proc.* V, iii (K II 495; Singer, p. 129).

4. The two belonging to the lowest ribs, again, constitute a pair; almost certainly the *serratus posterior inferior* of each side, described in *Anat. Proc.* V, iii (K II 498; Singer, p. 130) thus: "There is another pair of muscles [*serratus posterior inferior*] outside the thorax which, inserted along the last ribs, draws down this end of the thorax ... it draws down the last rib of the thorax along with the rib next to the last in most animals. ... I call the last rib, for the moment, not the small rib that is really false ... but the rib that comes next to it."

5. The three attached to the neck. Here, three on each side of the neck are intended. Kühn's Latin text actually has *utrinque* inserted

here. The three are probably the *scalenus anterior*, *scalenus longus*, and *serratus posterior superior*. In *Anat. Proc.* V, iii (K II 495; Singer, p. 129), Galen says, apparently of these: "These three pairs, then, of the higher muscles of the thorax are [among those] responsible for respiration."

6. The seven aligned with the spinal muscles. These set the most difficult problem. The odd number seven shows that we are to consider muscles of one side, which will of course be paired with seven on the other. If we count the common origin of the *sacrospinalis* or *erector spinae* (which is in fact Galen's spinal muscle) as one, we then have its three branches, the *iliocostalis lumborum*, *longissimus dorsi vel thoracis*, and *spinalis dorsi vel thoracis*; and, adding the *iliocostalis dorsi vel thoracis*, *semispinalis capitis* and *longissimus capitis*, we can make up the seven. We have had, however, to include the spinal muscle itself (identified from *Anat. Proc.* V, iii; K II 497; Singer, p. 130). With this the other muscles can be said to be aligned in the sense that they run in the same direction. Considering the extreme brevity of our text, this is at least a possible interpretation of the seven muscles in question.

7. The eight belonging to the 'abdomen. These are readily and certainly identifiable as the members of the four pairs made up of two of each of the following: *obliquus abdominis externus*, *obliquus abdominis internus*, *rectus abdominis*, and *transversus abdominis*. *Anat. Proc.* V, vi (K II 507–509, 518; Singer, pp. 134–36, 139).

Here it will be noticed, our text gives, not the number on each side of the body, but the total of both sides.

8. The muscle rather vaguely identified in our text as "the portion around the hollows of the shoulder" must be supposed to be the *serratus anterior*.

This plays some part in normal breathing, and is of great importance in forced breathing. The expression used in our text may well cover more than one muscle; particularly since a similar expression occurs in *Anat. Proc.* V, iii, where Singer identifies the muscle concerned as the *rhomboideus*, which would also be of importance in forced breathing; for the scapula must be fixed by this and by other muscles, so that the *serratus anterior* may play its full part in breathing, when breathing is forced.

So far, our text seems to be amenable to interpretation as it stands; but the sentence that begins with the last three words on Kühn's IV

467, seems to be quite impossible as it stands in the manuscript tradition: "Of the straight ones belonging to the neck, those which stretch to the collarbone draw in the ends of the cartilages which are there, as do the muscles aligned with the spinal roots of the ribs. . . ." There are no muscles of the neck that are "straight" in Galen's sense and stretch to the collarbone, except the *sternohyoid* and *sternothyroids*; and it would never have entered Galen's head to think that muscles so situated could alter the shape of any part of the thorax. Of the muscles "belonging to the neck," the only ones that could in any degree have this action are the *sternomastoid* and *cleidomastoid*, which also are more clearly "attached to the collarbone"; but these are explicitly said by Galen not to be "straight" (not to have their long axes parallel with the long axis of the neck); and, again, he says explicitly that they move the head and do not move the thorax (*Anat. Proc.* IV, ix; K II 464). This passage in our text (K IV 467–68) seems to be a garbled version of a part of *Anat. Proc.* V, iii, which immediately follows an account of the "three pairs of the muscles higher than the thorax," which we have already identified with the three (pairs of) muscles of the neck, of our text. Immediately before the passage of our text now under review, we find it stated that these three (pairs) attached to the neck "*draw up and at the same time expand the higher parts of the thorax*"; and in *Anat. Proc.* we find, just before the passage that I shall immediately quote, the statement that one of the three of the neck "is attached to ribs three to seven, and if you pull on it from the head you will see them [the ribs] *dragged upward and dilating the thorax.*" Not only the content of this passage from the *Anat. Proc.*, then, but also its placing justifies us in considering it as that which we must use in interpreting the doubtful portion of our text:

If the thorax be laid bare, you will see along it two other pairs of muscles along its length, one pertaining to the spine, and the other to the sternum. . . . That by the sternum [thoracic part of the *rectus abdominis*] is of membranous tissue . . . not like the other membranes in strength . . . it is a sort of flat tendon. . . . This tendon, as I have said, is continuous with the rectus in the region of the abdomen and overlies the ends of all the ribs that approach the sternum. It rises to the first rib. The other muscle [*iliocostalis dorsi*] has a similar action. It is . . . extended along the spine . . . when taut, it both protects and pulls in the ribs. Nature seems to want these, to contract the thorax vigorously at need, when the abdominal muscles also visibly act. (*Anat. Proc.* V, iii; K II 495–97; Singer, pp. 129–30.)

We may note that both in our text and in *Anat. Proc.*, the notion of "pulling in" ("draw in the ends of the cartilages" and "pulls in the ribs") is expressed in the Greek by the verb προστέλλειν.

The passage just quoted agrees well with the brief fragment of our text if we suppose that the words "belonging to the neck" (τῶν κατὰ τὸν τράχηλον) in our text are an interpolation. We can then read the words "of the straight ones" (τῶν δὲ ὀρθίων) as meaning "of the *rectus muscles*"; for the *recti abdominis* are among the few muscles to which Galen gave something approaching a standard technical name. This name occurs in the passage from *Anat. Proc.* just quoted: ἔστι δ', ὡς εἴρηται, συνεχὴς ὁ τένων οὗτος τῷ κατ' ἐπιγάστριον ὀρθίῳ μυΐ. The whole passage would read: "Of the *rectus* muscles, those which stretch to the collarbone draw in the ends of the cartilages that are there; the muscles aligned with the spinal roots of the ribs have a similar constricting action [on the thorax]."

This still requires some explanation: the expression "to the collarbone" must be interpreted as meaning "to the region of the collarbone"; since Galen says that a "tendon," which, however, has "a fleshy character," is continuous with the *rectus* and "rises to the first rib" (*Anat. Proc.* V, iii; K II 496–97; Singer, p. 130). What this tendon with a fleshy character is, it would be difficult to say, if we were concerned with human anatomy; but Galen says, in the same passage of the *Anat. Proc.*, that it is present in all animals; and if we consider some quadruped, such as the horse, we find that the *rectus abdominis* terminates on the fourth rib, and that a muscle of the same width and collinear with it (*transversus costarum*) arises here (on the fourth rib) and is attached to the first rib. Thus, if we take this muscle to be a continuation of the *rectus*, we achieve agreement with Galen's texts.

The muscles "aligned with the spinal roots of the ribs" are clearly identical with the muscle (and its partner on the other side of the body) identified by Singer with the *iliocostalis dorsi* (Singer, p. 103). Singer's interpretation, however, cannot be correct, because the *iliocostalis dorsi* (*vel thoracis*) terminates on the last rib, whereas Galen says that the lower end of the muscle he is concerned with "is inserted into the spinal muscle" (*Anat. Proc.* V, iii; K II 497; Singer, p. 103). Probably Galen is speaking of the *latissimus dorsi vel thoracis*, which is "extended along the spine" (Singer, p. 103), and is even better characterized as "aligned with the spinal roots of the ribs," which is the expression used in our text.

The passage we have referred to (*Anat. Proc.* V, iii) allows us to identify the "spinal muscle" as the lower part of the *sacrospinalis* or *erector spinae*, of which Cunningham says that it "possesses vertebral, vertebro-cranial, and vertebro-costal attachments. It consists of an elongated mass composed of separate slips extending from the sacrum to the skull. Simple at its origin [Galen's 'spinal muscle'], it becomes more and more complex as it is traced upward toward the head" (Cunningham, sixth ed., p. 379). Its most striking branch is the *longissimus dorsi vel thoracis*. This seems to be the only muscle "aligned with the spinal muscles" that can be identified in Galen's text of *Anat. Proc.* V, iii; it is only one, though the stoutest, of the seven mentioned in our text; which seven I have endeavored to identify above (numbered paragraph 6).

There remain problems in *Anat. Proc.* V, iii. These cannot be discussed here; but I may mention that it is possible that Galen, in describing the *rectus*, has alternated between describing what he found in his "ape" and what is common in quadrupeds.

9. In the brief description, given in our text, of the actions of the "straight muscles" (K II 468), we have another sentence requiring expansion: "Those belonging to the abdomen, being the seat of the diaphragm, assist the contraction of the thorax." The meaning is that the diaphragm is "seated" on the abdominal viscera, and, when the abdominal muscles contract they press upon the viscera, which are forced upward, and thus force up the diaphragm and constrict the cavity of the thorax.

Sigla

A = Marcian. 276; s. xii. f. 268 (expl. K IV 486.6)
R = Rom. Reg. Suec. 175; s. xiv. f. 240^v
M = Marcian. App. Cl. V 4; s. xv. f. 433
P = Parisin. 2165; s. xvi. f. 187
Z = Modena, Mutinens 237 (III G 18); s. xvi. f. 247^v
a = editio aldina 1525
Ch = editio Charteriana 1679

ΓΑΛΗΝΟΥ ΠΕΡΙ ΤΩΝ ΤΗΣ
ΑΝΑΠΝΟΗΣ ΑΙΤΙΩΝ

K465   Τὰ τῆς ἀναπνοῆς αἴτια ὁ προκείμενος ἀποδεῖξαι
λόγος ἐπαγγέλλεται. οὔτε γὰρ βεβαιώσασθαι τὴν ὑπό-
θεσιν τῆς ἀναπνοῆς, οὔτε παραποδιζομένην ἢ καὶ τέ-
λεον εἰργομένην ἐπανορθώσασθαι δυνατὸν τὰς αἰτίας
5 αὐτῆς ἀγνοοῦντα. ὁ γὰρ τὸ ποιοῦν φωράσας πρὸς ἀλή-
θειαν, οὗτος εἰδήσει μόνος καὶ τῆς βλάβης τὴν διαφοράν,
καὶ τῆς ἰάσεως τὸν τρόπον.

                     1. ὄντων δὲ τριῶν κατὰ γένος,
ὡς τύπῳ φάναι, τῶν αἰτίων τῆς ἀναπνοῆς, δυνάμεως προαι-
ρετικῆς, ὀργάνων τῶν ὑπηρετουμένων τῇ προαιρέσει, κἀπὶ
K466 τούτοις τῆς χρείας, δι' ἣν καὶ τῶν προκειμένων αἰτίων
δεόμεθα, ἡ μὲν χρεία τὸ κυριώτατόν ἐστι τῶν τῆς ἀναπνοῆς αἰτίων, τηροῦσα μὲν τὴν συμμετρίαν τῆς ἐμφύτου
θερμασίας, τρέφουσα δὲ τὴν οὐσίαν τοῦ ψυχικοῦ πνεύματος·
5 ἡ προαίρεσις δὲ διατάττει καὶ οἷον ῥυθμίζει τὰς ἀναπνευ-
στικὰς ἐνεργείας· τό γε μὴν τῶν ὀργάνων εἶδος πολυσχιδὲς
καὶ πολύτροπόν τι καθέστηκε. τὰ μὲν γὰρ τῇ παρακο-
μιδῇ τοῦ πνεύματος ἀνάκειται· τὰ δ' ὑποδέχεται τὸν ἀέρα·
τὰ δὲ τούτων ἐστὶ κινητικὰ τῶν κινούντων.

                     2. ἀρχὴ μὲν οὖν
10 διὰ τοῦ στόματος καὶ τῶν ῥινῶν ἑλκόμενος ἀήρ, ὕλη τυγ-
χάνων τῆς κατὰ τὴν ἀναπνοὴν χρείας, διχῇ μεριζόμενος,
θατέρῳ μέν, τῷ μείονι, διὰ τῶν ῥινῶν εἰς τὸν ἐγκέφαλον
φερόμενος, θατέρῳ δέ, τῷ πλείονι, διὰ τῆς τραχείας ἀρτηρίας εἰς τὸν πνεύμονα κομιζόμενος. αὐτή γε μὴν ἡ ἀρτηρία,
15 ὄργανον οὖσα φωνῆς, ὁδός ἐστιν ἀναπνοῆς. ὁ δὲ πνεύμων
οἷα βαθὺς γαστὴρ ὑπόκειται τῷ πνεύματι. τούτου δὲ τὰς
διαστολάς τε καὶ συστολὰς ὁ θώραξ οἰακίζει, μυσὶ κινούμενος, ὀστοῖς τε διαρθρούμενος. καὶ μὴν καὶ τὸ διάφραγμα·

K465
  1 ἀποδεῖξαι] ὑπο- MRZ
  2 ἐπαγγέλλεται] ὑπ'- MRZ
  5 ἀγνοοῦντα] -ας A   γὰρ τὸ] γάρτοι τὸ MRZ: γάρ τι τὸ a: γάρ τοι Ch

ON THE CAUSES OF
BREATHING

The following discourse proposes to demonstrate the causes of breathing. It is impossible either to confirm the hypothesis of breathing[1] or to put it [the breathing] right if it is impeded or completely stopped, without knowing its causes. He who has chased the cause[2] into the light of truth is the only one who will know the variety of disorders of breathing and the manner of healing them.

2. There are three kinds of causes of breathing, to speak summarily: the faculty of choice,[3] the organs that minister to choice, / and third, the use for which we need the former two. K466 The use is the most important of the causes of breathing: on the one hand, preserving the balance of the innate heat, on the other, nourishing the substance of the psychic pneuma.[4] Choice organizes and as it were sets the rhythm of the activities of breathing. The form of the organs is complex and various: some are assigned to the conveyance of pneuma, some receive the air, others serve to move these to perform their motions.

3. The beginning, then, is air drawn in through the mouth and nostrils, which is matter for the use that belongs to breathing. It is divided into two: one part, the lesser, goes through the nostrils into the brain;[5] the other, the larger, is carried through the rough artery [the trachea] to the lung. The artery itself, while serving as the organ of voice, is the path of breathing. The lung serves as a deep belly, so to speak, for the pneuma. Its expansions and contractions are controlled by the thorax, which is moved by the muscles and articulated by bones. Then

---

K466

4 δὲ om. A

9 τὰ δὲ] τὰ δὲ καὶ A

10 διὰ] ὁ διὰ ARZ

14 ἀρτηρία] τραχεῖα ἀρτηρία A

15 δὲ] μὲν A

17 συστολὰς] τὰς σ. A   ὁ om. AMRZ

K467 καὶ γὰρ δὴ καὶ αὐτὸ τοῦτο ἦν ὄργανον ἀναπνοῆς· κυκλοτε-
ρὲς δέ ἐστι, καὶ νευρῶδες μὲν περὶ τὸ κέντρον ἑαυτοῦ, σαρ-
κῶδες δὲ τὰ πέριξ.

3. οὕτω δὲ καὶ οἱ κατὰ τὰς πλευρὰς μύες,
οἱ μὲν ἐν ταῖς μέσαις χώραις αὐτοῦ δύο καὶ εἴκοσιν
5 τυγχάνουσιν, καὶ δύο μὲν οἱ τῶν πρώτων πλευρῶν, ἰσά-
ριθμοι δὲ τούτων οἱ τῶν ἐσχάτων δύο· καὶ πρὸς τούτοις
οἱ καθήκοντες ἐκ τοῦ τραχήλου τρεῖς· εἶθ' οἱ παρατεταμένοι τοῖς ῥαχίταις ἑπτά· σὺν αὐτοῖς δὲ οἱ κατ' ἐπιγάστριον
ὀκτώ. τοσοῦτοι μὲν οἱ ὑπηρετοῦντες μύες τῇ ἀναπνοῇ.

4. ἐνέρ-
10 γειαι δὲ καθ' ἕκαστον τούτων, τῶν μὲν τῶν φρενῶν, ἀβίαστον
ἐργάζεσθαι τὴν ἀναπνοήν, τῶν δὲ κατὰ τὰς πλευράς, διαστέλλειν τε καὶ συστέλλειν ἀκριβῶς τὸν θώρακα. διπλῶν δὲ
ὄντων αὐτῶν, οἱ μὲν ἐκτὸς τὴν ἐκπνοήν, οἱ δ' ἐντὸς
τὴν εἰσπνοὴν ἀποτελοῦσιν. καὶ τῶν μὲν πρώτων δυοῖν
15 ἐνέργεια μέν ἐστι διαστέλλειν μόνον τὸ ἄνω τοῦ θώρακος
μέρος, τῶν δ' ἐσχάτων συστέλλειν μόνον τὸ κάτω μέρος.
οἱ δ' ἐκ τοῦ τραχήλου καθήκοντες ἀνασπῶσί τε ἅμα καὶ
διαστέλλουσι τὰ τοῦ θώρακος ὑψηλὰ μόρια. τῶν δὲ ὀρθίων
K468 [τῶν κατὰ τὸν τράχηλον] οἱ μὲν πρὸς τὰς κλεῖς ἀνατεινόμε-
νοι προστέλλουσι τὰ ταύτῃ πέρατα τῶν χόνδρων, ὥσπερ
καὶ οἱ παρατεταμένοι ταῖς ῥαχίτισι ῥίζαις τῶν πλευρῶν. οἱ
δὲ κατ' ἐπιγάστριον, ἕδρα τῶν φρενῶν ὄντες, τῇ τοῦ θώ-
5 ρακος βοηθοῦσι συστολῇ.

5. διττῶν τοίνυν οὐσῶν κατὰ γένος τῶν
ἀναπνοῶν, ἀβιάστου τε καὶ βιαίας, εἶθ' ἑκατέρας αὐτῶν ἐχούσης οἰκεῖα μόρια β', τήν τε εἰσπνοὴν καὶ τὴν ἐκπνοήν, τέτταρα
τὰ σύμπαντα μόρια γίγνεται τῆς ἀναπνοῆς. καθ' ἕκαστον δὲ
τῶν τεττάρων ἰδία τις φύσις ὀργάνων ἐστί, ἀβιάστου μὲν
10 εἰσπνοῆς τὸ διάφραγμα, βιαίας δὲ ἥ τε κατὰ τὰ σιμὰ τῶν
ὠμοπλατῶν, ἥ τ' ἐντὸς τῶν μεσοπλευρίων μοῖρα· ὡσαύτως
δὲ καὶ τῆς ἐκπνοῆς, ἀβιάστου μὲν οἱ κατ' ἐπιγάστριον

K467
2 δέ ἐστι καὶ] ὡς A
7 εἶθ' οἱ παρατεταμένοι] οἱ θυπερι τεταγμένοι AZ
8 σύν] ἐπ' A
9 μὲν] μὲν οὖν M

there is the diaphragm— / for this too is after all an organ of K467
breathing; it is somewhat rounded, full of nervous tissue[6] toward the center, fleshy at the circumference.

4. Also there are the muscles belonging to the ribs: there are
twenty-two in their intermediate spaces; also two belonging to
the first ribs, and the same number, two, belonging to the
lowest; in addition there are three attached to the neck, seven
aligned with the spinal muscles, and eight that belong to the
abdomen. This is the number of muscles that serve respiration.[7]

5. The activities of these severally; those of the diaphragm,
to perform unforced breathing; those about the ribs, to expand
and contract the thorax exactly. These are double: the outer set
effects breathing out, the inner breathing in. The activity of the
first two is to expand only the upper part of the thorax, and of
the lowest, to contract only the lower part. Those attached to
the neck draw up and at the same time expand the high parts of
the thorax. Of the straight ones,[8] / those that stretch to the K468
collarbone draw in the ends of the cartilages which are there, as
do the muscles aligned with the spinal roots of the ribs. Those
belonging to the abdomen, being the seat of the diaphragm,
assist the contraction of the thorax.

6. Now, there are two kinds of breathing: forced and unforced; and each of these has its own two parts, breathing in
and breathing out; hence there are four parts altogether. There
is a special sort of organ for each of the four: for unforced
breathing in, the diaphragm; for forced breathing in, the portion
around the hollows of the shoulder blades and the inner lot of
the intercostal muscles; similarly for unforced breathing out, the

---

13 ἐκτὸς om. A   ἐκπνοήν] εἰς- A
14 εἰσπνοήν] ἐκ- A   καὶ om. A
15 διαστέλλειν μόνον] μένον A
16 μέρος . . . τὸ] μέρος κινῶν τῶν ἐσχάτων συστέλλειν τὸ A
17 τοῦ τραχήλου A: τῶν τραχήλων cett.
K468
1 τῶν κατὰ τὸν τράχηλον] seclusimus: v. comm.
2 ταύτῃ] πάντα A
6 expl. A
10 τὸ om. MRZ

μύες, βιαίας δὲ τῶν μεσοπλευρίων ἡ ἐκτὸς μοῖρα.

6. τὰ μὲν
δὴ κατὰ τοὺς μῦς ὧδ' ἔχει. τῶν δὲ νεύρων τὰ μὲν εἰς τὸ
15 διάφραγμα καθήκοντα, ἐκ τῆς μεταξὺ τετάρτου τε καὶ πέμ-
πτου τῶν ἐν τῷ τραχήλῳ σπονδύλων διαρθρώσεως ὁρμη-
θέντα, δύο ὄντα, εἰς αὐτὸ τὸ νευρῶδες αὐτοῦ μέρος κατα-
K469 φύεται· τὰ δ' εἰς τοὺς μεσοπλευρίους μῦς ἐκ τῆς ῥάχεως
διασπειρόμενα εἰς τὸ στέρνον φέρονται, οὔτ' οὖν ὀρθὰ κατὰ
τοῦ ζώου μῆκος ἐκτεινόμενα, οὔτ' ἐγκάρσια ὁμοίως τοῖς
μυσίν, ἀλλὰ λοξὰ φερόμενα, κεφαλὴν μὲν ἔχοντα τὸν ταύτῃ
5 σπόνδυλον, τελευτὴν δὲ τὸ στέρνον. καὶ μὴν καὶ τὰ εἰς
τοὺς ἄλλους μῦς τοὺς τῆς ἀναπνοῆς δημιουργοὺς φερόμενα
σχεδὸν ἅπαντα ἐκ τοῦ ῥαχίτου μυελοῦ βεβλάστηκε.

7. τοιού-
των οὖν καὶ τοσούτων ὑπαρχόντων τῶν τῆς ἀναπνοῆς αἰτίων, εὔδηλον τῷ γε μὴ παντάπασιν ἀνοήτῳ, τίνι διενήνο-
10 χεν ἕκαστον αὐτῶν. ἡ μὲν γὰρ προαίρεσις ἔοικε τῷ κινοῦντι
τὰς ἡνίας καὶ τοὺς ἵππους ἀναβάτῃ· ταῖς δ' ἡνίαις τὰ
νεῦρα ἐοίκασι, καθάπερ καὶ ἵπποις οἱ μύες· οὕτω δὲ καὶ
ἡ χρεία τὸ ἔσχατον ὀρεκτὸν καθέστηκε τῆς ἀναπνοῆς, ὥσπερ
ἡ νίκη τῆς ἡνιοχικῆς.

---

15 τετάρτου ... πέμπτου] -ης ... -ης MRZ
K469
1 τὰ] τοὺς MRZ
2 οὔτ' οὖν] οὔκουν MRZ

muscles belonging to the abdomen; for forced breathing out, the exterior lot of the intercostal muscles.

7. So much for the muscles. Of the nerves,[9] some are attached to the diaphragm, starting from the articulation between the fourth and fifth vertebrae of the neck. They are two in number [one on each side of the body; actually the phrenic nerves], and grow into the nervous tissue of the diaphragm. / Others disperse from the spine to the intercostal muscles and go K469 as far as the breastbone, being neither extended straight down the length of the animal, nor oblique, like the muscles, but going at an angle; their head is the vertebra here [in the relevant place] and their end is the breastbone. Moreover, the nerves that go to the other muscles that operate breathing almost all grow out of the spinal marrow.

8. This, then, is the number and kind of the causes of breathing, and it is clear to anyone who is not utterly stupid what is the different character of each. Choice is like a charioteer who moves the reins and the horses; the nerves are like the reins, and the muscles are like the horses; similarly the use is the desired end of breathing, as victory is of chariot racing.

---

3 τοῦ] τὸ RZ
4 κεφαλὴν] καλὴν Z   τὸν ταύτῃ] τοσαύτη Z
9 μὴ] μὴν Z   διενήνοχεν] δὲ ἐνήνοχεν M
13 τῆς] καὶ τῆς MRZa

NOTES TO TRANSLATIONS

ON THE USE OF BREATHING

1. For the earlier theories of breathing mentioned here, see Introduction, I.
2. Cf. *De locis affectis* VI 5 = K VIII 413, where Galen expresses impatience about the question whether ὑστέρα or μήτρα is the right word.
3. The three doctrines mentioned here are that breathing is for strengthening the innate heat, for fanning it, and for cooling it. Galen says that all three amount to the same thing, viz. preserving the innate heat. He thus appears to be distinguishing these from theories that say that the purpose of breathing is to replenish the substance of the soul; and there appears to be a *non sequitur* in saying that the theory of preserving the innate heat is difficult to discuss because we do not know the substance of the soul.

    It is possible that there is a lacuna in the text. But the connection is not too difficult to supply. In *De simplicium medicamentorum temperamentis ac facultatibus* (K XI 730–31) Galen recounts some words of Hippocrates that he understands to be about innate heat, "which we identify in each animal as pneuma, about which Aristotle also wrote.... And the Stoics believe this same pneuma to be the substance of the soul. For our part, we do not presume to make any statement at all about the substance of the soul, and we suppose it is irrelevant to the present context. However, we have already shown in *De placitis Hippocratis et Platonis* [VII 3] that even if the connate pneuma is not the substance of the soul, it is nevertheless its first instrument."

    So discussion of all theories (πασῶν αὐτῶν, 2.9), both those that mention innate heat and those that mention the soul, presents the same difficulty, that to understand them fully one would have to know the substance of the soul, because innate heat is so closely connected with soul. The same point reappears below in Chapter 5.

    Galen's modesty in disclaiming knowledge of the substance of the soul is noted by Dr. May (50 n. 211), who compares *De nat. fac.* I 4.

    Noll suggests reading δυσδιαίτητος for δυσδιαίρετος in 2, 9, comparing 12, 13 χαλεπὸν ... καὶ δυσδιαίτητον. But δυσδιαίρετος is attested also in Galen (K IV 400) and it seems best to let it stand. It does not affect the meaning.
4. The word "ποιότης," translated "quality," occurs first in Plato *Theaetetus* 182 b, with an apology for the neologism. The distinction between οὐσία (substance) and ποιότης became thoroughly familiar in Aristotle (*Categories* 8 b 25, etc.). Galen has some general remarks about quality in *De nat. fac.* I 2, where he refers to the authority of Hippocrates and Aristotle. The primary qualities are heat, cold, dryness, and wetness.
5. The physiology of Erasistratus is explained in the Introduction, I f; his theory here depends on the presumption that air is noncompressible and

nonexpandable. Note that Galen agrees with Erasistratus that in normal breathing air or pneuma is drawn from the lung by the heart through the pulmonary vein, which he calls "the venous artery." He disagrees with Erasistratus' view that the "venous artery" contains only pneuma (see *An in arteriis*). Galen distinguishes arteries from veins by the pulse in the former; this criterion is explained and defended in *De anatomicis administrationibus* VII 4.

6. The distinction between interspersed void and massed void seems to have been first worked out in the Peripatetic School, becoming particularly important in the generation after Aristotle. See Introduction, I f. The point of mentioning it here is that it would allow for rarefaction of the air contained in the lung. Note that it is brought up as an objection to Erasistratus' doctrine. From *De nat. fac.* II 6 (K II 99), it seems that Erasistratus did not rule out the possibility of interspersed void. It is not clear how he could have answered this objection.

7. Galen frequently uses the term "the Erasistrateans." Sometimes he means contemporaries of his own (cf. *De nat. fac.* II 2; K II 79); but probably the school of Erasistratus was continuous from the time of the founder to Galen's time, and Galen was acquainted with writings from various periods. He often accuses the Erasistrateans of holding views inconsistent with Erasistratus (see Lonie, "Erasistratus"), and sometimes describes differences among the Erasistrateans themselves (*De nat. fac.* II 5). Here the Erasistrateans are said to have produced arguments against the view that air can expand and contract, and against the interspersed void.

8. The manuscripts say that the Asclepiadean doctrines were refuted by Asclepiades, but if Galen really meant to say this, he would have expressed it with some emphasis. So it is probably a mistake. The name of Athenaeus was substituted by Noll, on the basis of two passages (*De symptomatum causis* II 3 [K VII 165] and *De tremore* K VII 615–16) in which Galen reports that Athenaeus criticized Asclepiades. Athenaeus of Attalia practiced in Rome in the 1st–2nd century A.D., and was one of the founders of the Pneumatic School (see Wellmann, *Pneum.*, pp. 5–11).

9. Elsewhere Galen concedes that it is possible for something to go back from the artery to the heart, in spite of the valve. See *De usu pulsuum* 5 and *De usu partium* VI 16 (K I 357): "We should think that Nature found means to prevent a large quantity of blood and pneuma from flowing past, but was unable to find anything to stop the flow altogether of the smallest possible quantity" (tr. May). For Erasistratus' own view, see the next paragraph.

10. This is a good argument against the Erasistrateans.

11. ἐκφύσησις is used of blowing the nose in *De usu partium* VIII 7 (K III 654–55). In *De usu pulsuum* 7, Galen uses the distinction between blowing and breathing out in introducing the proposition that the contraction of the pulse may be a natural relaxation after an active expansion.

12. Earlier editions print a comma before "$\mu\nu\rho\iota\alpha\kappa\iota\varsigma$," thus giving a meaning "breathe in very deeply a thousand times" (in Cornarius' Latin version "ut sescenties inspirationem faciat"), which is nonsense.

13. See Chapter 3, especially the analogy of an oven choked with smoke (§8).

14. The two groups are the Erasistrateans and their opponents.

15. Galen's own theory of the pulse is that it is transmitted through the coats of the artery from the heart. Erasistratus' theory was that the expansion of the artery at any point is due to the pneuma forced through it by the heartbeat, and its contraction is a return to the natural state after the pneuma has passed through. The argument against him is that according to Erasistratus' view of what happens when the breath is held, the pneuma has to pass through the artery twice, once outward bound, when the heart contracts, and once inward bound, when the heart expands; so according to his theory of the pulse, the expansions of the artery ought to occur twice as often when the breath is held as in normal breathing.

16. In Erasistratus' theory the pneuma is drawn in in breathing, distributed to the body through the arteries, and either expelled through the pores of the skin or else consumed by the tissues of the body.

17. The manuscripts and all earlier editors print "$o\dot{v}\ \mu\dot{\eta}\nu\ \delta$' $\ddot{\epsilon}\lambda\kappa\epsilon\sigma\theta\alpha\iota$" (except that K omits "$\delta$'"); "it is indeed emptied, but *not* drawn in again." This negative makes nonsense of the passage, and I believe it is a mistake, caused by a false analogy with the previous sentence, in which a positive was paired with a negative. The words "$o\dot{v}\ \mu\dot{\eta}\nu$" conceal something like "$\ddot{o}\lambda\omega\varsigma$," "entirely," or perhaps an adverb meaning "then." I print "$\ddot{o}\lambda\omega\varsigma$" *exempli gratia*.

18. Again the manuscript reading makes nonsense. I follow the early Latin translations, and Noll, in reading "$\dot{\epsilon}\sigma\tau\dot{\iota}\ \delta\nu\nu\alpha\tau\dot{o}\nu$" ("it is possible") for "$\dot{\epsilon}\sigma\tau\dot{\iota}\nu\ \dot{\alpha}\delta\dot{\nu}\nu\alpha\tau o\nu$" ("it is impossible").

19. Again it seems likely that the manuscript reading is based on a misunderstanding of the argument. According to the manuscripts, the text means "in spite of the valves being closed, the heart is able to draw no less." But the argument requires "although it can draw something, it draws less."

20. The Erasistratean might try to defend the usefulness of the thorax and lungs by saying that although the heart can draw pneuma from outside the body by way of the artery, it cannot draw so much as from the lungs. This escape route is blocked by Galen's observation that the size of the pulse is not diminished in these circumstances, thus proving that if pneuma is being transmitted through the artery to the heart from outside the body, a normal amount of pneuma is being transmitted. Galen then adds that, in fact, it is obvious that the valves would have to cause some diminution of the amount, so this whole explanation of why the pulse continues during suspension of breathing is inconsistent with the observation that there is no diminution in the size of the pulse.

21. Galen has now shown that during suspension of breathing, with the lungs full, the heart and the arteries must still have a plentiful supply of the substance of pneuma. The fact that we still suffocate in this condition shows that we need something other than the substance of pneuma from breathing. Asclepiades and Praxagoras (see K 471) both held that it is only the substance that is needed, according to Galen. Philotimus was a pupil of Praxagoras: see *Praxagoras*, ed. Steckerl, and Introduction, I e.

    In his book *De propriis libris* VIII (p. 105, 1–4 Mü.), Galen mentions eight books of his on the doctrines of Asclepiades, and another small one with the title "On the substance of the soul according to Asclepiades." These do not survive.

22. This is an example of the fifth type of undemonstrated argument in Stoic logic; see Mates, *Stoic Logic*, p. 73; Stakelum, *Galen*, p. 62; Galen, *Institutio logica* (ed. Kalbfleisch) VI 6, p. 16, 6.

23. "Bulimus: vehemens, frequentior, et nimium aucta fames, Franc. Sylvius 1; Pr. c. 5. Qui cum Galeno caussam in refrigeratione oris ventriculi et indigentia quaerunt, ex 1. i, *De causis symptomatum* 7, operam perdunt" (Bartholomaei Castelli, *Lexicum Medicum Graeco-Latinum*, Leipzig, 1713).

24. "The same appearances" are that we continue to breathe when very cold. Two opposing schools of thought draw support from this: i. some say breathing is for cooling, because we breathe less when chilled; ii. others say breathing is not for cooling, because we continue to breathe when chilled.

25. The Greek manuscript tradition is corrupt in this passage. The medieval Latin version makes better sense, and I follow Noll in emending the Greek accordingly.

26. The argument is clumsily expressed. Noll is probably right in supposing that "λέγοντας" has fallen out, by haplography, in line 1, but there is no need to mark a lacuna after this word, as he does. Those who oppose the cooling theory of breathing, Galen says, quote Hippocrates (*Prognostic* V) to the effect that very cold breath is a sign of approaching death. This condition, Galen adds, is presumably due to severe chilling of the organs of respiration. So these opponents argue that if breathing were for the sake of cooling, people in the condition described by Hippocrates would be better off if they did not breathe at all.

27. That is, in saying "breathing is for cooling," they would not have said anything directly about the use of breathing, which is on this supposition the kindling of which cooling is the efficient or productive cause.

28. Galen now goes back to the point he made in Chapter 1, that cooling, kindling, and strengthening all have a common element—the preservation of the innate heat.

29. A very prophetic remark: strange that about one and a half millennia elapsed between Galen's time and the discovery of oxygen.

30. Most of the following theory about fire can be found in Theophrastus *De igne* §§20–27. It is interesting that the extinction of a flame through putting a cover over it is described by Theophrastus with the words "if

one gives it no respiration (ἀναπνοή)." The analogy between the body's need for respiration and a fire's need for a draught was clearly a well-established one.

31. The strange notion that the direct rays of the sun can extinguish flames is not mentioned by Theophrastus, although it occurs elsewhere in Greek literature. Perhaps the mistake arose because a flame is sometimes made invisible by strong sunlight. The idea that fire can be extinguished by excessive cold belongs to Aristotle's theory that opposite qualities can blend only if each is present in a moderate degree: if one is much more powerful than the other, it overwhelms it and destroys it.

32. The Latin translation has "ex motibus contrariis, quorum alter alterum mutuo excipit et consequitur, alterum sine altero conservari impossibile est." Galen uses the same idea in *De tremore*, K VII 617: "Since the innate heat is always in motion (ἀεικίνητον), it moves neither inward nor outward alone, but the one motion always follows upon (διαδέχεται) the other. For the inward motion alone would soon end in immobility, and the outward motion would disperse and thus destroy the heat. But 'being quenched in measures and kindled in measures,' as Heraclitus used to say, it remains always in motion." Noll's suggestion that the manuscripts' "δεχομένων" should be emended to "διαδεχομένων" is probably right.

33. The Greek text is corrupt here, and I have adopted Noll's proposals for want of anything better.

34. According to *De usu partium* VI 7 (K III 436), the heart is "as it were the hearthstone and source of the innate heat" (οἶον ἑστία τέ τίς ἐστι καὶ πηγή). See also *ibid.* VI 15 (K 481), where the heart is compared to a lamp; and VII 9 (K 545), where the source of heat is said to be the left ventricle of the heart. In *De temperamentis* I 9 (K I 569–70), Galen says the blood itself derives its heat from the heart. This is hardly consistent with the statement in our text that the blood is the matter, or fuel, of the innate heat. The point is that the innate heat is not in fact a fire (see *De placitis Hippocratis et Platonis* VIII 7; K V 703), and the heart is not literally a lamp that burns fuel. Fire consumes its fuel, but the innate heat does not. This point is explained in a discussion of the causes of senility (*De marcore* 3; K VII 672–76): old age cannot be the gradual exhaustion of the fuel for innate heat, as some say, because it is the characteristic of the innate heat to restore and increase its matter, not to consume it.

35. There are two similes here. The lungs are compared to a cover of a lamp, which protects the flame from excessive draughts but allows the right amount of air to reach it, and also to a medical cupping glass (σικύα—literally a gourd, so called from its shape), which normally of course has no hole in it. See Niebyl, "Old Age, Fever, and the Lamp Metaphor."

36. Purging the smoky vapor is not the only way in which breathing serves the innate heat, of course; breathing in is the most important part.

37. The text of the last few lines is again corrupt. The articulation given here, as in the Aldine edition (*a*, fanning and cooling, and *b*, motion to evacuate smoke) is almost certainly correct, but some points remain obscure.

38. Galen refers to the formal arguments in *An in arteriis* as ἀποδείξεις (demonstrations). What his present arguments lack can be inferred by comparison.

39. This passage has been misunderstood in previous editions, possibly because the logical terms were interpreted wrongly. The "conditional proposition" (συνημμένον) is "if we breathe only for the sake of cooling, those who breathe the vapor of cauldrons must stifle." The "second premise" (πρόσληψις) is "but they do not stifle"; other editors have punctuated as though Galen asserted this, instead of quoting it.

    For the logic, see Mates, *Stoic Logic*, pp. 71 and 132–36, and Introduction, III. Galen assumes that his opponents use a type 2 argument:
    A. If the first, then the second.
    B. Not the second.
    C. Therefore, not the first.
    A is true, he says, but B is false, and therefore C does not follow. Now, since Galen does not assert "they do not stifle" but says this is false, there is no need to remove "ἧττον" from the text in the following sentence, as Noll does.

40. For Galen's theory of breathing through the pores of the skin, see *De usu pulsuum* 3 and Introduction, II.

41. The opponents believe that people faint at the baths through loss of pneuma. It is not clear whether they think that pneuma is lost from the body with sweat (or perhaps *is* sweat), or that the body breathes pneuma out but cannot breathe it in through the moisture (as with attempts to breathe through the nose and mouth under water), or that the pneuma becomes unduly thin because of the heat (see next paragraph).

42. This Chrysippus is not to be confused with the famous Stoic, Chrysippus of Soli, as in Kühn's index to Galen's works. Chrysippus of Cnidos is mentioned by Diogenes Laertius (VII 186) as well as by Galen (K XI 197) as being a teacher of Erasistratus. There were other doctors of the same name (Diogenes Laertius VIII 89), at least one other from Cnidos, but the teacher of Erasistratus appears to have been the one best known to Galen.

43. Charonian pits, named after Charon, the ferryman of the underworld, are caverns full of poisonous vapors. Such caverns near the Maeander River are referred to by Strabo, 12, 8, 17; 14, 1, 11; and 14, 1, 44. The same list of circumstances that affect breathing occurs in *De usu partium* VII 8 (K III 540).

44. Note the importance of density for Erasistratus.

45. The Greek text here and for the next few lines seems hopeless. For want of any better ideas, I have followed Noll's text from "ἡμεῖς δέ φαμεν" to "εὑρεθῆναι," although I am unable to explain why "αἰτίας" is not in

the accusative. In the next sentence it is at least clear that Galen must be *asserting* that the motions of the arteries are unchanged; the manuscript text is impossible, and so I have made two changes, "ϵi" to "$\overset{\text{"}}{\alpha}\lambda\lambda o$," and "$\tau o \hat{v}$" to "$\hat{\eta} \ \tau o$."

46. The manuscripts have "$\theta \alpha \lambda \acute{\alpha} \tau \tau \iota o \iota \ \zeta \omega \gamma \rho \epsilon \hat{\iota} s$," "men at sea who capture alive." This is unlikely, since "$\zeta \omega \gamma \rho \epsilon \acute{v} s$" is a noun not found elsewhere, and in any case they are harpooning the creature. The Latin translator probably found "$\zeta \hat{\omega} o \nu$" in his text, and I have adopted his reading. But there is a point in saying that the fish is still alive, as in Galen *De locis affectis* II 2 (K VIII 72): $\grave{\alpha}\phi\acute{\alpha}\mu\epsilon\nu o\iota \ \tau o\hat{v} \ \zeta \acute{\omega} o v \ \tau \hat{\eta} s \ \nu \acute{\alpha} \rho \kappa \eta s \ \overset{\text{"}}{\epsilon} \tau \iota \ \zeta \acute{\omega} \sigma \eta s$. Possibly Galen wrote "$\zeta \acute{\omega} \sigma \eta s$" here.

The torpedo fish excited much interest in antiquity. Meno says Socrates has torpedoed him, in a famous passage (Plato, *Meno* 80 a). Pliny, *Natural History* 32, 2(7) explains its power as coming from "what I may call the breath of the creature's body" (*quaedam aura corporis*). In *De locis affectis* VI 5, Galen uses the torpedo fish (along with the scorpion and the lodestone) as an example of the great power that can be exerted by a small thing, to make plausible his medical theory that the unwonted retention of semen may be a cause of many ills.

47. Cf. *An in arteriis* 6.

48. The "two schools" are the Erasistrateans, who think breathing is for the substance of the air breathed in, and the anti-Erasistrateans, who think it is for its quality. Much of the subject matter of the rest of Chapter 4 is also found in *De difficultate respirationis* I 7 (K VII 768ff.).

49. In Chapter 2.

50. Probably Galen is referring to *De causis pulsuum*, as also in Chapter 5, §2.

51. The ground for believing that exercise increases heat is presumably just observation.

52. Galen is still arguing primarily against Erasistratus' theory of breathing.

53. The manuscripts have "$\sigma \phi o \delta \rho o \grave{v} s$," and Noll therefore imports "$\tau o \grave{v} s \ \sigma \phi v \gamma \mu o \grave{v} s$" as subject to the infinitive "$\gamma \acute{\iota} \gamma \nu \epsilon \sigma \theta \alpha \iota$": "the *pulse* becomes vigorous." But there is no mention of the pulse in the second half of the sentence, and no need to import it in order to make an argument against Erasistratus. Galen's point is that if exercise caused faster breathing because it emptied more pneuma from the arteries, this effect ought to be noticed at once. I think the verb "$\kappa \iota \nu \epsilon \hat{\iota} \sigma \theta \alpha \iota$" was changed to "$\gamma \acute{\iota} \gamma \nu \epsilon \sigma \theta \alpha \iota$" by analogy with "$\gamma \acute{\iota} \gamma \nu \epsilon \sigma \theta \alpha \iota$" three lines before.

54. The (partial) analogy between the innate heat and a flame is presented in Chapter 3. See also Introduction, II.

55. A quotation from Hippocrates *Aphorisms* (IV 466 L).

56. Nourishment of the psychic pneuma is one of the uses of breathing, according to Galen (see Chapter 7), but it has hitherto not been mentioned in the course of the argument against Erasistratus' doctrine that breathing is only to keep up the supply of pneuma.

57. According to Galen's physiology, food is "worked up" by a series of stages into blood, which is nutriment for the tissues. Each stage of the

working up produces "surpluses" or "residues" (περίττωματα), which have to be expelled. See *De usu partium* IV 15.

58. See note 48.

59. See Chapter 1, and *De nat. fac.* I 4.

60. The manuscript reading, adopted also by earlier editors, makes the genitive "πνεύματος" depend directly on "κοιλίαι." It makes better sense and better syntax to suppose that a participle such as "στερηθεῖσαι" has fallen out.

61. See *De usu partium* IX 4 and *De placitis Hippocratis et Platonis* VII 3 (K V 600ff., especially pp. 605–609); also Introduction, II.

62. Cf. *De placitis Hippocratis et Platonis* II 8 (K V 281).

63. In fact, Galen does not explicitly say much about Erasistratus in *De causis pulsuum*; perhaps he is thinking of *De usu pulsuum*. The experiment referred to in the next sentence is described in the latter book. Chapter 1 §2.

64. *De usu pulsuum* 2. For the distinction between vital and psychic organs, see Temkin, "Pneumatology," and May, *Usefulness*, pp. 46–47.

65. *De usu pulsuum* 2 §3.

66. Galen's acceptance of such vague conclusions prevented him from progressing far in physiology.

67. Hippocrates *De alimento* (IV 108 L); the same quotation again in *De placitis Hippocratis et Platonis* II 8 (K V 281), where it is discussed at some length.

68. This is a very difficult passage, because the Greek text tradition evidently became corrupt at an early date. The most important question is this: is the bladder placed over the boy's mouth and nostrils (τῷ στόματι), as the manuscripts say, or over all the rest of his body except the mouth and nostrils (τῷ σώματι πλὴν τῷ στόματι), as Noll proposed? Fortunately this is easily answered. Noll must be wrong. Admittedly the passage cited by him, *De morborum causis* 3 (K VII 15–16) states that the arteries communicate with the outer air through the skin, as well as through the heart and pharynx, and considers the case in which the pores (στόματα) are blocked. But (a) Galen says that in this case the body dies (νεκρωθῆναι τὸ διατεθὲν οὕτω σῶμα), and (b) the experiment of putting the body in a bladder (supposing a big enough one could be found) would not prove what Galen wants, because he acknowledges that the arteries can get pneuma also through the heart and pharynx.

Of course, Galen knows that one stifles if prevented from breathing through the mouth and nostrils (see above, Chapter 2). So the point of the experiment must be (as it has usually been taken to be) to make the boy breathe the same air in and out all the time. If pneuma is expended into the arteries in the breathing process, one would expect the supply to be soon exhausted. The fact that the boy goes on breathing shows that pneuma is not so expended. (The bladder was clearly not totally airtight—see Introduction, III).

The next few lines (28.8–29.5 Noll) are concerned with the positive contribution that breathing does make to the psychic pneuma, in Galen's view. The transition seems very abrupt. So I am inclined to believe that there is a lacuna in the text—as Noll did, but for different reasons.

Kühn's text makes Galen say that the arteries in the body have little or no need of the qualities of the external air. This seems to be a contradiction of his real doctrine.

The text in the next sentence is very dubious. The logic of the passage seems certainly to require a distinction between substance and quality of the inspired air. Somehow the distinction has been obliterated in the corrupt manuscript tradition. The translation printed in < > is a guess.

69. Hippocrates *Epidemica* VI 6 (V 322 L); Galen *In Hippocratis Epidemica* VI (K XVII B 311ff.). He quotes the same line from Hippocrates in *De usu pulsuum* 2 §5 and 5 §2.

70. As suggested at the beginning of this chapter. Notice the cautious manner of expression in this passage.

71. Cf. *De temperamentis* II 3.

72. This refers back to p. 498 (Kühn) above, where Galen said that he had not found a necessary proof of his own theory, but only arguments more persuasive than any others.

73. "διαίρεσις" is not as a rule used to mean "disjunction"; it normally means "division." In *Institutio logica* 3, 4 Galen writes: "An expression like 'either it is day or it is night' is called a 'disjunctive proposition' (διεζευγμένον ἀξίωμα) by the more recent philosophers, a 'hypothetical proposition by division' (πρότασις ὑποθετικὴ κατὰ διαίρεσιν) by the older ones." The distinction appears to be between the Stoics ("the more recent") and the Peripatetics. See also Stakelum, *Galen*, pp. 29–30, and Kieffer, *Institutio*, index s.v. "disjunction."

74. The Greek tradition in this sentence is corrupt, and I have translated the Latin translation.

75. The argument becomes muddled at this point, perhaps because the manuscripts are wrong. It seems impossible to interpret the text so as to preserve a consistent distinction between the soul itself (or its substance) and its primary organ. Motion is presumably mentioned as a criterion of life: cf. *De placitis Hippocratis et Platonis* I 6 (K V 186). Perhaps there is some antithesis between "motion" and "unaffected" (ἀπαθῆ): to be the cause of change, it must preserve the substance of the soul unchanged (?).

76. Cf. *De usu partium* VII 9 (K I 396).

77. See *De usu partium* VI 15 (K III 481).

78. See *De instrumento odoratus* I 7 (K II 867) as well as *De placitis Hippocratis et Platonis* III 8; (K V 356). See also *De usu pulsuum* 2 §2.

79. But none of the editors has been able to find this discussion, including ourselves.

80. *De difficultate respirationis* I 7 (K VII 772).

BLOOD IN THE ARTERIES

1. The beginning of the treatise in the Arabic manuscripts is as follows:

Z 1 [83^b]

بسم الله الرّحـمٰـن الرّحيم

كتـاب حالينوس في

ان الدم محتبس في العروق الضوارب بالطّبع

ترجمة حنـن بن اسحق

إلى السريان وترجمـه عيسى بن يحيى

إلى العـربي

قال لـمّـا كنّـا نرى الدم يستفرع من أي العروق الضوارب سُـقّ

"In the name of God, the Compassionate, the Merciful:
The book of Galen concerning
that blood is contained in the arteries
naturally. The translation of Ḥunain ibn Ishaq
into Syriac and the translation of 'Īsa ibn
Yahyā into Arabic.
He said: Since we have [constantly] seen blood flowing out from whatever artery has been pierced. . . . "

Y 37^b

سم الله الرّحـمٰـن الرّحيم

كتاب حاليوس في أن الدم محتبس في العروق الصوارب بالطّبع

نقل ابى زيد حسين بن اسحق

الباب الأول في البرهان على أن الدم محتبس في العروق الضوارب بالطّبع قال جاليوس إنا لـمّـا نرى الدم الذي يستفرغ

من أي العروق الضوارب سُـقّ

"In the name of God, the Compassionate, the Merciful:
The book of Galen concerning that blood is contained
in the arteries naturally.
The translation of Abu Zaid Ḥunain ibn Isḥāq.
The first chapter in the proof that blood is contained in the arteries naturally. Galen said: Now since we have [constantly] seen the blood that flows from whatever artery is pierced. . . . "

2. The work opens *in medias res*. The chief target of the polemic is the theory of Erasistratus and his school. The only alternatives considered are the Erasistratean thesis that the arteries in their natural state contain only pneuma, and Galen's, that they contain blood and pneuma mixed.

3. Galen now changes from a common-sense argument to the schemata of Stoic logic. He states the last step in the argument first, and sets it out in full in the following paragraph. It can be represented schematically thus:

258

I. If the first, then the second.
The first.
Therefore the second.

If blood is observed escaping from wounded arteries, then either it was contained in the arteries, or it was transferred from elsewhere.
It is so observed.
Therefore, either it was so contained, or it was so transferred.

II. If the first, then the second.
Not the second.
Therefore not the first.

If blood is transferred from elsewhere, then pneuma is observed to be voided before blood.
But it is not so observed.
Therefore blood is not so transferred.

III. Either the first or the second.
Not the first.
Therefore the second.

Either blood is transferred from elsewhere, or it was contained in the arteries.
It is not so transferred.
Therefore it was so contained.

These are set out according to the schemata of "undemonstrated arguments" in Stoic logic. Argument I is of type 1, argument II of type 2, and argument III is of type 5 (see Mates, *Stoic Logic*, pp. 67–74, and Introduction, III).

4. There is some doubt about the tenses used here and in line 12. The manuscripts seem to have had present indicatives, and since this is usual in the examples given by our sources for Stoic logic, I think it is right. Albrecht prints imperfects.

5. For differences among later Erasistrateans, see *De usu respirationis* 2. Erasistratus did not believe that the arteries themselves have a pulsating faculty that might explain the expulsion of pneuma; Galen accuses him of treating the arteries as lifeless drains, in *De usu pulsuum* 5.

6. The precise point of the question is this. Supposing for the moment that the arteries in their natural state contain no blood but only pneuma, and that the reason for our not observing the escape of pneuma when an artery is punctured is that the pneuma is exceptionally swift to move and very fine, what is the cause of the escape of the pneuma from the puncture? The first alternative is that there is no external cause, but the pneuma moves because of some property of its own. Galen then assumes something like an Aristotelian theory of natural motions. The environment of the punctured artery is air—the ordinary atmospheric air around us. If the pneuma were of the same nature as the air, there would be no

explanation of its motion. So he considers two alternatives (he does not mention a third, that it might be heavier than air, presumably because it would then have to be observable): either it is like the matter of the heavens, aetherial; or it is fiery. In either case, it would naturally rise through air to the higher regions, according to the Aristotelian theory. But Galen now produces arguments to show that neither can be the case.

7. That is, the *vena pulmonaris*, which Galen calls the "venous artery"; see Introduction, I e.

8. The adjectives translated "composed of finer parts" and "more coarse-grained" (λεπτομερέστερον, παχυμερέστερον) are an interesting pair. They have an obvious meaning in the context of an atomic theory of matter, such as that of Epicurus or Asclepiades. It is not so clear what they mean in continuum theories. It is certain, however, that they were used in continuum theories, by the Aristotelians and Stoics, and their occurrence in any context should not be taken to indicate the influence of atomism.

9. See Introduction, I e, and *De usu respirationis* 2, §11. This is fragment 31 in Steckerl's collection of the fragments of Praxagoras, and he discusses the theory briefly (p. 19).

10. The idea that pneuma is the motor agency that produces the voluntary movements of the body is found in Aristotle, *De motu animalium* 10. The Epicureans used a similar idea (Lucretius 4, 889–906). See Solmsen, "Nerves" 176ff.

11. For the vapors in the arterial blood in Galen's theory, see *De nat. fac.* III 14, *De usu partium* VI 16. The point of the argument is that in Galen's view we can observe that arterial blood is hotter and more vaporous than venous blood; and this is equivalent to observing that it has pneuma in it.

12. By the principle of "refilling the void" (πρὸς τὸ κενὸν ἀκολουθία), which was one of the main tenets of Erasistratus' physiology. It is discussed and criticized at length in *De nat. fac.*, especially I 16–17. See also Introduction, I f.

13. Erasistratus and Galen both believed that the arteries are linked to the veins at their extremities by extremely fine, imperceptibly small, connecting channels. See *De usu pulsuum* 5.

14. The vital pneuma, originating in the heart, is to be distinguished from the psychic pneuma that originates in the brain. (See Temkin, "Pneumatology" for a discussion of Galen's theory.) The point of the argument is, of course, that an animal *can* live after bleeding from an artery.

15. For this use of διαίρεσις, see *De usu respirationis* 5 §7.

16. The insertion of "massed" (ἀθρόος) is due to the distinction between massed void and disseminate void. See *De usu respirationis* 2 §2, and Introduction, I f.

17. This criticism of Erasistratus is attributed to Asclepiades in *De nat. fac.* II 1 (K II 75).

18. The argument is of the fifth type in the Stoic system:

    Either the first or the second.
    Not the first.
    Therefore the second.

    "Not the first" is the minor premise ($\pi\rho\acute{o}\sigma\lambda\eta\psi\iota\varsigma$).

19. Albrecht conjectured that the impossible Greek of the manuscripts, "$\kappa\alpha\grave{\iota}$ $\delta\grave{\eta}$ $\mu\acute{e}\nu$ $\mu\text{o}\iota$," concealed a perfect participle. He supplied "$\delta\iota\eta\rho\eta\mu\acute{e}\nu\eta\nu$" because that verb is found in the same context at 7.22. This conjecture receives support from the Arabic version. Perhaps the infinitive "$\delta\epsilon\acute{\iota}\kappa\nu\upsilon$-$\sigma\theta\alpha\iota$" has fallen out also.

Z 7, lines 8–10

وينبيّن ما أقول إن ابتدأ بالبرهان من تسريح العروى الصوارب فاحطر لي الآن ببالك أن العرى الضارب المنقسم في اليد كلها
ثقب بإبرة دقيقه

"And what I say will become clear if I begin [or you begin] with the proof from the anatomy of the arteries. So imagine for me now that the artery distributed to the whole hand is pierced with a fine needle."

Y 41[b]: line 16 to 42[a] line 1.

وينبيّن لك ما أقول إن ابتدأتَ بالبرهان من تسريح العروى الصوارب المنقسمه في اليد كلها فأُحطر لي ببالك أن العرق الضارب
ثقب بإبرة دقيقة

"And what I say will become clear to you if you begin with the proof from the anatomy of the arteries distributed to the whole hand. So imagine for me that the artery is pierced by a fine needle."

20. For this translation of $\chi\epsilon\acute{\iota}\rho$, see May, *Usefulness*, p. 115 n. 8 (I owe this point to P. DeLacy).

21. Rather an odd use of "$\acute{o}\gamma\kappa\text{o}\varsigma$." Probably the whole of the animal's body is meant.

22. A fuller account of Erasistratus' doctrine is given in *De venae sectione adv. Erasistratum* 3 (K XI 152ff.).

23. Erasistratus' doctrine is described by Anonymus Londinensis XXI 23ff. (Jones, p. 83): "Erasistratus supposed that the primary bodies are observed only by reason, so that the perceived vein is composed of bodies observed only by reason, namely, vein, artery, sinew." (So Jones; but the word "$\nu\epsilon\hat{\upsilon}\rho\text{o}\nu$," which originally meant "sinew," was used for "nerve" after the discovery of the nerves. See Solmsen, "Nerves" 188). According to the pseudo-Galenic *Introductio*, Erasistratus held that all the tissues of the body are composed of the three elements, the $\tau\rho\iota\pi\lambda\text{o}\kappa\acute{\iota}\alpha$ of vessels: nerves, veins, and arteries (K XIV 697). Presumably the network is here taken by Galen to be so fine that even a pinprick necessarily punctures one of each type of vessel.

24. The reading of the Greek manuscripts makes no sense here, and an attempt has been made to supply something that might have been trans-

lated as the Arabic version has it. The Arabic is more long-winded than the proposed Greek original, but there are other instances where the translator adds "we say that this is so" or the equivalent. Earlier editors supplied "$\delta\iota\alpha\pi\nu\circ\hat{\eta}\varsigma$" (transpiration) as the noun modified by "invisible."

Z 10, lines 3–7: Y 43^b, lines 3–8

¹فينثقب الجلد الذي على الساعد المغسى للعرق الضارب الذى فى الابط ²ويستفرغ الروح الذى فى العرى الضارب الخفى عن
البصر ونضع أن ذلك كذلك ³لأن ارسسطراطس ⁴احبّه ⁵فلِأن المشقوق عرق ضارب يجب أن يستفرغ الروح ويستفرغ معه
ما يتّصل به من الروح الذى فى العرق الصارب العظيم الذى تحته وهو ⁶الذى يمرّ بالابط

¹فلينثقب   ²ليستفرغ   ³لا أن
⁴احـمه   ⁵قال   ⁶الذى فى الابط

"So let the skin which is on the arm and covering the artery that is in the armpit be pierced, and let the pneuma that is in the hidden artery be emptied out; and we concede that that is so because Erasistratus will have it [so]; then, because what is pierced is an artery, the pneuma must necessarily be emptied out and there will be emptied out with it what is contiguous with it of the pneuma that is in the large artery that is beneath it, and that is the one running through the armpit."

25. K 712–13.
26. Exactly the same simile appears in *De nat. fac.* II 2 (K II 79–80), where the floored wrestlers are also Erasistrateans, and the subject is their theory of bile secretion.
27. Some Erasistrateans attempt to mitigate the paradoxes of Chapter 4 by saying that a wound to an artery does not empty the entire arterial system of pneuma and fill it with blood. Blood enters the wounded artery from the nearest junction with the veins—and that is, presumably, enough to stop the rest of the pneuma from escaping. Galen's answer is (a) that this is contrary to what Erasistratus wrote, and (b) that a wound to the arterial system in the abdominal wall can be seen to have emptied the pneuma from the arteries of the mesentery, which are acknowledged by Erasistratus himself to be not "near," in the relevant sense, to those of the abdominal wall.
28. Cf. *De anatomicis administrationibus* VII 16 (K II 648–49).
29. There is a similar comparison of the arterial system to a tree in *De placitis Hippocratis et Platonis* VI 3 (K V 524ff.).
30. The following two paragraphs really belong to Chapter 6.
31. "To fall from a donkey" is a proverbial phrase, apparently punning on the similarity between "$\dot{\alpha}\pi'\;\ddot{o}\nu\circ\nu$" (from a donkey) and "$\dot{\alpha}\pi\grave{o}\;\nu\circ\hat{\nu}$" (from sense). It means to talk complete nonsense. Cf. Aristophanes *Clouds* 1273, with K. J. Dover's note, and Plato *Laws* 701 c.
32. Galen may be thinking of his *De sectis* (K I 64ff.) or his *De optima secta* (K I 106ff.), or possibly his (now lost) *De demonstratione*. In the first two he distinguishes three sects, whom he called the Empiricists, the Rationalists, and the Methodists. What he says about the Empiricists and

Rationalists is consistent with what he says here about the Sceptics and the Dogmatists, respectively.

33. The Eleatics, especially Zeno, used arguments "against motion." But it is more likely that Galen is thinking of the later Megarian philosopher Diodorus Cronus, whose arguments are reported by Sextus Empiricus, *Adv. Math.* I 311–12, X 93ff.

34. Aristotle *De caelo* A 6, 271 a 33 (and elsewhere): "God and nature do nothing in vain." This teleological slogan was reiterated by Erasistratus as well as by Galen. For a discussion of Erasistratus' position, see *De nat. fac.* II 3, and for Galen's explanation of the two kinds of blood vessel, see *De usu partium* VI 10 and 17.

35. The Arabic version suggests that L's ἄπορα must be preferred to V's ἄπειρα, and that an optative νομισθείη is more likely than the (counterfactual) aorist participle νομισθέντα.

Z 14, 3–5; Y 46ᵃ, 10–12

فإنّ هذه الاشياء انــها هي مسائل ١يحب المسائله والبحث عنها مفرده على حد ٢نها وحلبى أن يتوقّم بعض الناس أن فيها موضع شَكّ وتحيّر إلآ أه ليس يبلغ من ذلك أن يُبطل معها ما يظهر للحس

١تحب المسائله   ٢عنها والبحث مفرده

"Now indeed those things are questions that have to be asked and investigated each separately and by itself; and perhaps someone will suspect that there is in them an occasion for doubt and perplexity; however, this does not go so far as to nullify there what appears to the senses."

36. Cf. Aristotle *De partibus animalium* III 14, 674 a 29: animals have several stomachs if their food is thorny and woody and not easy to concoct, or to compensate for a lack of teeth.

37. *De usu partium* VI. The Greek manuscripts are ambiguous about the tense of the verb; but Kühn's past tense is confirmed by the Arabic version, which has *qad waṣaftuhā fī kitāb āḫar* (Z 14, lines 12 and 13; Y 46ᵛ, line 4).

38. At this point, "ἀλλὰ πῶς, φασι ...," there begins a section where the Arabic translator worked with a text radically different from that of the surviving Greek manuscripts and the Latin translations; and it is clear beyond doubt that the Arabic version is right.

In the Western tradition, two passages appear in reverse order: ἀλλὰ πῶς, φασι (K 724.5, A 14.2)–ὅπως αἱ κατὰ προαίρεσιν (K 725.4, A 14.16) appears *after* αἱ κατα προαίρεσιν (K 723.6, A 13.14)–αἵματος μεστάς (K 724.5, A 14.2). Since the two passages are of almost equal length (the first has 126 words, the second 125), it is likely that the mistake occurred through a leaf of the text being removed and reinserted with verso preceeding recto. This hypothesis is confirmed by the double appearance in the Western tradition of the words "αἱ κατὰ προαίρεσιν": they were no doubt "turn over" words at the bottom of the recto side.

The proof that the Arabic version is right and the Western tradition wrong is twofold:

(a) The Western tradition has a text with two bad anacolutha (K 723.6; A 13.14, and K 725.4; A 14.2), which editors have tried to mend by positing lacunae.

(b) Only the Arabic version presents a coherent argument. Galen lists four problems at the beginning of Chapter 6 (A 12.17–25): (i) Why has Nature made two kinds of vessel to contain the same material? (ii) How will pneuma be conveyed to the whole body if the arteries contain blood? (iii) How will voluntary motions be carried out if pneuma is not so conveyed? (iv) How can we explain the regular motions (the pulse) of the arteries, if there is blood in them? According to the Arabic version, Galen deals with these problems in order: in the Western tradition they are treated in a jumbled and confused way.

For the important difference this restoration of the text makes to the logic of Galen's experiment, see note 43. We have published a note on this passage in *Classical Review* NS XXII (1972) 164–67.

39. According to Galen's own physiology, some pneuma passes from the lung to the heart, and then goes with the blood from the left ventricle of the heart into the arteries. Cf. *De usu partium* VII 8 (K III 542): "The outer air drawn in by the rough arteries receives its first elaboration in the flesh of the lungs, its second thereafter in the heart and the arteries, particularly those of the retiform plexus, and a final one in the ventricles of the encephalon, where its transformation into psychic pneuma is complete." His difference with Erasistratus appears to be a quantitative one, but one would hardly guess it from his manner of expression here.

40. The reading of the Greek manuscripts, "σκοπούμενοι καὶ πάντες ὁμοῦ ζητοῦντές τε καὶ πράττοντες," is plainly wrong: a finite verb is required to complete the clause beginning "ὅσοι." The Arabic version has:

Z 14, line 19 to 15, line 2; Y 46^b, lines 11–14

على أنه قد كان يبغي لهم أن يبحثوا عمه مفردًا على حدته كما علنا نحن وجميع مَن يسلك ما يبحث عنه من الاشياء الطريق
المستقيم ولا يبحث عن جميع الاسياء معًا ويخلط بعص ذلك بعض

"Although it was incumbent upon them that they should investigate it alone and by itself, as we ourselves have done, and all those who follow in their investigations the right way [that is, the correct method], and do not investigate everything together and mix up one part of it with another."

ταράττοντες, for the MSS reading πράττοντες, is a suggestion offered by P. DeLacy; it seems plainly right, and I adopt it gratefully.

41. *De usu respirationis* 2.

42. For the text, see note 38.

43. According to Galen's account of Erasistratean theory, the act of cutting away the tissues to expose a great artery would be enough to cause the

evacuation of the pneuma and the filling of the artery with blood. This was explained by Galen in the last paragraph of Chapter 4. It follows that the mere act of ligaturing an artery in two places, cutting the middle section and showing it to contain blood, has in itself no force whatever against the Erasistratean position. It was a great weakness of the text preserved in the Western tradition that this appeared to be the only point that Galen was making.

With the text restored according to the Arabic version (note 38), we can see that the point is that the arteries, being full of blood, nevertheless continue to pulsate regularly. This is effective against the Erasistrateans, who maintained that the pulse was inexplicable if the arteries contained blood.

44. Something was omitted from the Greek in the Western tradition when the order of the pages was confused. In the Greek manuscripts the end of the sentence "$\alpha\ddot{\iota}\mu\alpha\tau\sigma\varsigma\ \mu\epsilon\sigma\tau\acute{\alpha}\varsigma$" is followed at once by the beginning of a new one, "$\dot{\alpha}\lambda\lambda\grave{\alpha}\ \pi\hat{\omega}\varsigma,\ \phi\alpha\sigma\iota\ \ldots$." Presumably the missing words were omitted because they had no syntactical role. I have filled in the gap according to the Arabic version:

Z 15, lines 17–18; Y 47ᵃ, lines 13–15

فاذا اقرّوا بأن العروق الضوارب ١المكسوفة محوى الدم بيّنـا لهم بعـد ذلك أنها تتحـرّك بلا تعـذّر وأن البصر يدلّ على ذلك فضلاً عن حسّ اللمـس

١المكسفة

"So when they agree that the exposed arteries contain blood we demonstrate to them, after that, that they move without impediment and that sight shows that, to say nothing of [or as well as] the sense of touch."

45. The two premises ($\lambda\acute{\eta}\mu\mu\alpha\tau\alpha$) are: A. The arteries contain blood; B. The arteries are expanded by being filled from the heart. The Erasistrateans accept A only in the pathological condition. The conditional is: if A and B, then C—the order of their movements will be destroyed. The consequent is C. Kalbfleisch's emendation in line 15, "$\lambda\acute{\eta}\gamma\sigma\nu\tau\sigma\varsigma$" for "$\lambda\acute{\eta}\mu\mu\alpha$-$\tau\sigma\varsigma$," must be right.

46. A type 2 undemonstrated argument (see Introduction III):
   If the first, then the second.
   Not the second.
   Therefore not the first.

47. Pyrrho of Elis (ca. 360–270 B.C.), generally regarded as the founder of scepticism. His followers are commonly called "boorish": cf. K XIV 628.

48. For the relation between Erasistratus and the Peripatetics, see Introduction, I f, and De nat. fac. II 4.

49. The Arabic translator takes $\tau\acute{\iota}\ \pi\lambda\acute{\epsilon}\sigma\nu\ \ddot{\alpha}\nu\ \pi\epsilon\rho\alpha\acute{\iota}\nu\sigma\iota\tau\sigma$ to mean "what benefit is achieved." This leaves the comparative genitive "$\tau\sigma\hat{\nu}\ \sigma\dot{\nu}\chi\grave{\iota}\ \kappa\alpha\grave{\iota}$ $\alpha\ddot{\iota}\mu\alpha$" $\kappa\tau\lambda$. in line 9 (depending on $\pi\lambda\acute{\epsilon}\sigma\nu$, as I take it), without any

obvious construction. The translator takes it in apposition to τοῦ λόγου, making the whole passage incoherent.

50. This is another place where the Arabic version is from a better text than the Western tradition.

The Greek manuscript tradition presents the following argument:

If (A) the arteries, being full of blood, pulsate regularly, etc.,

then (B) either: (a) they pulsate through being filled with pneuma or (b) through some other cause.

But the first (A).

Therefore the second (B).

But this is nonsense, since B is a truism.

Western editors have attempted to mend matters by inserting a negative in the second premise:

If A, then B (either a or b).

But *not* the first (a).

Therefore the second (b).

But this is a mistake. The logical pattern requires the *assertion* of the first clause (A) of the conditional.

The Arabic version has it right: in the text of B, the translator clearly read not "ἤ ... ἤ (either ... or)," but "οὐ ... ἀλλά." B now reads, "They pulsate *not* through being filled with pneuma but through some other cause," and the logical pattern is correct:

If A, then B.

But A.

Therefore B.

Here is the Arabic text, beginning immediately after the passage quoted in the last note:

Z 18, line 15–19, line 1; Y 49ʳ, 2–6

وإن احببتُ ايضًا ادكـرْتُـك بعقب ذلكِ ما ملْتُـهُ ما تـقـدّم فسألتُـك ١مايةُ هذه المسئلة إن كانت العروق الضوارب مملوّة دمًا وحركاتها لأزِمة لِلنظام ولم يكن ذلك مما يمنع الحركات التي يحدث عنها أن تحدث على ما كانت عليه فليس السبب في بٰضها أنها تمتلى من الروح الذى في القلب لاكن عِلّه احرى والاوّل حـنّ والثاني ٢ادا حـنّ

٢ادں   ملئه [٢]١

"And if I wished I might also remind you [singular], following upon that, of what I said before, and I would propose to you again the problem: If the arteries are filled with blood and their movements remain orderly and there is nothing preventing the movements that arise from them from occurring as they did before; then the cause of their pulse is not that they are filled with the pneuma that [was] in the heart, but some other cause; and the first is true, so the second is true."

51. See *De usu pulsuum* 5.

52. For example, *De placitis Hippocratis et Platonis* VI 7 (K V 560 ff.).

53. This is explained further in *De usu pulsuum*.

54. See Introduction 1 c and e. For Diocles, see W. Jaeger's monograph.

55. For Galen's use of the word "faculty" ($\delta\acute{\nu}\nu\alpha\mu\iota\varsigma$—often also translated "power"), see especially *De nat. fac.* I 2 and 4. The faculty is relative to an activity ($\dot{\epsilon}\nu\acute{\epsilon}\rho\gamma\epsilon\iota\alpha$). We first identify an activity, and then posit the faculty as its cause. "And so long as we are ignorant of the substance of the activating cause, we call it a faculty, saying that in the veins there is a bloodmaking faculty, in the stomach a peptic faculty, in the heart a pulsating faculty, and so on" (K II 9).

See also Introduction IV, on "Use and Activity."

56. Especially *De placitis Hippocratis et Platonis* VI and *De usu pulsuum.*

57. See *De usu pulsuum* 5, §4.

58. Galen makes the same point against the Erasistrateans, on the subject of the heart (not the arteries), in *De placitis Hippocratis et Platonis* VI (K V 549).

59. In the Arabic version there is no equivalent for the Greek words $\dot{\alpha}\tau\rho\epsilon$-$\mu\epsilon\acute{\iota}\eta$ $o\dot{\upsilon}$ $\kappa\iota\nu\epsilon\hat{\iota}\sigma\theta\alpha\iota$: instead we have "by which the pulse occurs in the arteries." Moreover, the Arabic has no "$\mu\grave{\epsilon}\nu$ ... $\delta\acute{\epsilon}$." The Greek of the manuscripts does not make sense, and I have substituted what the Arabic translator might have had before him.

Z 20, lines 18–19; Y 50^a, lines 8–9

معنى البيّن أن ذلك لـمّا كان لا يوجد أن العضو التي يكون بها سض العروق 'الصوارب تبعث اليها من القلب في طبقاتها
فتجميع ما قاله ارسسطراطس في حركات العروق الضوارب كذباً .

'الصوارب

"Since it is clear, that not being the case, that the power by which occurs the pulse of the arteries is transmitted to them from the heart through their coats [or walls], then everything that Erasistratus said about the motions of the arteries is false."

The Arabic is as given; the English attempts to render what was probably the meaning of Hunain's Syriac. On the experiment itself, see Introduction III. There is a description of it in *De anatomicis administrationibus* VII 16 (K II 646–49). See also the article by M. Peter Amacher.

60. From here to the end the Greek manuscripts are corrupt. The Arabic translation again seems to preserve a better tradition and I have tried to restore the Greek according to it. Here is the Arabic text in full:

Z 21, line 16–22, line 6, plus colophon on three lines; Y 50^b, lines 9–17, plus colophon of two lines

الا اني اعلم انك 'إن لم تضع ما قاله ارسسطراطس وسعته وضعًا 'كما من عاده ارسسطراطس أن يعول 'صـح عندك يعيّنًا أن
ما قصدنا له قد تبيّن وإن أنت عسكّتَ بما قالوه محتّه للفله وجبَ صرورةً ألا ينفعك شيءً 'ما 'قلناه ولا غره من الراهن إلا أن
ارسسطراطس مع ساير ما هذى به لم يكذبْ على ما °يظهر في التسريح
وامّا شيعته فكتبوا اصنافا كثيرة من التسريح يتصمّمون فيها أن يبيّنوا أن العروق الضوارب حاليـة من الدم وليس يُوجد واحـد

منها حــقّا وذلك اىه لــوْ كان فيها سىْ واحد ٬حــقّا لم يكى ارسسطٰراطس ليدع ذِكْـرَهُ ومعه مِـس القـوّة اكر كثيراً مما مع [هؤلاء
الذيں نجدهم يكدبوں على التسريح بمحه واهدام الا أں] ارسطراطـس لم يبلغ مِـس قحته هذا المقدار كلّـه حتى يكتب ما ٨لا عكنه
أں يبيّـه

		٣عدك صحّ	٢كمــا	١إں
	٨لا	٦حـق	٥يطهر	٤قلا

Colophon Y

تـمّ القٰول فى أں الـدم
محتبس فى العـرٰوں الضٰوارٰب
بالطبع بمل حـسـيں
والحٰمد للّٰه ربّ العلٰمـں

Colophon Z

تـمّ كتـاب حاليـٰوس
فى أں الدم محتبٰس فى العـرٰوى
الضٰوارٰب بالطبـع
وللّٰه الحٰمـد

"Now I know that if you have not posited what Erasistratus and his school have said, *as it was the custom of Erasistratus to say,* then you must certainly have realized for a fact that what we intended has already been proved; but if you have clung to what they say, from a desire of victory, necessarily nothing of what we have said will profit you, nor any other proof; but Erasistratus, with all his other follies, did not tell lies about what is manifest in anatomy.

"As for his followers they have written many kinds of anatomies in which they claim to prove that the arteries are empty of blood; and not one of them is found to be true; for if any one thing in them were true, Erasistratus would certainly not have omitted to mention it; and he was possessed of much greater power [of intellect] than they, whom we find telling lies about anatomy with impudence and forwardness. Yet Erasistratus did not achieve that full measure of impudence which would permit him to write down what he could not demonstrate [*probably* give ocular demonstrations of]."

Z
"[Here] ends the book of Galen
concerning that blood is contained in
the arteries naturally.
And to God the Praise."

Y
"[Here] ends the discourse concerning that blood
is contained in the arteries

naturally. The translation of Ḥunain.
And Praise be to God, the Lord of the Worlds."

[*Note: This phrase is certainly misplaced. The reading of "Erasistratus" for "Aristoteles" would easily occur, in Arabic, to a scribe who had already copied the first many times.]

The expression θέσιν διαφυλάττειν is used by Aristotle (N.E. I 5, 1096 a 2; De caelo III 7, 306 a 12) to mean "to maintain a thoroughly paradoxical thesis just to prolong the argument." Kalbfleisch's conjecture that the negative μή should be moved from φυλάττοντι in A 21.1 to φυλάττοι[το] in A 20.25 is confirmed by the Arabic.

61. The Greek manuscripts make nonsense of this sentence. The Arabic version (quoted in note 60) suggests that several words have dropped out of them.

62. The Arabic translation (see note 60 above) specifies that the subject is the followers of Erasistratus, and attaches the epithet "many" to the kinds of Anatomies. So perhaps the Greek should read πολυτρόπους τινὰς ἀνατομὰς αἷς, leaving the subject of γεγράφασι to be understood (this is a suggestion made by P. DeLacy).

63. The neuter οὐδὲν ... ἀληθές seems to be better than the masculine, to supply a subject for the next sentence. One Greek manuscript has the neuter ἀληθές, and the Arabic confirms this reading.

64. The Greek manuscripts lack any noun with the adjective μείζονα. The Arabic has "he was possessed of greater power," which suggests that the Greek manuscript reading "ἐξ·ν" ("ἐξ ὧν" in V) conceals an accusative noun: perhaps ἐξουσίαν.

65. The Greek manuscripts and the Arabic translation both say that Erasistratus would not have been so shameless as to write what it was impossible to observe. But he did, and Galen knew well that he did. So I have adopted a suggestion made by P. DeLacy.

ON THE USE OF THE PULSE

1. The beginning of the treatise in the Arabic manuscript is as follows:

بسم الله الرّحْمْن الرّحِيم

مقاله حاليوس في منفعه النص

احراج ابی زید حنین بن اسحق

إنه قد يجب علينا أن نظر ما منفعه النبض هل هي منفعه التنفّس بعينها على ما راى الفلاسفة والاطبّاء كلّهم في اكثر الامر
او هي غيرها

"In the name of God, the Compassionate, the Merciful:
The treatise of Galen on the Use of the Pulse,
The _ikrāj_* of Abu Zaid Ḥunain ibn Isḥāq

"Now it behoves us to consider what is the use of the pulse. Is it exactly the same as the use of breathing, as virtually all philosophers and physicians have thought, or is it something else?"

*Note: The word _ikrāj_ is not usual in the sense of "translation," which would normally be _naql_, as in the colophon of this manuscript, or _tarjama_, as in the title of manuscript A.S. 3631[8].

2. The Greek "παρὰ ταύτην" might mean either "in addition to this" or "instead of this."

3. Voluntary motion, according to Galen's theory, is effected by the psychic pneuma; and it is one of the uses of breathing to keep up the supply of this pneuma. However, he is presenting a dialectical argument here, because voluntary motion and feelings are effected by the nerves in his theory, and the pulse has no direct connection with them.

4. "Connected affection" (συμπάθεια) is not a concept much used by Galen. It is more prominent in Stoicism: See (e.g.) Sambursky, _Physics of the Stoics_, p. 41.

5. That is, if the pulse, like breathing, conveys something essential to life.

6. See Introduction, II.

7. Once the diagnostic value of the pulse had become recognized, doctors claimed to notice many distinctions in the pulse, in addition to its frequency. For example, see Archigenes' list of ten categories, reconstructed by Wellmann (_Pneum._ pp. 70–71). Galen's full analysis is given in his _De pulsuum differentiis_ (K VIII). In the present list of three, "quickness" is distinguished from frequency by the pause between expansion and contraction mentioned below (K 163); the pulse is quick if the time between expansion and contraction is short; it is frequent if the time between two expansions is short.

8. The Greek manuscripts omit πρὸς before τὸν πρὸ τῆς τροφῆς, and Kühn adopted their text. The insertion of πρός, necessitated by the

sense, is noted as a correction in both of the older manuscripts and is now confirmed by the Arabic translation:

وقولنا في هدا الموضع في السص بعد تناول الطعام أنه متفاوب ليس هو ادا قسّاه ما كان عليه مل تناول الطعام وذلك أنه أسـدّ نواترًا منه لاكى بالعياس إلى التنفّس

"And what we say here about the pulse after taking food, that it is spaced out,* does not mean, when we compare it with what it was before taking food, for it is more frequent than that, but by comparison with breathing."

*Note: for this meaning of the sixth form of the verb *fāta*, see Hava.

9. That is, it does harm of a greater order.

10. See *De usu partium* VIII 3, with May's note 14 on p. 390, listing relevant passages from Hippocrates. Galen gives more credit for precision on the subject to the Hippocratic writings than they necessarily deserve. However, it is clear that *De natura pueri* 12 (VII 486–89 L) states that in-breathing is necessary for cooling; and *De alimento* 28–30 (IX 108–09 L) says that breathing is for nourishment. See also Introduction, I c.

11. The "breathing" of the brain is described in *De usu partium* VIII 6 (K III 650), where Galen says Hippocrates agreed (see *De morbo sacro* 7). See also *De usu respirationis* 5.

12. Perhaps *De placitis Hippocratis et Platonis* II 8 (K V 279ff.).

13. The Greek manuscripts are nonsensical here. The Arabic translation is as follows:

ملعّا رايتّه عند ذلك يَعْدُو مـدّه من الزمان طوبله سم يصسر ناحره إلى أن لا يعدر يعْدو رايبُ أن أحب ايضًا عن السبب الدى له صار عكنه أن يعْدو زمانًا طويلاً وذلك اى رايبُ أنه عجب ألاّ عكث يَعْدُو زمانًا طويلاً لاكى يسترحى على المكان عند ما ينفس منه الروح النعساني

"So when I saw him on that occasion running a long interval of time, then finally becoming unable to run, I decided to seek out also the cause by which it was possible for him to run a long time; because I [had] thought he could necessarily not go on running for a long time, but that he would slump down at once as soon as the psychic pneuma was dissipated from him."

This makes reasonably good sense, and I have emended the Greek text accordingly.

To some extent, the error in the Greek manuscripts can be explained. We might suppose that the text was once written thus:

1   ἐπεὶ δὲ μέχρι μὲν πολλοῦ

2 καλῶς ἔτρεχε, μέχρι παντὸς δ' οὐκ ἠδύνατο,

3 ζητεῖν ἐδόκει τὴν αἰτίαν δι' ἥνπερ μέχρι πολλοῦ

4 καλῶς ἔτρεχε, χρῆναι γὰρ οὐδὲ μέχρι

5 πολλοῦ διαρκεῖν

The lines were then jumbled up, so that line 2 followed a confusion of lines 3 and 4. The words "πάλιν αὐτό," which appear in the Manuscript

271

and the Aldine but seem to have no equivalent in the Arabic version, are perhaps some corrector's comment on the repetition, which has vanished from the manuscripts, of "μέχρι πολλοῦ καλῶς ἔτρεχε."

Kühn prints the following text: ἐπεὶ δὲ μέχρι μὲν πολλοῦ καλῶς ἔτρεχε, μέχρι παντὸς δὲ οὐκ ἠδύνατο, ζητεῖν ἐδόκει χρῆναι, διότι μέχρι μὲν πολλοῦ ἔτρεχε, μέχρι παντὸς δὲ οὐκ ἠδύνατο, καὶ πάλιν αὐτὸ μέχρι πολλοῦ οὐ διαρκεῖν ... This corresponds with Linacre's Latin version. The Arabic version is to be preferred, since the puzzle is not why the animal could run for a while but not indefinitely, but rather why it could go on running even for a while. The manuscript "οὐδὲ," which has disappeared from the Aldine and Kühn's text, must be preserved. (I am grateful to Mr. G. Pope for suggestions about this passage.)

14. See *De placitis Hippocratis et Platonis* VII 3 (K V 607ff.) and *De usu partium* IX 4, with May's notes.

15. "Concoction" (πέψις) is Aristotle's word for the physiological processes of transforming food and other materials into substances useful for life. See *De generatione animalium*, *passim*, and A. L. Peck's introduction, §§61ff. The agent is the innate heat.

16. The work of the netlike plexus in providing nourishment out of the vaporous blood in the arteries for the psychic pneuma is different from the process mentioned above (note 11) by which the psychic pneuma in the brain is nourished directly by breathing through the nostrils into the brain. I have not found any passage in which Galen discusses the relation between these two processes. In the present paragraph he seems to have forgotten about the former one, as also in the chapter of *De placitis Hippocratis et Platonis* referred to in note 12.

17. The same quotation in *De usu respirationis* 5: see note 69, on p. 257.

18. That is, the body of the cupping glass. The Greek could mean the body of the patient, but this seems unlikely.

19. The manuscripts have "οἷον προαναπνοή," which must mean "as it were a preliminary stage of breathing." But this seems unlikely to be right. I think all Galen means is that the pulse is to the parts whose warmth is preserved by it as breathing is to the heart. The noun "προαναπνοή" occurs only here, according to the lexicon (LSJ); the verb "προαναπνέω" occurs, but only in the sense "to draw breath before ...." The Arabic version is:

56^b line 6

على طريق التنفّس

"according to the manner of breathing" or "something like breathing." This is perhaps not too remote from the Greek emended in the simplest possible way: οἷον πρὸ ἀναπνοῆς, "as it were, in the place of breathing."

It is difficult to be sure what sense the Arabic had for Estefan, but the choice of preposition and the *status constructus* make it hardly credible that he meant "on the way to breathing."

20. After "those who fight in single combat" (μονομάχους) the manuscripts have "monarchs" (μονάρχους) and this is printed in Kühn's edition. I guess that at some point in the tradition a mistake was made in writing "μονομάχους," it was later corrected and by accident both words were then copied. Galen had plenty of experience with wounded gladiators in Pergamum, and with wounded soldiers and huntsmen; but it is doubtful if wounded monarchs "often" crossed his path. There is no trace of them in the Arabic version. See Nutton, "Chronology."

21. See note 15 above. Again, Galen says nothing about the pneuma drawn in directly by the brain in respiration; he appears to be thinking here, when he says respiration "concocts" the psychic pneuma, of the work done on the pneuma in the lungs and heart, before it is distributed to the arteries.

22. Chapter 3.

23. Note that although Galen knew of the valves, and therefore knew that the direction of motion of whatever is in the arteries must be from the heart (at least predominantly), tradition was so strong that he did not think the increased volume of the arteries in diastole could be filled entirely from the heart. He retained the theory that the arteries draw air into their extremities through pores in the skin. See Introduction, II. For the comparison between the innate heat and a fire, and between blood and fuel, see *De usu respirationis* 3, with note 34.

24. See Wellmann, *Pneumatische Schule*, pp. 19–22.

25. The reading of the Greek manuscripts makes no sense, and the emendation of κἂν ... to κατ᾽ ... is confirmed by the Arabic version:

58ᵃ lines 1 and 2

ليس في شيء من ساير الاعضاء سوىَ اقاصى طرف المنحرَيُـنِ العضر وفيَيُـنِ

"not in any other part of the body except the two cartilaginous tips of the nostrils."

26. The omission of μή by the Greek manuscripts is clearly a mistake. The Arabic version has it right:

58ᵃ lines 12 to 16

هلـوْ كان يكنهم أن يبيّنـوا أن هذه الحاري انعسها تنعص عنـد الاستنشاى لكانوا سير بحـوں سينا من هذا المثـال الذى ذكروه
هاد كانوا لا يعـدرون على أن يبيّنـوا ذلك فمع أنهم لم يربحـوا مِـن ذكرِهِ سينا قـد جلبوا به على انفـسهم مِـن موضع حجّـة وذلك
انّـا نقول لهم

"Now if it were possible for them to show that those channels themselves contract during inbreathing, then they would gain something from this comparison they have adduced. Since, however, they were not able to prove that, then, together with their not profiting by adducing it, they have produced an argument which, in one point, can be turned against them; for we shall say to them ...."

27. *De placitis Hippocratis et Platonis* VI 3 and 7.

28. Erasistratus believed that the heart is responsible for the pulse, but only in the sense that the heart propels the pneuma through the arteries and this causes the pulse. See also *An in arteriis* 8, and Introduction I f.

29. See *De usu partium* VI 15 for the further description of the faculties of the heart.

30. Galen seems to be imagining that he is lecturing, and points to the skin. For the theory of arteries breathing through pores in the skin, see Introduction, I a and II. For the so-called "vents," see below, note 34.

31. The Greek manuscripts are obviously corrupt at this point. Galen is considering *all* the openings in the arteries through which matter can pass. He has mentioned some that are not obvious—the "pores" in their coats—and now mentions others that are obvious, namely, their origins. Each artery has its origin either in the heart or in a larger artery. If the Arabic version is correct, he expresses this point by saying that the inner coats of the arteries are all joined ultimately to the heart.

    I cannot make any sense of the expression in the Greek manuscripts μᾶλλον δὲ εὐρυχωρίας ἁπάσας ("or rather, [by] all wide spaces"). So I suggest, tentatively, emending the last two words to κατὰ τοὺς ἔνδον χίτωνας ἅπαντας, following the Arabic:

    59ᵃ lines 5 to 7

    وبالقلب محـار عظيمه اعـي الطعمه كلّها التي في 'داحلها وهي ايضًا تتصل بالعروق عير الضوارب لاكنها ليس تتصل بها بمحـار في هدا المقدار من العظم

    'داحلهـا

    " ... and to the heart by great channels, or rather [*lit.* I mean] by the whole of the tunic that is within them; and they [the arteries] are joined also to the veins, but they are not joined to them by channels of this degree of magnitude."

    The intrusive words in the previous line might then be explained as being derived from a marginal gloss κατ᾽ αὐτὰς τὰς ἀρτηρίας ("that is, by the arteries themselves").

32. Galen's physiology included the propositions that blood comes from the heart into the arteries, that blood enters the heart from the veins, both of these motions being controlled by valves, and that the venous system is connected with the arterial system by invisible "anastomoses." But the possibility that blood circulates through the body apparently did not occur to him.

    Harvey says that Galen established, in connection with the human subject, that "even if a very small artery is divided, the whole mass of the blood, within the space of half an hour or less, will be withdrawn from the veins as well as the arteries throughout the body" (*De motu cordis* 9, tr. Franklin). Galen says here that he wounds "many of the large arteries"; so perhaps Harvey is thinking of another passage that I have not found, or is confusing this passage with something like *An in arteriis* 4 (K IV 712).

33. See *De usu respirationis* 5 and n. 69.

34. This is an interesting sentence. In *De usu partium* VI 10 (K III 447), the coats of arteries are described as "thick, dense and altogether impenetrable" (παχέσι καὶ πυκνοῖς καὶ πάντη στεγανοῖς), precisely in order to prevent pneuma from escaping prematurely. I have not found any other description of these supposed openings in the coats. But Galen's theory does in fact call for the possibility of matter passing through the coats, if the arteries are to serve their nutritional purpose. In *De nat. fac.* II 6–7, in a polemic against Erasistratus on the subject of attraction (ὁλκή), Galen discusses the problem of how a nerve gets nutriment. Erasistratus held that it gets it from adjacent vessels, the nutriment being attracted "through the sides of the vessels" (κατὰ τὰ πλάγια). Galen says he accepts this part of Erasistratus' theory: the nerve can take nutriment through its sides from the adjacent vein.

In *De usu partium* IV 15 (K III 318–19), he refers to this discussion but gives it a more general reference: "If I was right when I demonstrated in my book *On the natural faculties* that every part receiving nutriment attracts it from the adjacent vessels, then it is reasonable that the thinner nutriment is attracted from the arteries and the thicker from the veins. For the coat [of the arteries] is denser than that [of the veins] and the blood contained in them is thinner and more spirituous" (May, *Usefulness*, p. 233). That is why the spleen, which needs thin nutriment, has many arteries in its neighborhood.

Evidently Galen's doctrine requires that at suitable points the arteries have "vents" (ὀπαί) in them, through which nutriment is drawn by the neighboring parts.

35. More than once Galen compliments Erasistratus for his work on the heart valves (*De placitis Hippocratis et Platonis* I 10; K V 206; and VI 6; K V 548). The existence and function of the valves was first discovered about the time of Erasistratus, if not by Erasistratus himself.

36. The Greek manuscript tradition, followed by Kühn, has collected a redundant full stop and a conjunction. The Arabic version is correct:

60ᵃ lines 1 and 2

فلستُ أشكّ أنه يَرِدُهُ لا محالة سىءٌ عند الامر الغليظ العنيف ينزل بالحيوان

"So I do not doubt that something unquestionably comes to it, when some [*lit.* the] violent and distressing state afflicts the animal."

37. *De usu partium* VI 16.

38. The vague generalization, borrowed from the Hippocratic corpus, that "the whole body breathes and flows together" leads Galen into some very loose thinking.

39. *An in arteriis*.

275

40. If the pulsation of the arteries were due to pneuma being forced through blood along the arteries by the heart, or to the movement of blood itself from the heart, the motion should take a measurable time as it passes along the vessels. But that is not observed to be the case.

41. In *De usu partium* VII 20 (K III 594), Galen refers to his *De causis respirationis* for a full demonstration of the thorax and its motions. The work printed below under this title is probably a résumé of a longer book.

42. Cf. *De placitis Hippocratis et Platonis* II 4–5.

43. The Prado manuscript appears to have the words χαλεπώτερον δή τι τὸ τῆς εὑρέσεως (which make no sense as they stand) erased; they are faint but legible, and in the same hand as the original. The Cambridge manuscript had a gap, in which these same words have been written, in a different hand from the original. I am unable to solve this problem satisfactorily, but I have followed the Latin of Linacre in the supposition that a full stop must be inserted somewhere.

This is confirmed by the Arabic:

61ᵃ line 7 to 61ᵇ line 4

لاكن لــمّا كان الفاعل للنبض العـوّة الحيوانية التي مدأها من القلب والفاعل ١للتنفّس على ما بيّنـا القوّة النفسانية التي مدأها من الدماع فليس نقدر أن تستخرج مما فيـلَ في ٢التنفّس سيئًا يصلح لهـذا البحـث الذي نحن بسبيله وما يزيد في ٣معونة ادراك هذا الامر أنـا ليس نجد العروق الضوارب بعد الموت كما حد العروق غير الضوارب مطبية اجراءها بعضها على بعض, وذلك أن العروق غير الضوارب اذا خَـلَتْ من الدم تجتمع اجزاؤها بعضها إلى بعض, فيبطى ما علا من طـقاتها على ما بحته حتى يلزمه وامّا ٤العروق الضوارب فانّـا نجدها تلبث دايمّـا واجزاؤها مفارق بعضها لبعضٍ, سبب احدى طبعتيها وهي الصلبة ٥مهمـا على ان هومًّا قالوا ان ذلك إنـما يعرض لها بعد الموت لانها تجمد من البرد لا لانها كذلك في طبيعتها وقوم اخرون لـمّا الصوها في ماءٍ حارٍ وراوّاها قد لَيسَتْ بعد ذلك ايضًا اجزاؤها مفارق بعضها ٦من بعضٍ, صحّ عندهم أنها قبل الموت كانت كذلك

| | | ٢العبس | ١للبس |
| ٤العروق غير الضوارب | ٥مها | ٦من بعص | ٣معونة صعوبة |

"But, since the active agent in respect of the pulse is the animal faculty, the origin of which is from the heart, and that of breathing is, as we have proved, the psychic faculty of which the origin is from the brain, we cannot infer from what is said about breathing anything appropriate to this investigation in which we are now engaged; but what increases the help* of comprehending this matter is that we do not find the arteries after death in the same state as the veins, their parts superimposed the one upon the other. For in the case of the veins, when emptied of blood, their parts come together the one to the other; so that their walls which were above are applied to those below so as to cleave to them; while, as for the arteries, we find them remaining as they were, their parts separated the one from the other, because of one of their two coats, and that is the hard one.

"Although there are some who say that that only happens to it after death, because [then] it hardens on account of the cold, and not because it is so by its nature, others, when they have cast them into hot water and see that their parts remain then also separate the one from the other, are assured that they were so before death."

*Note: the text clearly says "help"; but, as I have indicated in the apparatus, this could be a miscopying of a word meaning "difficulty." [J.S.W.]

44. That is, that the artery is uncollapsed and rigid.

45. Galen acknowledges that one can blow the breath out forcibly; but this is different from merely breathing out. See the next chapter, and *De usu respirationis* 2.

46. Presumably Galen has in mind *De nat. fac.* III 6 (K II 160), in which it is argued that "in everything" (*sic*) there is a power of attraction and a power of repulsion.

47. *De difficultate respirationis* I 7 (K VII 769).

48. See above, Chapter 1, with n. 7.

49. The manuscripts have "ἐν τοῖς κάμνουσι κοιμωμένοις" ("in those who are ill when asleep"). The two participles are unlikely to be both right, and I suspect that one is a correction of the other. The Arabic translation has no mention of those who are ill.

50. I have not been able to guess what this is.

51. I have failed to track down this reference.

52. "We use the word 'habitus' (ἕξις) in all cases of that which is durable and indestructible" (*De bono habitu*, K IV 750). Thus ἕξις is generally distinguished from διάθεσις, which denotes a more temporary disposition. The word was used by Aristotle (e.g. *N.E.* II 5) in a threefold classification of the properties of psyche: emotions, faculties, and dispositions (πάθη, δυνάμεις, ἕξεις). The Stoics created a more technical sense for it: it was that which gave identity to a non-living subject, in the way that its nature (φύσις) did for a plant, and its psyche did for an animal. There is perhaps a reminiscence of the Stoic doctrine in the mention of τόνος ("spring," "tension") below. However, the concept of ἕξις plays no very great role in Galen's theory.

ON THE CAUSES OF
BREATHING

1. That is, one's hypothesis about how breathing works.
2. "τὸ ποιοῦν" is often the *causa efficiens* in the technical sense. Here it is used in an extended sense as equivalent to αἴτιον—which itself (as is well known to students of Aristotle) means something more like "explanatory factor" than "cause" in the modern sense.
3. This refers to the traditional distinction between voluntary and involuntary motions, for which see Aristotle, *De motu animalium* 11.
4. See *De usu respirationis*, Chapter 5.
5. See Introduction, II.
6. One of Galen's achievements was to attain greater clarity on the distinctions between nerve (νεῦρον), ligament (σύνδεσμος), and tendon (τένων). There was still some confusion remaining, however, with regard to the tendon of insertion of a muscle, which he thought of as composed of both nerve and ligament (see May, *Usefulness*, p. 22, and *De usu partium* XII 3). When he calls the diaphragm "νευρῶδές," he means that it is of the same character as the tendons.
7. For the identification of these muscles, see our Introduction to *De caus. resp.*, above.
8. The phrase "τῶν κατὰ τὸν τράχηλον" ("those of the neck") in Kühn's text appears to be a mistake (see our Introduction to *De caus. resp.*, above.), and should be omitted. In the previous sentence, the manuscripts except A have the plural "τραχήλων" in mistake for the singular. It may be that at some time a correction had been written in the margin, and a form of it later incorporated into the text here.
9. See note 6.

BIBLIOGRAPHY

Note: The short title used for reference to the work is in parentheses.

Collections and Reference Works

Diels, H. *Doxographi Graeci*. Berlin, 1879; repr. Berlin: De Gruyter, 1958. (DG)

———, and Kranz, W. *Die Fragmente der Vorsokratiker*. 6. verbesserte Auflage. Berlin: Grunewald, 1951–1952. (DK)

Liddell, H. G., and Scott, R. *A Greek English Lexicon*. Revised and augmented throughout by Sir H. S. Jones. Oxford: Clarendon Press, 1968. (LSJ)

Wellmann, W. *Fragmentsammlung der griechischen Aerzte I: Die Fragmente der Sikelischen Aerzte*. Berlin: Weidmann, 1901. (Sikel)

Classical Texts

Aëtius. *Placita. See* H. Diels, *Doxographi Graeci*.

Anonymus Londinensis. *Medical Writings*. Edited by W.H.S. Jones. Cambridge: Cambridge University Press, 1947: repr. Amsterdam: Hakkert, 1968.

Aristophanes. *The Clouds*. Edited by K. J. Dover. Oxford: Clarendon Press, 1968.

Aristotle. *De anima*. Edited with introduction and commentary by Sir D. Ross. Oxford: Clarendon Press, 1961. (DA)

———. *De caelo*. Edited with an English translation by W.K.C. Guthrie. London: Heinemann, Loeb Classical Library, 1939. (DC)

———. *De generatione animalium*. Edited with an English translation by A. L. Peck. London: Heinemann, Loeb Classical Library, 1943. (GA)

———. *De generatione et corruptione*. Edited with an English translation by E. S. Forster. London: Heinemann, Loeb Classical Library, 1955. (GC)

———. *De motu animalium*. Edited with an English translation by E. S. Forster. London: Heinemann, Loeb Classical Library, 1937.

———. *De motu animalium*. Edited with translation, commentary, and interpretive essays by Martha Craven Nussbaum. Princeton: Princeton University Press, 1978. (MA)

———. *De partibus animalium*. Edited with an English translation by A. L. Peck. London: Heinemann, Loeb Classical Library, 1937. (PA)

———. *De respiratione. See Parva Naturalia*.

———. *Historia animalium*, books I–VI. Edited with an English translation by A. L. Peck. London: Heinemann, Loeb Classical Library, 1965–1970. (HA)

————. *Historia animalium*. Translated by D'Arcy Thompson in *The Works of Aristotle*, vol. IV. Oxford: Clarendon Press, 1910.

————. *Meteorologica*. Edited with an English translation by H.D.P. Lee. London: Heinemann, Loeb Classical Library, 1952. (Meteor)

————. *Parva Naturalia*. Edited by Sir David Ross. Oxford: Clarendon Press, 1955. (PN)

————. *Physics*. Edited by Sir David Ross. Oxford: Clarendon Press, 1950. (Ph)

Celsus. *De medicina*. Edited with English translation by W. G. Spencer. Cambridge, Mass: Harvard University Press, 1935–1938.

Diogenes Laertius. *Lives of Eminent Philosophers*. Edited with an English translation by R. D. Hicks. London: Heinemann, Loeb Classical Library, 1958–1959.

Galen. Complete text in *Medicorum Graecorum Opera quae Exstant*, vols. I–XX. Edited by Karl Gottlob Kühn. Leipzig, 1821–1833. Repr. with bibliography by K. Schubring in vol. I; Hildesheim: Olms, 1965. (K)

————. *Scripta minora*. Edited by G. Helmreich, J. Marquardt, and I. Müller. Leipzig: Teubner, 1884–1893. Repr. Amsterdam: Hakkert, 1967.

————. *An in arteriis natura sanguis contineatur*. Edited by F. Albrecht. Marburg: Chatti, 1911.

————. *De anatomicis administrationibus*, books I–IX⁵. Translated by C. Singer in *Galen on Anatomical Procedures*. Publications of the Wellcome Historical Medical Museum, n.s. no. 7. Oxford: Oxford University Press, 1956.

————. *De anatomicis administrationibus*, books IX⁵–XV. Translated by W.L.H. Duckworth, M. C. Lyons, and B. Towers, *Galen on Anatomical Procedures: The Later Books*. Cambridge: Cambridge University Press, 1962.

————. *De naturalibus facultatibus*. Translated by H. J. Brock, *Galen on the Natural Faculties*. London: Heinemann, Loeb Classical Library, 1916.

————. *De placitis Hippocratis et Platonis*. Edited by I. Mueller. Leipzig, 1874.

————. *De placitis Hippocratis et Platonis*. Edition, Translation, and Commentary by Phillip DeLacy. First Part, books I–V. Corpus Medicorum Graecorum V 4, 1, 2. Berlin: Akademie, 1978.

————. *De temperamentis*. Edited by G. Helmreich. Leipzig: Teubner, 1919.

————. *De usu partium*. Edited by G. Helmreich. Leipzig: Teubner, 1907. Repr. Amsterdam: Hakkert, 1968. Translated by Margaret Tallmadge May, *On the Usefulness of the Parts of the Body*. Ithaca: Cornell University Press, 1968.

————. *De usu respirationis*. Edited by R. Noll. Marburg, 1915.

————. *Institutio Logica*. Edited by C. Kalbfleisch. Leipzig: Teubner, 1896.

Hero of Alexandria. *Pneumatica*. Edited by W. Schmidt. Leipzig: Teubner, 1899.

Hippocrates. *Oeuvres complètes*. Edited by A. Littré. Paris: Baillière, 1839–1861. (L)

————. Select texts with an English translation by W.H.S. Jones and E. T. Withington. London: Heinemann, Loeb Classical Library, 1923–1931.

BIBLIOGRAPHY

Plato. *Opera omnia*. Edited by J. Burnet. Oxford: Oxford Classical Texts, n.d.
———. *Timaeus*. See F. M. Cornford, *Plato's Cosmology*.
Pliny. *Natural History*. Edited with an English translation by H. Rackham, W.H.S. Jones, and D. E. Eichholz. London: Heinemann, Loeb Classical Library, 1938–1962.
Praxagoras. *The Fragments of Praxagoras of Cos and his School*. Edited with an English translation by Fritz Steckerl. Leiden: Brill, 1958.
Sextus Empiricus. *Adversus Mathematicos*. Edited with an English translation by R. G. Bury. London: Heinemann, Loeb Classical Library, 1933–1949. (Math)
Strabo. *Geography*. Edited with an English translation by H. L. Jones. London: Heinemann, Loeb Classical Library, 1917–1959.
Theophrastus. *De igne*. Edited with an English translation by V. Coutant. Assen: Vangorcum, 1972.
———. *De sensibus*. See H. Diels, *Doxographi Graeci*, pp. 499–527.

Postclassical Works

Abel, K. "Die Lehre vom Blutkreislauf im Corpus Hippocraticum," *Hermes* 86 (1958), 192–219. Repr. in *Antike Medizin*, edited by H. Flashar (Darmstadt, 1971) with a "Retraktatio" dated 1969.
———. "Plato und die Medizin seiner Zeit." *Gesnerus* 14 (1957), 94–118.
Amacher, M. Peter. "Galen's Experiment on the Arterial Pulse and the Experiment Repeated." *Sudhoff's Archiv für Geschichte der Medizin* 48 (1964), 177–80.
Balme, D. M. *Aristotle's De partibus animalium I and De generatione animalium I*. Oxford: Clarendon Press, 1972.
Bardong, Kurt. "Beiträge zur Hippokrates- und Galenforschung." *Nachrichten der Akademie der Wissenschaften in Göttingen*, Phil.-Hist. Klasse, 1942, 7, pp. 577–640.
Birch, Thomas. *The History of the Royal Society of London*. London, 1756.
Bollack, Jean. *Empédocle*, vols. I–III. Paris: Éditions de Minuit, 1965–1969.
Booth, N. B. "Empedocles' Account of Breathing." *Journal of Hellenic Studies* 80 (1960), 10–15.
Cooper, Sir Astley. *Guy's Hospital Reports*. 1836, 1, pp. 457–60.
Cornford, F. M. *Plato's Cosmology*. London: Routledge and Kegan Paul, 1937.
Daremberg, C. V. *Histoire des Sciences Médicales*. Paris, 1870.
———. *Oeuvres anatomiques, physiologiques, et médicales de Galien*. Paris: Baillière, 1854–1856.
Darwin, Charles. *The Origin of Species*. 6th. ed. London, 1880.
Deichgräber, Karl. "Galen als Erforscher der menschlichen Pulses." *Sitzungsberichte der deutschen Akademie der Wissenschaften zu Berlin*. Klasse für Sprachen, Literatur und Kunst. 1956, 3.
———. *Die griechische Empirikerschule: Sammlung der Fragmente und Darstellung der Lehre*. Berlin: Weidmann, 1930.

281

DeLacy, Phillip. "Galen's Platonism." *American Journal of Philology*, 93 (1972), 27–39.

——. *See* Galen, *De placitis Hippocratis et Platonis.*

Diels, H. "Handschriften der antiken Aerzte I." *Abhandlungen der preussischen Akademie der Wissenschaften zu Berlin. Philosophisch-Historische Klasse*, 1905.

——. "Ueber das physikalische System des Straton." *Sitzungsberichte der königlichen preussischen Akademie der Wissenschaften zu Berlin*, 1893, 1, 101–27.

Diller, H. "Die Lehre vom Blutkreislauf, eine verschollene Entdeckung der Hippokratiker?" *Archiv für Geschichte der Medizin* 31 (1938), 201–18. Repr. in his *Kleine Schriften zur antiken Medizin*, edited by G. Baader and H. Grensemann. Berlin: De Gruyter, 1973, p. 31–45.

——. "Stand und Aufgaben der Hippocratischen Forschung." *Jahrbuch der Akademie, Mainz*. 1959, pp. 271–87. Repr. in his *Kleine Schriften zur antiken Medizin*, edited by G. Baader and M. Grensemann. Berlin: De Gruyter, 1973, pp. 89–105; and in *Antike Medizin*, edited by H. Flashar. Darmstadt: Wissenschaftliche Buchgesellschaft, 1971.

Duckworth, W.L.H. *See* Galen, *De anatomicis administrationibus.*

Durling, Richard J. "A Chronological Census of Renaissance Editions and Translations of Galen." *Journal of the Warburg Institute* 24 (1961), 230–305.

Edelstein, Ludwig. "The Genuine Works of Hippocrates." *Bulletin of the History of Medicine* 7 (1939), 236–48. Repr. in *Ancient Medicine: Selected Papers of Ludwig Edelstein*. Edited by Owsei Temkin and C. Lilian Temkin. Baltimore: Johns Hopkins Press, 1967, pp. 133–44.

——. "Hippocrates." Pauly-Wissowa, *Realencyclopädie* suppl. vol. 4, 1935, cols. 1290–1343.

——. Περὶ ἀέρων *und die Sammlung der Hippocratischen Schriften. Problemata IV.* Berlin: Weidmann, 1931.

Fleming, Donald. "Galen on the Motions of the Blood in the Heart and Lungs." *Isis* 46 (1955), 14–21.

——. "William Harvey and the Pulmonary Circulation." *Isis* 46 (1955), 319–27.

Fraser, P. M. "The Career of Erasistratus." *Rendiconti dell' Instituto Lombardo* 103 (1969), 518–37.

Frede, Michael. *Die stoische Logik. Abhandlungen der Akademie der Wissenschaften in Göttingen, Phil.-Hist. Klasse* 3, LXXXVIII. Göttingen: Vandenhoeck und Ruprecht, 1974.

Fredrich, C. *Hippokratische Untersuchungen*. Berlin: Weidmann, 1899. *Philosophische Untersuchungen*, edited by A. Kiessling and U. von Wilamowitz-Moellendorff, vol. 15.

Fritzsche, R. A. "Der Magnet und die Athmung in antiken Theorien." *Rheinisches Museum* 57 (1902), 363–91.

Fuchs, Robert. *Erasistratea*. Leipzig: Fock, 1892.

Furley, David J. "Empedocles and the Clepsydra." *Journal of Hellenic Studies* 77/1 (1957), 31–34. Repr. in *Studies in Presocratic Philosophy*, edited by

R. E. Allen and David J. Furley. London: Routledge and Kegan Paul, 1975. Vol. 2, pp. 265–74.

———. Review of Sir David Ross, *Aristotle's Parva Naturalia. Classical Review* 6 (1956), 225–28.

Furley, David J. with Wilkie, J. S. "An Arabic Translation Solves Some Problems in Galen." *Classical Review* 22 (1972), 164–67.

Gabrieli, G. "Ḥunayn ibn Ishāq." *Isis* 6 (1924), 282–92.

Gatzemeier, Matthias. *Die Naturphilosophie des Straton von Lampsakos: zur Geschichte des Problems der Bewegung im Bereich des frühen Peripatos.* Meisenheim am Glan: Hain, 1970.

Gottschalk, H. B. "The Authorship of *Meteorologica* IV." *Classical Quarterly* 11 (1961), 67–79.

———. *Strato of Lampsacus: Some Texts.* Proceedings of the Leeds Philosophical and Literary Society, Literary and Historical Section, 11/6, pp. 95–182. Leeds: Mani, 1965.

Guthrie, W.K.C. *A History of Greek Philosophy.* Cambridge: Cambridge University Press, 1962–in progress.

Hall, A. Rupert. "Studies on the History of the Cardiovascular System." *Bulletin of the History of Medicine* 34 (1960), 391–413.

Harris, C.R.S. *The Heart and the Vascular System in Ancient Greek Medicine.* Oxford: Clarendon Press, 1973.

Harvey, William. *De motu cordis: Movement of the Heart and Blood in Animals.* Translated by Kenneth J. Franklin. Published for the Royal College of Physicians. Oxford: Blackwell, 1957; Springfield, Ill.: Charles C. Thomas, 1957.

———. *Opera Omnia.* E Coll. Med. Lond. edita. 1776.

———. *Works.* Translated into English by R. Willis. London: Sydenham Society, 1847.

Heidel, W. A. "The ἄναρμοι ὄγκοι of Heracleides and Asclepiades." *Transactions and Proceedings of the American Philological Association* 40 (1909), 5–21.

Hurlbutt, Frank R., Jr. "*Peri kardies*: A Treatise on the Heart from the Hippocratic Corpus: Introduction and Translation." *Bulletin of the History of Medicine* 7 (1939), 1104–13.

Jaeger, Werner. *Diokles von Karystos.* Berlin: De Gruyter, 1963.

———. "Das Pneuma im Lykeion." *Hermes* 48 (1913), 30–74.

Kieffer, John Spangler. *Galen's Institutio Logica.* English translation, introduction, and commentary. Baltimore: Johns Hopkins Press, 1964.

Kneale, William and Martha. *The Development of Logic.* Oxford: Clarendon Press, 1962.

Kudlien, F. "Die Pneuma-Bewegung: ein Beitrag zum Thema Medizin und Stoa." *Gesnerus* 31 (1974), 86–98.

Landels, J. G. *Engineering in the Ancient World.* London: Chatto and Windus; Berkeley and Los Angeles: University of California Press, 1978.

Lloyd, G.E.R. *Polarity and Analogy.* Cambridge: Cambridge University Press, 1966.

Lonie, I. M. "*The ἄναρμοι ὄγκοι of Heraclides of Pontus.*" *Phronesis* 9 (1964), 156–64.

———. "Erasistratus, the Erasistrateans, and Aristotle." *Bulletin of the History of Medicine* 38 (1964), 426–43.

———. "The Paradoxical Text on the Heart." *Medical History* 17 (1973), 1–34.

Mates, Benson. *Stoic Logic.* 2nd ed. Berkeley and Los Angeles: University of California Press, 1961.

May, Margaret Tallmadge. *Galen on the Usefulness of the Parts of the Body.* Ithaca: Cornell University Press, 1968.

Moraux, P. "Quinta Essentia." Pauly-Wissowa, *Realencyclopädie* 24 (1963), cols. 1171–1263.

Niebyl, P. H. "Old Age, Fever, and the Lamp Metaphor." *Journal of the History of Medicine* 26 (1971), 353–68.

Noll, R. "Zu Galens Schrift εἰ κατὰ φύσιν ... " *Berliner Philologischer Wochenschrift* 33 (1913), 1246–47.

———. *See* Galen, *An in arteriis.*

Nutton, V. "The Chronology of Galen's Early Career." *Classical Quarterly* 23 (1973), 158–71.

———. "Galen and Medical Autobiography." *Proceedings of the Cambridge Philological Society* 198 (1972), 50–62.

Nuyens, François. *L'Évolution de la Psychologie d'Aristote.* Louvain: Institut Supérieur de Philosophie, 1948.

O'Brien, D. "The Effect of a Simile: Empedocles' Theories of Seeing and Breathing." *Journal of Hellenic Studies* 90 (1969), 140–79.

Pagel, Walter. *William Harvey's Biological Ideas.* New York: Hafner, 1967; Basel: Karger, 1967.

Partington, J. R. *A Short History of Chemistry.* 3rd ed. London: Macmillan, 1957.

Peck, A. L. *See* Aristotle, *De partibus animalium; De generatione animalium; Historia animalium.*

Platt, Arthur. "Aristotle on the Heart." *Studies in the History and Method of Science*, edited by C. Singer. Oxford: Clarendon Press, 1921. Vol. 2, pp. 521–32.

Pringle, J.W.S. "The Gyroscopic Mechanism of the Halteres of Diptera." *Philosophical Transactions of the Royal Society of London.* Series B, 233, pp. 347–84.

Ritter, Helmut, and Walzer, Richard. "Arabische Uebersetzungen griechischer Aerzte in Stambuler Bibliotheken." *Sitzungsberichte der preussischen Akademie der Wissenschaften: Phil.-Hist. Klasse* 26 (1934), 801–46.

Sambursky, S. *Physics of the Stoics.* London: Routledge and Kegan Paul, 1959.

Schmekel, A. *Die positive Philosophie in ihrer geschichtlichen Entwicklung* I. Berlin: Weidmann, 1938.

Seeck, G. A. "Empedocles B 17.9–13, B 8, B 100 bei Aristoteles." *Hermes* 95 (1967), 28–53.

Sezgin, F. *Geschichte des arabischen Schrifttums*, vol. 3. Leiden: Brill, 1972.

Shaw, James Rochester. "Models for Cardiac Structure and Function in Aristotle." *Journal of the History of Biology* 5 (1972), 355–88.

Siegel, Rudolph E. "Galen's Experiments and Observations of Pulmonary Blood Flow and Respiration." *American Journal of Cardiology* 10 (1962), 738–45.

———. *Galen's System of Physiology and Medicine.* 1: *An Analysis of His Doctrines and Observations on Bloodflow, Respiration, Humors, and Internal Diseases.* Basel: Karger, 1968.

———. "The Influence of Galen's Doctrine of Pulmonary Bloodflow on the Development of Modern Concepts of Circulation." *Sudhoffs Archiv für die Geschichte der Medizin* 46 (1962), 311–32.

Sieveking, J. "Herophilus." In Pauly-Wissowa, *Realencyclopädie* 15 (1912), cols. 1104–10.

Singer, Charles, ed. *Studies in the History and Method of Science.* Oxford: Clarendon Press, 1921.

Solmsen, Friedrich. "Greek Philosophy and the Discovery of the Nerves." *Museum Helveticum* 18 (1961), 150–67 and 169–97.

Staden, H. von. "Experiment and Experience in Hellenistic Medicine." *Bulletin of the Institute of Classical Studies* (University of London) 22 (1975), 178–99.

Stakelum, James W. *Galen and the Logic of Propositions.* Rome: Angelicum, 1940.

Steckerl, Fritz. *See* Praxagoras.

Strohmaier, G. *Galen: Ueber die Verschiedenheit der homoiomeren Körperteile.* Berlin: Akademie, 1970.

———. "Ḥunayn b. Ischāk al-'Ibādī." *Encyclopaedia of Islam*, new ed., Vol. 3. Leiden: Brill, 1971. pp. 578–81.

Temkin, Owsei. "On Galen's Pneumatology." *Gesnerus* 8 (1951), 180–89.

Timpanaro Cardini, Maria. "Respirazione e Clessidra." *Parola del Passato* 12 (1957), 250–70.

Towers, B. *See* Galen, *De anatomicis administrationibus.*

Uexküll, J. von. "Studien über Tonus I." *Zeitschrift für Biologie* 44 (1903).

Ullmann, Manfred. *Die Medizin im Islam.* Leiden: Brill, 1970.

Walzer, R. *Galen: On Medical Experience: Arabic Text with an English Translation.* Oxford: Clarendon Press, 1944.

———. *See* Ritter, Helmut.

Wellmann, M. "Asclepiades von Preusa." *Geschichte der griechischen Literatur in der Alexandrinerzeit.* Edited by Franz Susemihl. Leipzig: Teubner, 1891–92. Vol. 2, 428–40.

———. "Erasistratos." Pauly-Wissowa *Realencyclopädie* 6/1 (1907), cols. 333–50.

———. *Die pneumatische Schule bis auf Archigenes in ihrer Entwicklung dargestellt.* Philosophische Untersuchungen 14. Berlin: Weidmann, 1895.

Wellmann, W. *See Fragmente der Sikelischen Aerzte.*

Westenberger, Hans. "Zu Galens Schrift Περὶ χρείας ἀναπνοῆς." *Hermes* 80 (1952), 124–45.

Whitteridge, Gweneth, ed. *The Anatomical Lectures of William Harvey*. Edinburgh and London: Livingston, 1964.

————. *William Harvey and the Circulation of the Blood*. London: McDonald, and New York: American Elsevier, 1971.

Wilkie, J. S. *See* David J. Furley with J. S. Wilkie.

Wilson, Leonard G. "Erasistratus, Galen, and the Pneuma." *Bulletin of the History of Medicine* 33 (1959), 293–314.

INDEX NOMINUM

INDEX OF PASSAGES
CITED IN INTRODUCTION
AND COMMENTARY

Library of Congress Cataloging in Publication Data

Galen.
  Galen on respiration and the arteries.

  "An edition with English translation and commentary of De usu respirationis,
An in arteriis natura sanguis contineatur, De usu pulsuum, and De causis
respirationis."
  Text in Greek and English; commentary in English.
  Bibliography: pp. 279–286.   Includes index.
  1. Respiration—Early works to 1800. 2. Blood—Circulation—Early works to
1800. I. Furley, David J. II. Wilkie, James S. III. Title. [DNLM: WZ 290 G153]
QP121.G18213 1984   599'.011   81–47130

ISBN 0–691–08286–3 (alk. paper)

Ingram Content Group UK Ltd.
Milton Keynes UK
UKHW022131100323
418392UK00005B/309